10
tenth edition

DENTAL ANATOMY

A Self-Instructional Program

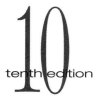

10
tenth edition

DENTAL
ANATOMY

A Self-Instructional Program

Nancy Shobe Karst, CDA, RDH, MS
Assistant Professor
Dental Programs
Missouri Southern State College
Joplin, Missouri

Sarah K. Smith, DDS
Owens Technical College
Toledo, Ohio

Kevin Minear
Illustrator

APPLETON & LANGE
Stamford, CT

Copyright© 1998 by Appleton & Lange
A Simon & Schuster Company
Copyright© 1982 by APPLETON-CENTURY-CROFTS
First through Eighth Editions © 1963, 1965, 1967, 1968, 1969, 1970, 1971, 1972; Revised Edition © 1974; Second Revised Edition © 1977
Teaching Research, A Division of the Oregon State System of Higher Education

98 99 00 01 02 / 10 9 8 7 6 5 4 3 2 1

Prentice Hall International (UK) Limited, *London*
Prentice Hall of Australia Pty. Limited, *Sydney*
Prentice Hall Canada, Inc., *Toronto*
Prentice Hall Hispanoamericana, S.A., *Mexico*
Prentice Hall of India Private Limited, *New Delhi*
Prentice Hall of Japan, Inc., *Tokyo*
Simon & Schuster Asia Pte. Ltd., *Singapore*
Editora Prentice Hall do Brasil Ltda., *Rio de Janeiro*
Prentice Hall, *Upper Saddle River, New Jersey*

Library of Congress Cataloging-in-Publication Data

Karst, Nancy Shobe.
    Dental anatomy : a self-instructional program. — 10th ed. / Nancy Shobe Karst, Sarah K. Smith; Kevin Minear, illustrator.
       p.   cm.
    Rev. ed. of: Dental anatomy / Teaching Research, a Division of the Oregon State System of Higher Education. c1982.
    ISBN 0-8385-1492-8 (pbk. : alk. paper). — ISBN 0-8385-1492-8 (pbk. : alk. paper)
    1. Teeth—Anatomy—Programmed instruction.   2. Teeth—Anatomy—Atlases.   I. Smith, Sarah K.   II. Title.
    [DNLM: 1. Tooth—anatomy & histology—programmed instruction.   WU 18.2 K18d 1997]
RK280.K37 1997
611'.314—dc21
DNLM/DLC
for Library of Congress
                              96-36841

ISBN 0-8385-1492-8

9 780838 514924   90000

Acquisitions Editor: Kimberly Davies
Production Editor: Sondra Greenfield
Designer: Janice Barsevich Bielawa

PRINTED IN THE UNITED STATES OF AMERICA

CONTENTS

Chapter 2   Permanent Anterior Teeth   121

Chapter 3   Permanent Premolars   249

Chapter 4 Permanent Molars   353

Chapter 5   The Primary Dentition   485

PREFACE

Dental Anatomy: A Self-Instructional Program, can be used either as a self-instructional textbook or as a required text in the dental curriculum. Many dental, dental hygiene, and dental assistant instructors require incoming students to purchase and work through the book prior to the beginning of their professional education. Mastery of the information will give the student a head start in the dental profession.

The book's organization in this tenth edition has been improved and, as a result, the student will be able to assimilate the information for each tooth with greater ease. The information has been reorganized to include the anatomy of the roots, pulp chambers, crown contours, contacts, and embrasures associated with the crowns of their respective teeth. This allows the student to learn and master facts about one tooth at a time. An added feature is a summary of the anatomical information presented for each tooth.

The tenth edition of this self-instructional program represents the latest in computer graphics technology. Over 1100 new illustrations replace the line drawings previously used in this text. All the illustrations are a production of the 3-D studio program. The software was produced by Viewpoint Datalabs for the graphics.

ACKNOWLEDGMENTS

The original text and its several revisions were written by the Teaching and Research Division of the Oregon State System of Higher Education. They were devoted to this project for several years and produced a well-written self-instructional program to assist with learning tooth anatomy information required in the pursuit of further education in the various professional dental programs.

The computer technology used to produce the illustrations in this text were a result of the efforts of Don Schultz of the Computer-Assisted Manufacturing Technology Department of Missouri Southern State College. Through his efforts the Viewpoint program was selected and instituted. Additionally, Don located a superb computer graphics operator, Kevin Minear. Kevin's tenacity and many hours of computer operation coupled with his creative abilities have provided the outstanding illustrations used in this text. These illustrations are more easily read and interpreted than the original line drawings.

The proofreading and diligent support of my husband, Larry, has been absolutely essential to meeting the deadline for this text. Additionally, he has been understanding of the many essential hours spent with the illustrator in the production of the illustrations.

Two other people who have been very supportive and helpful in this project were my brother, Les Shobe, and Joe Enders. Joe was instrumental in selection of the electronic transfer program so the large files created in the process of illustrating this text could be successfully transported. Les has provided encouragement and support throughout the revision project.

DIRECTIONS FOR THE STUDENT

The objective of this text is to help you master the terminology and basic facts of dental anatomy. This self-instructional text has been tested on a large number of students over many years. It has been demonstrated that when students use the text according to directions and diligently answer the embedded questions and review tests, they effectively learn dental anatomy.

Because this is a self-instructional program, you will find that it deviates from traditional textbooks in several ways:

- In addition to reading, you will be answering questions that are embedded in the text. Questions appear in nearly every "frame" of the text. Frames are separated by dotted black lines.
- You will be using the illustrations to help answer questions.
- Answers appear in the shaded answer column. You will reveal an answer only after you have tried to answer it on your own.
- You will use the Answer Mask packaged with the book to cover each answer in the answer column until you have answered the question. See directions at the top of the next page for using the mask.
- Once you have mastered the content in each section, repeat the section and summarize each frame with a one- or two-word summary. This will reinforce the learning and provide a quick synopsis heading for locating information at a later time. Information learned in the first chapter will be background information for new material in later chapters. Having your written descriptions on each frame may assist in locating that information.
- You are given review tests at regular intervals throughout the book to help you check your understanding of each section of material presented. These review tests help you measure whether you have mastered each section and are ready to proceed to the next section or whether you need to review. Mastery of each section is important because later parts rely on your knowledge of earlier parts. Also, these tests help you to prepare for exams in classes as well as national, regional, and state boards.

The illustrations used in this self-instructional text are a product of software from Viewpoint Datalabs. The images are a product of model teeth scanned into the program. Not all model teeth are anatomically perfect. Individual teeth will vary somewhat from person to person as model teeth will vary from model to model. There can be as many anatomical differences between teeth as there are differences between people. The anatomy is explained by text and illustration in this volume; however, the illustration may vary somewhat from the explanation due to the differences that may occur between real teeth and model teeth. The student who excels will take the time to check other references and compare illustrations and explanations between textbooks because each author will emphasize different aspects of the subject.

HOW TO USE THE MASK

1. Place the mask over the complete column of answers before you begin each new page of question frames. Align the top of the mask with the top dotted line. Do not reveal the answer below the dotted line.
2. Try to answer the first question. Jot your answer on the answer line or answer the question to yourself.
3. Lower the mask in the answer column far enough to reveal only the answer of the question you have just attempted.
4. Proceed to the next question frame using the above directions (2 and 3) until you have attempted to answer all the questions on that page.

Introduction to Dental Anatomy

Every tooth has two basic parts, a **crown** and a **root.** The part of a tooth which is visible in the mouth is the **clinical crown.** The part which is not visible in the mouth is the **clinical root.**

To the clinician, then, the supportive soft tissue that surrounds the tooth forms the boundary between the _____ _____ and the _____ _____ of a tooth.

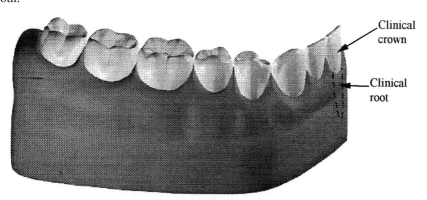

Clinical crown

Clinical root

When examining a tooth outside of the mouth, a clinical crown and root cannot be defined because there is no soft tissue to form a boundary. However, an **anatomical crown** and **anatomical root** can be defined by the type of hard tissue covering the tooth. **Enamel** is a very hard, whitish, translucent tooth tissue that covers and defines the anatomical crown. Another hard tooth tissue called **cementum,** covers and defines the anatomical

_____ .

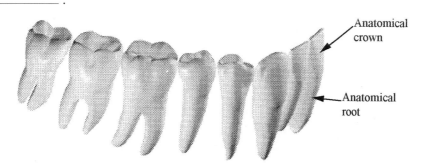

Anatomical crown

Anatomical root

anatomical

The part of a tooth covered with cementum that connects the tooth to surrounding tissue is termed the _____ root.

B

The boundary between the anatomical crown and root is the **cervical line** (SIR vik ul—the word is related to *cervix,* the neck). On actual teeth, the cervical line is the division between the enamel and cementum and it may be faint or distinct. You will see it drawn as a line separating the crown and root in illustrations in this text. Identify the cervical line in the drawing—is it A, B, or C? _____

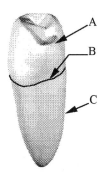

b

Eruption is the movement of the tooth through the surrounding tissues so that gradually more of the tooth becomes visible in the mouth. If a tooth in the mouth of a child is *partially* erupted, then which of the following is true? _____

a. The clinical crown includes all of the anatomical crown.
b. Part of the anatomical crown may not be included in the clinical crown.

If you said *a,* you were incorrect. If a tooth is partially erupted, only a small portion would be visible and the clinical crown would not include all of the anatomical crown. Some of the anatomical crown would be still covered by supportive soft tissues.

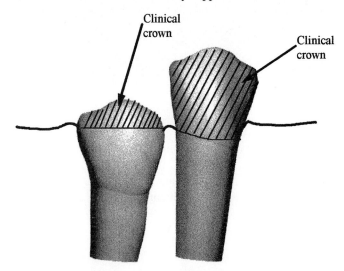

If you said *b,* you were correct. Note the distinction between the boundaries of the anatomical and clinical crowns. The boundary of the anatomical crown never changes. However, the boundary of the clinical crown and clinical root can change with the position of the tooth and position of the supportive soft tissues around the tooth.

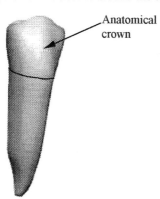

Anatomical crown

An adult with a normally developed **dentition** (full set of teeth) has 32 teeth. Each of these 32 teeth has a crown. However, the crowns may not resemble each other. Teeth are classified into four groups: **incisors** (in SIZE urs), **canines, premolars,** and **molars.** Teeth in each classification have similarities of form, location, and functions.

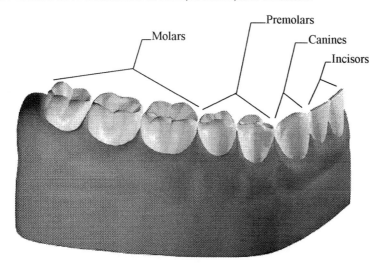

Molars

Premolars

Canines

Incisors

1.1.1

incisors

INCISORS

In the adult dentition, 8 of the 32 teeth have crowns with relatively straight edges, which are well designed to cut through foods. A term similar to "cut" is "incise." The associated noun is *incisor.* An instrument used to make an incision could be called an incisor. Teeth that have this shape are called _____ .

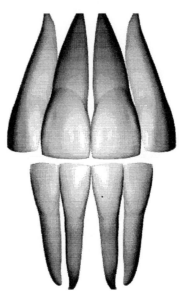

A

Those eight teeth whose crowns are so well adapted to cutting are the incisors. Their cutting edges are termed **incisal** (in SIZE ul) edges. Identify the incisal edge in this drawing of an incisor (A, B, or C?). _____

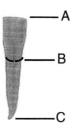

CANINES   1.1.2

Canines are another classification of teeth. Of the 32 teeth in an adult dentition, 4 are canines. We associate the word "canine" with the dog family. We can use this association to aid our memory. In dogs, the canine is usually a prominent tooth. The long, pointed canine of a snarling dog can be frightening.

These teeth are frequently called **"cuspids,"** a term that indicates the presence of one cusp. They are also commonly referred to as **"eye teeth,"** but the preferred term is canine. They are highlighted black in the drawing.

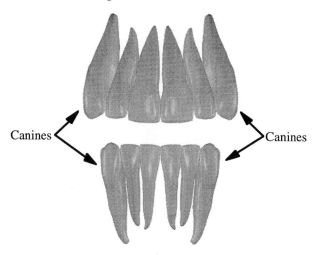

Canines   Canines

In humans, the canine is somewhat pointed. The incisal edge is not straight like the incisors, but spear-shaped. The point is called a **cusp.** A cusp is a pointed projection or mound on a tooth's crown.

The cusp shape and the well-developed root of the canines make them very powerful teeth, able to concentrate forces into a small area. The canines can function as wedges, to pierce and hold foods. The strength and shape of canines aids the tearing and breaking action accomplished by the coordination of the teeth with the movement of fingers, wrist, and arm. In eating a crisp apple, for instance, we grasp or hold the apple with our teeth, then, with a motion of the fingers, wrist, and arm, we break or tear the food into pieces of a size suitable for chewing. Another example of canines in action would be in the eating of a tough steak where the canines would help to _____ and _____ the meat.

pierce, hold

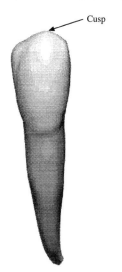

Cusp

cusp

The piercing and holding function of the canine teeth is made easy by the pointed shape of their crowns. The point on the crown of these teeth is called a _____ .

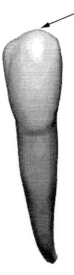

incisal

Both the cutting edge of an incisor and the piercing edge of the canine cusp are termed _____ edges.

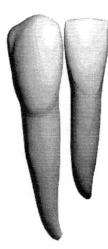

cusp

The process of chewing food is called **mastication** (mass tuh KAY shun). The incisal edge of a canine and its pointed _____ are involved in mastication.

The cusp of a canine tooth provides an example of a convex surface. All tooth surfaces are either *flat, concave,* or *convex.*

Some students have trouble with the terms *convex* and *concave.* Convex means bulging or arching outward like the surface of a ball. Concave means being shaped like a hollow or recess. A mental clue is that the word concave suggests something cavelike.

Which figure has a convex top? _____
Which figure has a concave top? _____

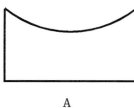

A

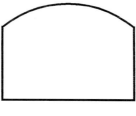

B

Therefore, when we say that the incisal edge or cusp of the canine is convex, we mean that it bulges or arches _____ (toward/away from) the root.

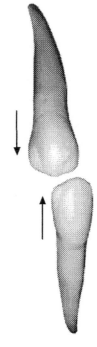

incisors, canines

The overall crown and root length of canines make them the longest teeth in an adult's mouth. The long root gives the canines pronounced stability. Because of their firm anchorage and location in the mouth, the canines contribute importantly to the stability of all the teeth.

The tissue that surrounds the root structure receives its contours from the shape of the root and in turn affects the contours in the person's face, particularly around the corners of the mouth. Thus, canine teeth have a major influence on a person's facial appearance.

The two classifications of teeth which have been discussed in the program so far are _____ and _____ .

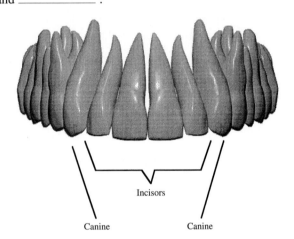

Incisors

Canine   Canine

mastication

The incisors and the canines, two of the four classifications of teeth, are both wedge-shaped in appearance from a side view of their crowns.

Both incisors and canines have edges suitable for cutting or piercing food. The incisal edges of both are involved in the process of chewing, which is called _____ .

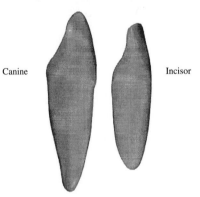

Canine   Incisor

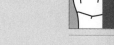

The incisors and the canines have two of the following four characteristics in common: _____

Choose the pair of letters of the two correct statements:

a. Both have incisal edges.
b. The incisal edge on each is relatively straight and sharp.
c. There are four teeth in each classification.
d. Both are relatively wedge-shaped in appearance when viewing the crown from the side.

a and b
b and c
a and c
a and d
c and d

a and d

If you chose another answer, go back and review beginning at page 1. For your own benefit and increased learning, you should evaluate your answers to questions in this text in a critical and honest way. You should now be able to describe the differences between incisors and canines on the basis of what has been presented so far. If you can do this, it will help you identify these teeth and communicate with other professional people. If you cannot yet do this, please review from page 1.

PREMOLARS   1.1.3

The next classification of teeth to be considered consists of as many teeth as the incisors. These teeth are called **premolars.** There are how many premolars? _____ .

eight

Eight teeth of the adult dentition are premolars. These teeth are sometimes called **bicuspids,** because they generally have two _____ .

cusps

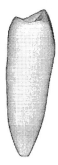

The term *bicuspid* has been used because these teeth usually have only two cusps. However, since two of the eight premolars vary in that they may have either two or three cusps, the term "bicuspid" is not technically accurate. While this program will use the term premolar, the student should be aware of other common terms so that he can recognize and identify the appropriate teeth from any typical word usage.

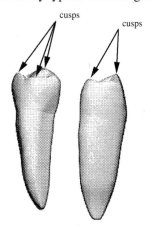

cusps   cusps

in front of

In the accompanying drawing, the premolars and molars are identified. We use the name premolars because these teeth are _____ (in front of/behind) the molars.

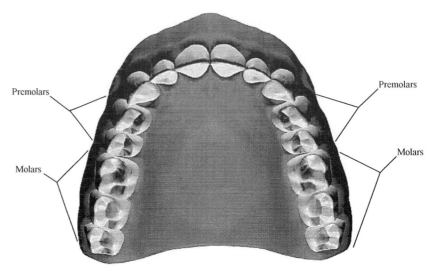

canine

The premolars and molars have larger masticating surfaces than do the incisors and canines to facilitate the crushing and grinding of foods. Premolars have characteristics of both the canines and the molars. Premolars have similarities to molars but they differ from molars in the number of cusps, their form, and arrangement. Premolars have smaller masticating surfaces and more pointed cusps, which concentrate the forces exerted on foods. In this respect, premolar cusps resemble the form of the cusps on _____ teeth. The cusps of the premolars are indicated with circles in the illustration.

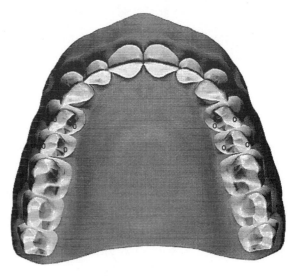

MOLARS   1.1.4

There are twelve **molars.** The molars have more cusps and a larger masticating surface than the other classifications of teeth. They are located in the back of the mouth where the muscles of the jaw can apply strong forces, making the molars effective in crushing and grinding. In the picture, the six lower molars are indicated. There are also _____ molars on the upper arch.

six

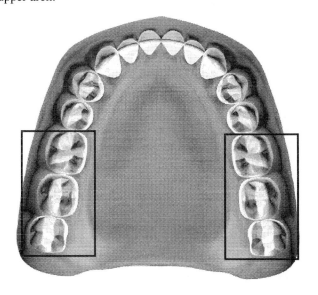

Molars are distinguished from one another by their position in the mouth, the shape of the crown, and the number of cusps. Molars may have from three to five cusps, depending on their location in the mouth and normal variations which occur. The apex, or point, of each cusp is called a cusp tip. The number of cusps may easily be determined by counting the cusp tips (marked as small circles in the illustration). How many cusps are there on the tooth marked with the arrow? _____

four

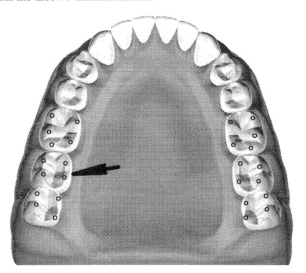

TURN TO THE NEXT PAGE AND TAKE REVIEW TEST 1.1.

REVIEW TEST 1.1

1. Supply the name for the teeth corresponding to the following anatomical forms:

   Tooth name   **Form**

   a. _____   one cusp
   b. _____   usually two cusps
   c. _____   straight incisal edge

2. During the development of teeth in adolescence, the clinical crowns of teeth gradually become longer. What is the name for this process?

   a. mastication
   b. eruption
   c. cusp development

3. How many teeth in the adult dentition are molars?

   a. 4   c. 12
   b. 8   d. 2

4. Which two classifications of teeth have a wedge-shaped crown from a side view?

   a. incisor   c. premolar
   b. canine   d. molar

5. Which of the following would never be seen in a visual inspection of the mouth, by definition?

   a. anatomical crown
   b. anatomical root
   c. clinical root

6. Which teeth are the longest and have a major influence on the shape of a person's facial appearance?

   a. central incisors   d. premolars
   b. lateral incisors   e. molars
   c. canines

7. Which teeth are located in front of the molars?

   a. incisors
   b. canines
   c. premolars

8. The premolars generally have _____ cusps (although some have three).

   a. one   c. three
   b. two   d. four

CHECK YOUR ANSWERS IN APPENDIX A.

ARRANGEMENT OF TEETH

1.2.0

maxillary

Each tooth is fixed in its relative position in the supporting bone to form the dentition. The dentition is divided into two arches, the upper and lower. The teeth belonging to the upper arch are supported in the **maxilla** (MAX uh luh) or **maxillary** (MAX uh larry) bone. They are therefore called _____ teeth.

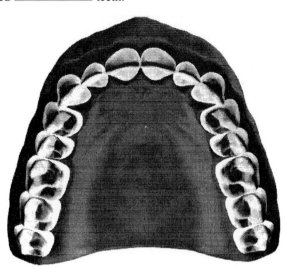

The maxillary teeth account for one half of the total number of teeth. The total number of teeth in the adult maxillary arch is _____ .

sixteen

The upper jaw is the maxilla. Another name for the maxillary set of teeth is the _____ set of teeth.

upper

maxillary arch

The lower jaw is the **mandible** (MAN duh bull), and therefore the set of teeth attached to the mandible makes up the **mandibular** (man DIB u lur) arch.

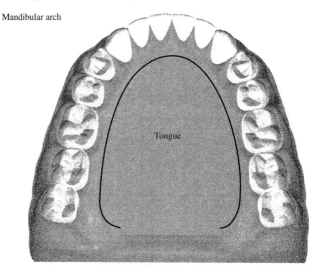

Mandibular arch

Tongue

Mandre means to chew. The mandible is the movable jaw used for chewing. As the mandible is raised, the teeth in the mandibular arch are brought into contact with those of the _____ .

posterior

The incisors and canines are positioned in the *front* part of the mouth and are called anterior teeth. Premolars and molars are located in the *back* of each dental arch and are called _____ teeth.

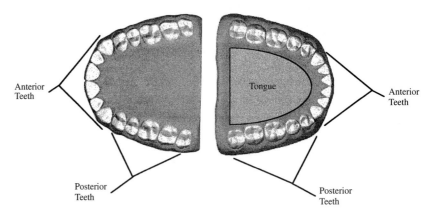

Anterior Teeth

Tongue

Anterior Teeth

Posterior Teeth

Posterior Teeth

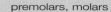

The grinding or chewing surfaces of maxillary and mandibular posterior teeth come into contact when the mouth is closed. These surfaces are termed **occlusal** (ah CLUE zul) surfaces. Which two classifications of teeth have occlusal surfaces? _____ and _____

The teeth with incisal edges are collectively called anterior teeth. The teeth with occlusal surfaces are collectively called _____ teeth.

posterior

Which group of teeth have masticating surfaces called incisal edges? _____

anterior

The masticating surfaces of the posterior teeth are termed _____ surfaces.

occlusal

Which of the following are anterior teeth? _____

a. incisors and canines
b. premolars and molars

a. incisors and canines

right

To identify a tooth as a maxillary canine, for example, is not sufficient to identify a specific tooth since two such teeth are normally present. Not only is the dentition divided into maxillary and mandibular arches, but also into right and left quadrants.

The technical term for the dividing line between the right and left sides of the body is **midsaggital** (mid SAHJ juh tull) plane. Dentally, this is called the midline or median line of the dental arches. The midline equally divides both the maxillary and mandibular arches, falling between the central incisors. Each half of each segment then becomes a quadrant, or one-fourth of the complete dentition. Normally, there are eight permanent teeth in a quadrant.

The order of arrangement of the eight teeth is identical in each of the four quadrants. The diagram shows the maxillary arch as seen if you were looking into a patient's mouth. Indicating either the right or left quadrant is always in reference to the patient's right or left, not in reference to the viewer's right or left.

The labeled teeth in the diagram represent an occlusal view of the maxillary _____ (right/left) quadrant.

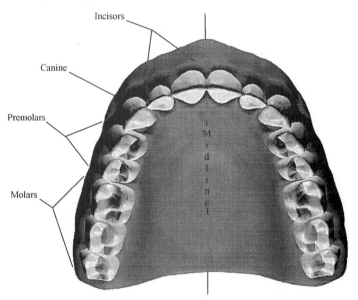

The human dentition is composed of several kinds of teeth, serving a variety of functions. The term to denote this is **heterodont dentition** (*hetero* means "different," *-odont* means "tooth"; thus heterodont means literally "different teeth"). It is used to refer to "having teeth of different shapes."

In some species, only one type of tooth is found throughout the arches. This is known as **homodont dentition** (*homo* means "the same").

Human dentition is also described as **diphyodont** (die FI oh dont; *di* equals "two," *phyo* means "to produce," *-odont* means "tooth"; meaning "to produce two sets of teeth"), because during his lifetime, man has two different sets of teeth, the *primary* (deciduous) teeth, and the *permanent* teeth. In contrast, fishes, amphibians, and reptiles continue to replace teeth throughout their lifetime, so with respect to replacement, their dentition is described as **polyphyodont** (*poly* means "many"; meaning "to produce many sets of teeth").

We have discussed two terms that describe human dentition. When we speak of the variety of teeth in a dental arch, we use the term _____ . When we speak of the fact that humans have primary teeth and then permanent teeth, we use the term _____ .

heterodont, diphyodont

The first set of teeth may properly be called primary, which obviously means first; or deciduous, which means falling away and refers to the fact that, like the leaves of deciduous trees, they will fall away when their function has been fulfilled.

These teeth are also often called "baby," "temporary," or "milk teeth," but these terms are technically unacceptable.

A complete set of the primary dentition includes only twenty teeth. Each arch of primary dentition therefore contains how many teeth? _____

Ten is correct. This means that there are six less teeth in an arch of primary dentition than in the same arch of permanent dentition. As the skull grows and develops along with the development and growth of the body, the increased size of the maxilla and mandible accommodates the eruption of three permanent molar teeth in each quadrant posterior to the primary molars.

In each quadrant, five permanent teeth (incisors, canine, and premolars) succeed or take the place of the five primary teeth. They are therefore called succedaneous (SUCK sa DANE nee us; *succedo* means "to follow") teeth. Three permanent molars do not succeed primary teeth (in each quadrant); therefore, they are nonsuccedaneous teeth.

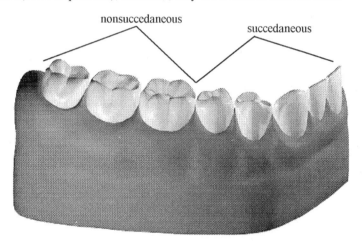

Each quadrant of the primary dentition includes two incisors (2 I), one canine (1 C), and two molars (2 M). There are no primary premolars. Since there are four quadrants, the primary dental formula is 2 I plus 1 C plus 2 M = 5; 5 × 4 = 20. There is also a permanent dentition dental formula. Try it on scratch paper and compare your answer with the one in the next frame.

2 I plus 1 C plus 2 P plus 3 M = 8; 8 × 4 = 32

(In each quadrant, two incisors plus one canine plus two premolars plus three molars, totaling eight, times four quadrants, totaling 32 teeth.)

Teeth are identified by their arrangement relative to the median line. In the primary dentition beginning at the midline, the teeth are arranged in the following order: central incisor, lateral incisor, canine, first molar, and second molar. In the permanent dentition, following the same order relative to the median line, the arrangement of the teeth is central incisor, lateral incisor, canine, first premolar, second premolar, first, second, and third molars. All of the twenty original teeth will be replaced by permanent teeth. Because all the original primary teeth will be replaced with permanent teeth, these permanent teeth are called

succedaneous

nonsuccedaneous

Teeth that come up in their own space are called _____ .

32

Eventually there will be _____ (how many) permanent teeth?

20

There were originally _____ (how many) primary teeth?

1.2.1   TOOTH NAMING AND CODING

primary maxillary
right canine

We have covered several items of tooth arrangement. By putting these together, one is able to identify a particular tooth with accuracy, confident of being understood by a colleague.

When identifying a specific tooth, we list the dentition, arch, quadrant, and tooth name in that order. An example would be permanent mandibular left first molar or primary mandibular left lateral incisor. The order in which these terms have been given has become standard and should be learned in that manner.

Rearrange the description of the following tooth by placing the words in proper order.

right   maxillary   primary   canine
_____   _____   _____   _____

primary, permanent

Which terms name the dentition? _____ and _____ .

maxillary, mandibular

Which terms name the arch? _____ and _____

right, left

Which terms name the quadrant? _____ and _____

List the eight permanent teeth in order starting at the midline (anterior to posterior order).

_____   _____
_____   _____
_____   _____
_____   _____

central incisor,
lateral incisor, canine,
first premolar,
second premolar,
first molar, second
molar, third molar

Throughout this text, the drawings will be labeled with the correct names, in the correct order, for the tooth (or teeth) shown in the illustrations.

To communicate with colleagues and to keep records of patients' teeth, a coding system for designating teeth is helpful and widely used. There are several different coding systems. One of the most commonly used systems in the United States is the military or universal coding system. This code will be used throughout the remainder of this program.

Arabic numbers one through thirty-two (1–32) are used for permanent teeth; letters A through T are used for the twenty primary teeth. Assuming the two arch segments form an elliptical circle, then a diagram can represent the complete dentition, and the pattern for the number and letter code can be readily seen.

Try to use some key numbers to help you remember these codes. For example, 8 and 9 are the maxillary central incisors and 24 and 25 are the mandibular central incisors. You might think of the groups of teeth such as 3, 14, 19, 30 representing all the first molars and 6, 11, 22, 27 representing the canines. Using these landmark numbers may help you to recall the ones in between.

Permanent   Universal Coding System
Maxillary
Mandibular
OCCLUSAL

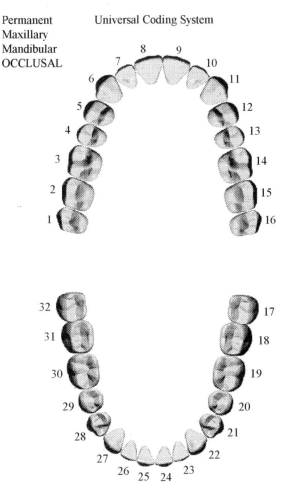

maxillary right

Notice that the right and left is in reference to the patient, not the viewer. When coding the teeth, you always begin lettering or numbering with the posterior tooth in the _____ _____ quadrant. (Be sure your answer words are in the correct order.) The primary teeth labeled in this drawing are identified with the letters A through T.

Primary
Maxillary
Mandibular
OCCLUSAL

Universal Coding System

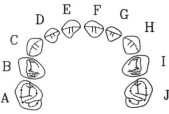

Right   Left

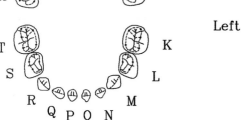

C, 20, 16, J, P

List the code letter or number for each of the following teeth.

_____ primary maxillary right canine
_____ permanent mandibular left second premolar
_____ permanent maxillary left third molar
_____ primary maxillary left second molar
_____ primary mandibular right central incisor

---

a

Which one of the following tooth identifications uses the correct order? _____

a. Permanent mandibular left central incisor
b. Permanent left mandibular central incisor

For each of the following code letters and numbers write the name of the tooth, being careful to place the terms in standard order.

5 _____

30 _____

K _____

26 _____

D _____

9 _____

Q _____

16 _____

5, permanent maxillary right first premolar
30, permanent mandibular right first molar
K, primary mandibular left second molar
26, permanent mandibular right lateral incisor
D, primary maxillary right lateral incisor
9, permanent maxillary left central incisor
Q, primary mandibular right lateral incisor
16, permanent maxillary left third molar

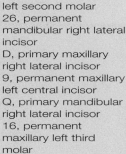
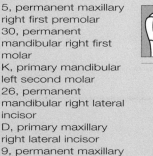

There are several other coding systems used to identify teeth. Listed below are three main types:

1. Quadrant symbols: (⌋) maxillary right, (∟) maxillary left, (Γ) mandibular left, (⌐) mandibular right, are combined with numbers (1–8) for the teeth in each permanent quadrant, or letters (a–e) for the teeth in each primary quadrant, beginning with the central incisor. This system is known as "Palmer notation." Following are some examples:

<table>
<tr><td>Maxillary right</td><td>Maxillary left</td></tr>
<tr><td>a⌋</td><td>⌊a</td></tr>
<tr><td>b⌋</td><td>⌊b</td></tr>
<tr><td>c⌋</td><td>⌊c</td></tr>
<tr><td>d⌋</td><td>⌊d</td></tr>
<tr><td>e⌋</td><td>⌊e</td></tr>
</table>

2. Quadrant abbreviations: Abbreviations for upper and lower, right and left quadrants (UL, UR, LL, LR) are combined with numbers or letters.

3. International system: A system that is useful for computer processing and foreign language translation of tooth codes has been approved by the International Federation of Dentistry. In this system, each tooth is given two numbers which may be separated by a dash (as 1–8).

The first number identifies the quadrant. The permanent quadrants are numbered from 1 (maxillary right) to 4 (mandibular right) following the standard elliptical diagram of teeth in a clockwise direction. The primary quadrants are numbered from 5 (maxillary right) to 8 (mandibular right) in the same way. The permanent teeth are numbered from 1 (central incisor) to 8 (third molar) in each quadrant. The primary teeth are numbered from 1 to 5. See pages 22 and 23 for illustrations of this system.

INTERNATIONAL CODING SYSTEM

permanent teeth

Permanent
Maxillary
Mandibular
OCCLUSAL

International Coding System

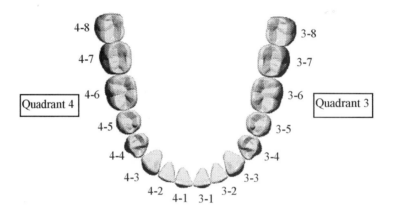

Quadrant 1

Quadrant 2

Quadrant 4

Quadrant 3

primary teeth

Primary
Maxillary
Mandibular
OCCLUSAL

International Coding System

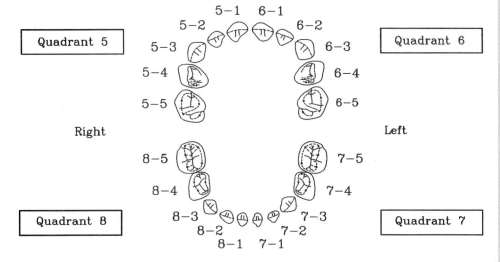

Study the charts on page 22 and top page 23 to answer the following questions.

The first digit of the international code identifies the quadrant and whether the tooth is permanent or primary. Below is a list of the first digit numbers and quadrants. Fill in the missing elements by writing the dentition and quadrant name in the blank space.

First digit of the international code:

1—Permanent maxillary right
2—Permanent maxillary left
3— _____ _____ _____
4— _____ _____ _____
5—Primary maxillary right
6— _____ _____ _____
7—Primary mandibular left
8—Primary mandibular right

The second digit of the international code identifies the individual teeth within each quadrant. Below is a list of the second-digit codes with some missing elements. Fill in the missing tooth names.

Second digit of International Code:

1—Permanent or primary central incisor
2—Permanent or primary lateral incisor
3—Permanent or primary canine
4—Permanent first premolar or primary _____ _____
5—Permanent second premolar or primary second molar
6— _____ _____ _____
7—Permanent second molar
8—Permanent third molar

Although the international system is probably the code of the future, it is not currently in wide use in the United States.

Throughout the remainder of this program, the military (universal) code of 1–32 and A–T will be used, because of its popularity and because the introduction of two codes throughout the text would be confusing. From time to time you will be asked to remember the correct universal code for certain teeth. A table of code conversions can be found in Appendix B, however, a system of learning the codes should be considered. It is often suggested to learn the codes by grouping such as:

UNIVERSAL CODES FOR THE PERMANENT DENTITION

		Right	Left
Central incisors	maxillary	8	9
	mandibular	25	24
Lateral incisors	maxillary	7	10
	mandibular	26	23
Canines	maxillary	6	11
	mandibular	27	22
First premolars	maxillary	5	12
	mandibular	28	21
Second premolars	maxillary	4	13
	mandibular	29	20
First molars	maxillary	3	14
	mandibular	30	19
Second molars	maxillary	2	15
	mandibular	31	18
Third molars	maxillary	1	16
	mandibular	32	17

UNIVERSAL CODES FOR PRIMARY TEETH

		Right	Left
Central incisors	maxillary	E	F
	mandibular	P	O
Lateral incisors	maxillary	D	G
	mandibular	Q	N
Canines	maxillary	C	H
	mandibular	R	M
First molars	maxillary	B	I
	mandibular	S	L
Second molars	maxillary	A	J
	mandibular	T	K

TOOTH SURFACES 1.2.2

occlusal

After having designated a particular tooth, it becomes necessary to be able to designate any one of the surfaces on the tooth. The tooth surfaces receive their name either because of function, relationship to the midline, or anatomical structure.

The crown of a tooth may be visualized as a cube or a wedge. One surface is occupied by the root end. Incisors and canines are roughly wedge-shaped with the narrow portion of the wedge corresponding to the incisal edge. Molars and premolars can be visualized as cubes with the top surface of the cube called the _____ surface.

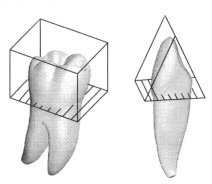

Even though teeth are not exact cubes or wedges, it is helpful to imagine them in this way in order to learn the names of each surface.

The premolars and molars are collectively called _____ teeth, being _____ (same word) to the incisors and canines.

posterior (in both cases)

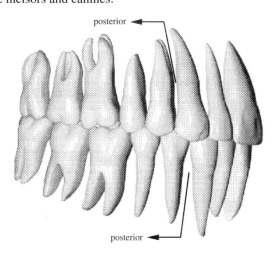

posterior ←

posterior ←

The posterior teeth do not have incisal edges. Instead, their masticating surface is in the form of an occlusal "table," with interspaced valleys and projecting mounds called _____ .

cusps

mesial

Two surfaces of each tooth receive their name from the position relative to the midline of the face. The **mesial** (MEE zee ul) surface is toward or adjacent to the midline. The distal surface is away from the midline. The surface indicated at the arrow is the _____ surface.

Permanent
Maxillary
OCCLUSAL

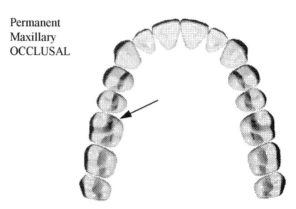

mesial-mesial

The dental arch is made up of teeth which contact one another, the mesial surface of one tooth contacting the distal surface of the next tooth in most cases. However, the contact between the central incisors (at the midline) is an exception. Is this area, indicated in the circles, mesial–distal, mesial–mesial, or distal–distal? _____

Permanent
Maxillary
Mandibular
INCISORS

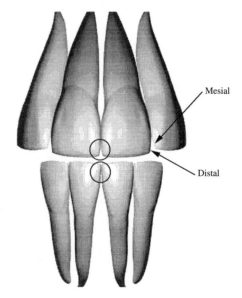

Mesial

Distal

Question Frame

The two frames following this question are labeled Frame A and Frame B for ease in location.

Teeth contact one another **interproximally** (inter PROCK sim ma lee), except the distal of the third molars. Therefore, each tooth normally has _____ contacting surfaces.

two . . . . GO TO FRAME A.
three . . . . GO TO FRAME B.

>**Frame A**

You are correct. Of course, you realize that the occlusal surface is a contacting surface also. But for now the contact between teeth belonging to different arches will not be considered. By limiting the use of the words "contacting surface" to those surfaces where contact remains constant, only the proximal (PROCK sim ul) surfaces are contacting surfaces. In this context, the _____ surface of one tooth ordinarily contacts the _____ surface of the adjacent tooth (use the technical words).

two is correct

distal, mesial (in either order)

>**Frame B**

You are counting the surface contacting the tooth on the mesial side (toward the midline), the surface contacting the tooth on the distal side (away from the midline), and the masticating surface (incisal or occlusal, as the case may be). You are right. These three surfaces normally do make contact with another tooth surface.

RETURN TO THE QUESTION FRAME AND ANSWER AGAIN.

three is incorrect

For the present time, the contact between teeth belonging to different arches will not be considered. By limiting the use of the words "contacting surfaces" to those surfaces where contact remains constant, only the proximal (PROCK sim ul) surfaces are contacting surfaces. Considering one arch only, the _____ surface of one tooth ordinarily contacts the _____ surface of the adjacent tooth (use the technical words).

distal, mesial (in either order)

The distal surface of one tooth ordinarily contacts the mesial surface of the adjacent one, or vice versa. However, there are four teeth whose distal surface does not contact another tooth. These four teeth all belong to the same family; in fact, they are all _____ _____ .

third molars

Permanent
Maxillary
Mandibular

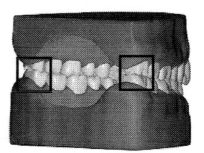

central incisors

Also, there are four teeth whose mesial surfaces contact mesial surfaces. These four teeth are all _____ _____ .

Permanent
Maxillary
Mandibular
Central Incisors

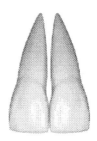

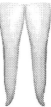

distal

Except for the mesial surfaces of the central incisors and the distal surfaces of the third molars, the mesial surfaces make contact with adjacent distal surfaces. Surfaces facing toward adjacent teeth are known as proximal surfaces. The term proximal cannot be used collectively to describe all mesial and distal surfaces because the _____ surface of the third molar does not face an adjacent tooth.

proximal

However, both the mesial and distal surfaces of most teeth are correctly termed _____ surfaces.

c

In truth, a proximal surface does not contact the adjacent tooth throughout its entire wall, but instead touches only in a well-defined, distinct contact area.

If normally developed teeth do not make contact on their proximal surfaces, the resulting space between the proximal surfaces is known as a **diastema** (die ASS tim uh). This condition occurs frequently between the maxillary central incisors.

Which of the following could correctly be termed a diastema? (select one of the following)

a. the space due to a missing central incisor lost in a fight
b. the space due to the natural loss of a primary tooth
c. neither of these

Lingual (LING wull) refers to the tongue (lingua). The lingual surfaces of maxillary and mandibular teeth are those tooth surfaces adjacent to the tongue. **Facial** (FAY shull), of course, refers to the face and names those surfaces opposite the lingual surfaces and adjacent to the face. The surfaces indicated with the line in the drawing are the _____ surfaces.

Permanent
Maxillary
OCCLUSAL

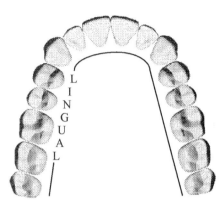

The term "facial" is generally the accepted term, however, the facial surfaces are often further distinguished as to whether they are facial surfaces of anterior teeth or posterior teeth. The facial surfaces of anterior teeth (incisors and canines) are sometimes called **labial** (LAY bee ul), or near the lip, while the facial surfaces of the posterior teeth (premolars and molars) are sometimes called **buccal** (pronounced like "buckle"), or near the cheek. The cheek is where a muscle called the **buccinator** (BUCK sin nate ur) is located. Even though the terms labial and buccal are often used, it is proper (and simpler) to use facial for all teeth. For this reason, the remainder of this program will emphasize facial surfaces. However, the student should remember each term.

Permanent
Maxillary
OCCLUSAL

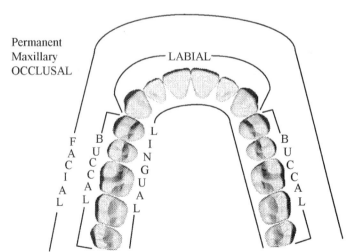

Question Frame

The two frames following this question will be labeled Frame A and Frame B for ease in location.

Whether the facial surface is called labial or buccal and whether the functional surface is incisal or occlusal corresponds to whether the tooth is _____ or _____ .

maxillary or mandibular . . . . GO TO FRAME A.
anterior or posterior . . . . GO TO FRAME B.

---

maxillary or
mandibular is incorrect

>Frame A

The terms maxillary and mandibular are very common terms in dental anatomy. If you are not sure about their meaning, they are defined in frames on pages 13 and 14. They primarily refer to the upper (maxillary) and lower (mandibular) arches. The other technical words in the item were anterior and posterior. The prefixes "ante" (before) and "post" (after) suggest the usage of the words. Anterior refers to things in front and posterior to things behind.

RETURN TO THE QUESTION FRAME AND ANSWER AGAIN.

---

anterior or posterior is
correct
mesial, distal, facial,
lingual

>Frame B

If a tooth is an anterior tooth, labial applies; if it is a posterior tooth, buccal applies. Four tooth surface names are the same for all teeth, whether anterior or posterior. These four are _____ , _____ , _____ , and _____ .

---

facial

That tooth surface that is positioned toward and adjacent to either the cheek or lip is termed the _____ .

---

facial

When a person smiles, you will see his teeth from a _____ view.

---

lingual

That tooth surface which is opposite the facial surface and positioned toward the tongue is termed the lingual surface.

The term *lingual* is a Latin-derived word from which also comes the word *linguist*. In viewing a tooth from the tongue side, one sees the _____ surface.

---

opposite

A tooth's facial surface is _____ (adjacent to/opposite) its lingual surface.

cervical third

For precise communication about tooth surfaces, a scheme of division into thirds is used. The figures in the next two frames represent the arbitrary division into thirds. The particular third spoken of is designated the facial third, lingual third, occlusal third, cervical third, etc.

Vertical divisions of the crown from a facial view (figure 1) are distal third, middle third, and mesial third (anterior or posterior teeth). From the proximal view (figure 2), the vertical divisions are facial third, middle third, and lingual third (anterior or posterior teeth). From the facial view (figure 3), the horizontal divisions are incisal third, middle third, and cervical third for anterior teeth (occlusal third, middle third, and cervical third for posterior teeth).

What name is given to the division labeled "A" in figure 3? _____ _____

Permanent
Maxillary
Right
Central Incisor
1. & 3. FACIAL
2. MESIAL

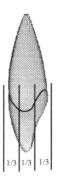
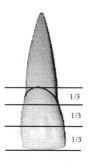

1   2   3

In terms of the horizontal divisions of the crown (figure 4), the incisal edge would be located in the _____ third.

incisal

Permanent
Maxillary
Right
Central Incisor
4. & 5. MESIAL
6. FACIAL

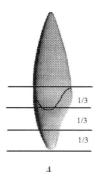
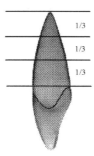
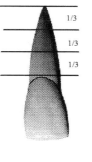

4   5   6

---

apical

Only horizontal divisions (figures 5 and 6) are necessary for tooth roots. These are the cervical third, middle third, and **apical** (APE ik ul) third. The third containing the end of the root would be designated the _____ third.

It should be emphasized that there are no existing anatomical boundary lines for the exact division into thirds. The division is arbitrary.

mesial, middle, distal

Review by answering the following:

Vertical divisions of a posterior tooth viewed from the lingual aspect would divide the crown into divisions called the _____ , _____ , and _____ thirds.

occlusal, middle,
cervical

Horizontal divisions of the same tooth viewed from the lingual aspect would divide the crown into divisions called the _____ , _____ , and _____ thirds.

always

If the crown of any tooth is divided into thirds horizontally from any view, the cervical line is _____ (always/sometimes) in the cervical third.

b. horizontal thirds

The root of any tooth is divided into

a. vertical thirds
b. horizontal thirds
c. both vertical and horizontal thirds

GO TO THE NEXT PAGE AND TAKE REVIEW TEST 1.2.

REVIEW TEST 1.2

1. Maxillary and mandibular identify the two _____ of the dentition.

   a. arches
   b. quadrants
   c. diphyodonts

2. Choose the most correct statement for normal dentition.

   a. All mesial and distal surfaces are contacting surfaces.
   b. Distal surfaces that contact mesial surfaces are proximal surfaces.
   c. All contacting surfaces are mesial against distal.

3. Which two of the following are horizontal divisions of both crowns and roots?

   a. apical third   c. middle third
   b. cervical third   d. lingual third

4. Which of the two arches in the illustration is the maxillary arch?

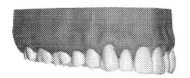   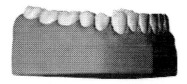

         B   A

5. Give the full names for the teeth indicated by the universal codes below:

   18 _____
   I _____
   3 _____
   M _____

6. Which tooth is indicated at the arrow in the drawing?

   a. 32
   b. 18
   c. 10
   d. 13

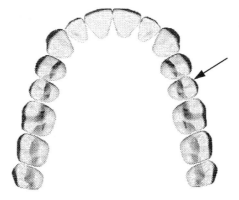

TURN PAGE

7. The tooth identified in question 6 is the

    a. permanent maxillary right second premolar
    b. permanent mandibular right second premolar
    c. permanent maxillary left second premolar
    d. permanent mandibular left second premolar

8. Two statements of the following four are correct. Identify them.

    a. Facial and lingual surfaces are the occlusal surfaces of two different types of teeth.
    b. Some tooth surface names depend on the position of the tooth in the dental arch.
    c. All posterior teeth have occlusal surfaces.
    d. Every tooth has an incisal surface.

9. Which of the following selections indicate teeth with incisal edges?

    a. 1, 16, 17, 32
    b. 5, 12, 21, 29
    c. 7, 10, 23, 26
    d. 4, 13, 20, 28

10. Which of the following has an occlusal surface?

    a. 6
    b. 3
    c. 8
    d. 25

11. Which of the following indicate teeth with occlusal surfaces?

    a. C, H
    b. M, N
    c. B, I
    d. O, P

12. Of the following selections, which selection is a listing of teeth with labial surfaces?

    a. E, F, O
    b. I, J, K
    c. A, B, T
    d. S, L, K

13. The teeth labeled A in the drawing are the _____ teeth.

    a. succedaneous
    b. nonsuccedaneous

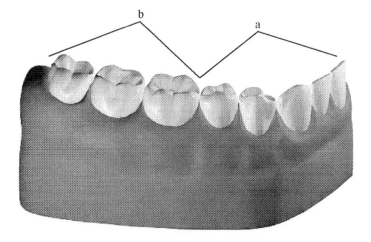

14. Which of the following selections indicate teeth with occlusal surfaces?

    a. 7, 10, D, G

    b. 26, 23, N, Q

    c. 6, 11, 27, H

    d. 12, 5, B, 30

15. The incisors, canines, and premolars are _____ teeth.

    a. succedaneous

    b. nonsuccedaneous

CHECK YOUR ANSWERS IN APPENDIX A.

ROOT STRUCTURE OF TEETH

cervical

Whereas the crown is the superstructure of the tooth, the root is its substructure. The basic function of the root is the same for all the teeth; that is, to support the crown so that the tooth may function adequately.

Recall that the clinical root is defined as that portion of the tooth which is not visible in the mouth. The anatomical root is that part of the tooth from the apical end of the root to the _____ line.

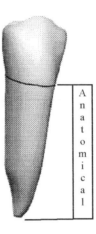

apical foramen, apex

At or near the end or **apex** (A pex; plural: apices) of a root, nerves and blood vessels enter the tooth through one or more openings, the **apical foramen** (pronounced, foe RAY men; plural: **foramina,** four RAM i na).

When examining a specimen tooth, one could insert a very fine probe through the _____ _____ (apex/apical foramen) located near the _____ (apex/apical foramen) of the tooth.

three

Some teeth have only one root. Other teeth characteristically have two or three roots. Where there are two roots, the roots are said to be **bifurcated** (BUY fur kate ted; *bi* means "two," *furca* means "to fork"). **Bifurcation** (buy fur KAY shun) is the division of one into two branches. Some teeth have **trifurcated** (TRY fur kate ted) roots, a condition where there are _____ roots in number.

As shown in the table below, incisors, canines, and some premolars commonly have only one root. The remaining teeth are commonly bifurcated or trifurcated (third molars are variable from one to several roots). Maxillary premolars may be either single-rooted or bifurcated (the maxillary first premolar is the one most often bifurcated). In rare instances, mandibular canines occasionally have bifurcated roots. Maxillary molars are trifurcated and mandibular molars are bifurcated. Which premolar is most often bifurcated?

_____   _____   _____

NUMBER OF ROOTS COMMONLY FOUND ON PERMANENT TEETH

	Incisors	*Canines*	*Premolars*	*Molars**
MAXILLARY	single	single	single or bifurcated	trifurcated
MANDIBULAR	single	single (or bifurcated)	single	bifurcated

*Third molars are variable.

Which of these teeth illustrates single roots? _____

Trifurcation? _____

Bifurcation? _____

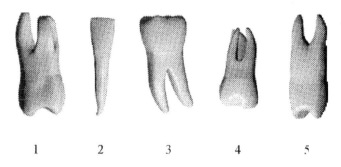

1   2   3   4   5

For simplification, the anatomical definition for the root of a tooth will be used in the following section of this chapter.

Root anatomy is of particular concern in surgical procedures, fixed and removable bridge design, treatment and maintenance of the supporting tissues, treatment of the root canal, and other dental procedures.

Alveolar (al VEE o lar) bone supports the teeth. The bone cavity or socket that holds a root is called an **alveolus** (al VEE oh luss; plural, **alveoli,** al VEE oh lie). The apex and apical foramen are found at or near the base (deepest point) of the _____ .

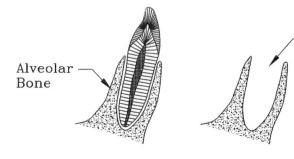

Alveolar Bone

Alveolus

apical

Some of the significant features of root anatomy that you will learn are the number and location of the roots of each tooth, the relative length of the roots, and the usual convex and concave areas on the root surfaces.

Teeth have many variations in their crown and root forms. There is great variability found near the end of the root, that is, in the _____ third of the root.

maxillary first premolar

Incisors, most canines, and most premolars have a single root. The mandibular canine is infrequently bifurcated. On which of these teeth is a multiple root most common (see illustration)?

_____ _____ _____

(arch)   (tooth name)

Permanent
Maxillary
Mandibular
Right
Incisors
Canines
Premolars

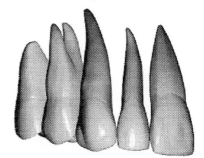

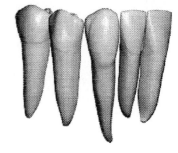

Premolars   Canines   Incisors

root trunk

The root of a multi-rooted tooth includes a root trunk and two or more terminal roots. That portion of a multi-rooted tooth located between the cervical line and the division is called the _____ _____ .

Permanent
Maxillary
Right
First Premolar
MESIAL

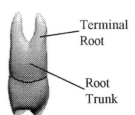

Terminal Root

Root Trunk

Maxillary molars generally have three roots. When a tooth has three roots, the root portion of that tooth has one root trunk and three _____ _____ .

Permanent
Maxillary
Right
First Molar
1. FACIAL
2. DISTAL

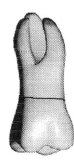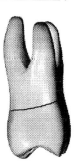

1   2

Although the curved contours of the roots do not present distinct surface boundaries, the terms facial, lingual, mesial, and distal are used to indicate root surfaces and directions.

Of the three terminal roots on maxillary molars, one is located toward the lingual and two toward the _____ .

Permanent
Maxillary
Right
First Molar
1. FACIAL
2. DISTAL

D   M   L   F

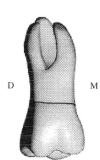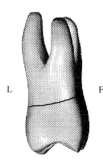

1   2

Terminal roots are named for the position they occupy in relation to the surfaces of the crown. Root A is the distofacial root, B is the _____ root, and C is the _____ root.

Permanent
Maxillary
Right
First Molar
1. FACIAL
2. DISTAL

A   C   C   A
         B   B

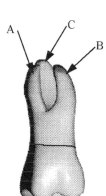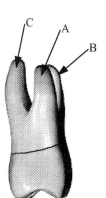

1   2

mesial, distal

Mandibular molars generally have two terminal roots, the _____ and _____ .

Permanent
Mandibular
Right
First Molar
1. FACIAL
2. MESIAL

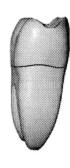
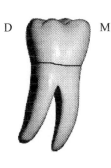

D M

1   2

facial, lingual

The maxillary first premolar is usually bifurcated. The terminal roots are named the _____ and _____ roots.

Permanent
Maxillary
Right
First Molar
1. FACIAL
2. DISTAL

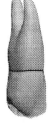
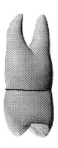

1   2

maxillary first premolar,
mandibular canine

Of the anterior and premolar teeth, the only tooth that is commonly bifurcated is the _____ _____ _____ . The anterior tooth that is less frequently bifurcated is the _____ _____ .

Question Frame

The three frames following the question in this frame are labeled A, B, and C for ease in reference.

Remembering the number and relative position of the roots of the permanent teeth, which one of the following surfaces would not generally occur?

a. The lingual surface of the mesiofacial root of the maxillary second molar
.... GO TO FRAME A.

b. The mesial surface of the mesial root of the mandibular first molar
.... GO TO FRAME B.

c. The mesial surface of the facial root of the maxillary canine
.... GO TO FRAME C.

a is incorrect

>**Frame A**

A mesiofacial root is usually present on all maxillary molars. Also there is a distofacial root and a lingual root. Each of these terminal roots has a lingual surface.

Permanent
Maxillary
Right
First Molar
1. LINGUAL
2. MESIAL

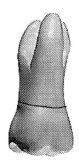
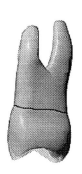

1   2

RETURN TO THE QUESTION FRAME AND ANSWER AGAIN.

>**Frame B**

b is incorrect

The mandibular first molar has two terminal roots, the mesial and distal. Each of these has a broad mesial surface.

Permanent
Mandibular
Right   D   M
First Molar
MESIOFACIAL

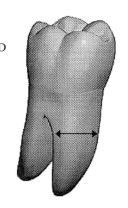

RETURN TO THE QUESTION FRAME AND ANSWER AGAIN.

>**Frame C**

c is correct (The maxillary canines are single rooted and would not have a "facial root".)

Which premolar is frequently multi-rooted, and what are the names of the two roots?

_____   _____   _____ , _____

(arch)   (tooth name)   (root names)

maxillary, first
premolar, facial, lingual

A

Descriptions of teeth involve curvatures in the longitudinal and horizontal directions. For instance, the long dimension of the root (cervical line to apex) is referred to as the cervicoapical or longitudinal dimension. In the drawing, the longitudinal dimension of the root is indicated by line _____ (A/B/C).

Permanent
Maxillary
Right
Central
MESIAL

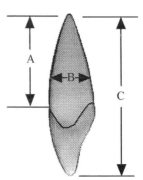

mesiodistal

The width of a tooth is described in either of two directions—mesiodistal or faciolingual. If you look at the lingual surface of a tooth, the width of the root will be seen in a _____ direction.

Permanent
Maxillary
Right
Central Incisor
1. LINGUAL
2. MESIAL

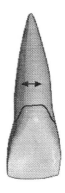   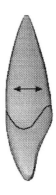

1   2

Fig. 2

Internal tooth anatomy is frequently described and illustrated by showing either a longitudinal section or a cross section. Which drawing represents a cross section? (A cross section is taken horizontally.) _____ _____ (Fig. 1; Fig. 2; Fig. 3)

Permanent
Maxillary
Right Canine

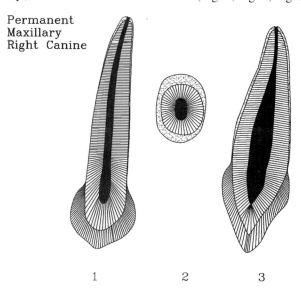

1   2   3

The concept of cross section and longitudinal section is simple, but often the vocabulary makes it confusing. A longitudinal section can be taken in two ways: a mesiodistal longitudinal section or a faciolingual longitudinal section. The drawing illustrates a cut made through the tooth in the mesiodistal longitudinal direction.

Permanent
Maxillary
Right Canine
DISTOFACIAL

D   M

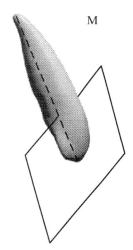

mesiodistal

This representation would be the longitudinal section in the _____ (mesiodistal/faciolingual) direction.

Permanent
Maxillary
Right Canine

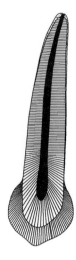

The faciolingual longitudinal section will show the cervicoapical curvature of the facial and lingual surfaces. In this drawing, the distofacial view of the maxillary right central incisor, a cut through the tooth in a faciolingual direction is illustrated.

Permanent
Maxillary
Right Canine
DISTOFACIAL

D   M

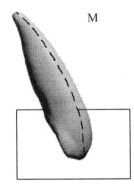

The resulting longitudinal section is a representation of the _____ (mesiodistal/ faciolingual) longitudinal section.

Permanent
Maxillary
Right Canine

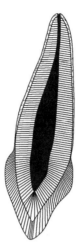

Which type of section reveals the outline of each of the four root surfaces of the maxillary canine in both the mesiodistal and faciolingual directions? _____ _____ .

cross section

Permanent
Maxillary
Right Canine

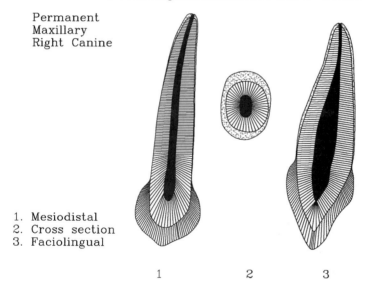

1. Mesiodistal
2. Cross section
3. Faciolingual

     1   2   3

NOW TURN THE PAGE AND TAKE REVIEW TEST 1.3.

REVIEW TEST 1.3

1. The term "alveolus" refers to
   a. part of the root
   b. the apex
   c. socket in the bone supporting a tooth

2. Which list gives the universal code numbers of three teeth that are likely to be bifurcated?
   a. 3, 21, 15
   b. 31, 5, 19
   c. 5, 32, 8

3. Although permanent teeth may have one, two, or three roots, each tooth has only one
   a. root trunk
   b. terminal root

4. In this volume, the term "root" refers to the anatomical root of a tooth, i.e., that part of a tooth
   a. embedded within the alveolar bone
   b. between the cervical line and the apex

5. Which of the following teeth are commonly trifurcated?
   a. lateral incisor
   b. maxillary canine
   c. mandibular molar
   d. maxillary molar
   e. maxillary premolar

6. Which of the following are names of longitudinal sections of roots?
   a. mesiodistal
   b. mesiofacial
   c. faciolingual
   d. distofacial
   e. all of the above

7. Which root, a, b, or c, is the lingual root in the accompanying drawing?

Permanent
Maxillary Right
First Molar

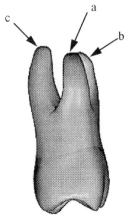

8. Which figure, a or b, represents a faciolingual longitudinal section?

Permanent
Maxillary
Right Canine

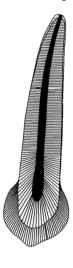 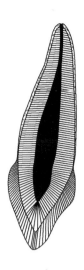

a   b

9. Which of the following are commonly bifurcated?

   a. maxillary canine
   b. maxillary first premolar
   c. mandibular first premolar
   d. mandibular molar

10. The maxillary molars are

   a. bifurcated
   b. trifurcated
   c. single rooted

CHECK YOUR ANSWERS IN APPENDIX A.

1.4.0 ## INTRODUCTION TO TOOTH TISSUES

A tooth is composed of both hard and soft tissues. The hard tissues will be discussed first. The hard tissues are **enamel, cementum,** and **dentin** (DEN tun, not "dentyne"). Enamel is the tooth's hardest tissue and forms the shell of the anatomical crown. The enamel ends where it meets the cementum. The cementum covers the anatomical root. Where the crown and root join, the cementum and enamel form the cementoenamel junction, also called the cervical line or the CEJ.

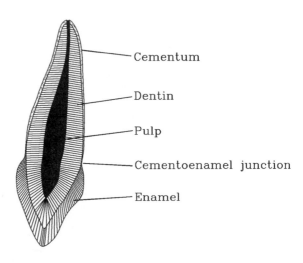

Permanent
Maxillary
Right Canine
FACIOLINGUAL
LONGITUDINAL
SECTION

Cementum

Dentin

Pulp

Cementoenamel junction

Enamel

crown

Together, the enamel and cementum form the outer shell of the tooth. The *enamel* covers the anatomical _____ of the tooth.

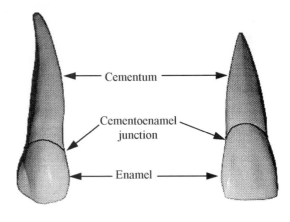

Permanent
Maxillary
Right
1. CANINE
2. CENTRAL INCISOR

Cementum

Cementoenamel junction

Enamel

1   2

root

The *cementum* covers the anatomical _____ of the tooth.

The cementoenamel junction is found where the _____ and _____ meet.

cementum (root), enamel (crown)

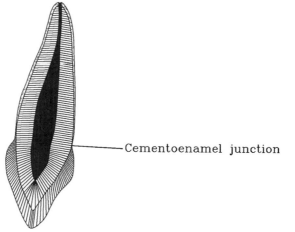

Permanent
Maxillary
Right Canine
FACIOLINGUAL
LONGITUDINAL
SECTION

——— Cementoenamel junction

Another name for the cementoenamel junction or CEJ is the _____ line.

cervical

The *dentin* is the third hard tissue of the tooth. Dentin forms most of the root and a major portion of the crown. The dentin is covered by the enamel on the crown and the cementum on the root. Within the dentin is a cavity, which begins at the apical foramen and terminates in the crown. Within the crown, the cavity is termed pulp chamber; within the root, root canal. The pulp chamber follows the general contours of the tooth, causing the chambers to terminate in conical-shaped peaks. These are called pulp horns. The pulp horns, pulp chamber, and root canal make up the cavity in the _____ .

dentin

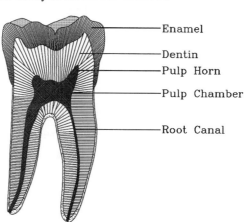

Permanent
Mandibular
First Molar
MESIODISTAL
SECTION

——— Enamel

——— Dentin

——— Pulp Horn

——— Pulp Chamber

——— Root Canal

1.4.1   PULP ANATOMY

The cavity in the dentin is filled with soft tissue called pulp. Both the pulp chamber and root canal are filled with pulpal tissue. The pulp chamber is lined with cells called odonto-blasts (dentin-forming cells). Throughout the pulp is a rich network of blood vessels and lymphatic vessels.

The pulp has several functions. Its primary function is to form dentin throughout the life of the tooth. The pulp also supplies nutrients to the tooth through its network of blood vessels, and responds defensively to any injury to the tooth.

Permanent
Maxillary
Canine
FACIOLINGUAL
   LONGITUDINAL
     SECTION

Permanent
Maxillary
First Premolar
FACIOLINGUAL
   LONGITUDINAL
     SECTION

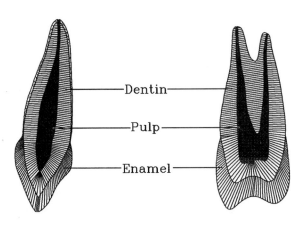

Dentin — Pulp — Enamel

dentin

The pulp cavity is the central cavity within each tooth. The hard tissue that completely surrounds the pulp cavity is the _____ (enamel/dentin/cementum).

Permanent
Mandibular
First Molar
MESIODISTAL
SECTION

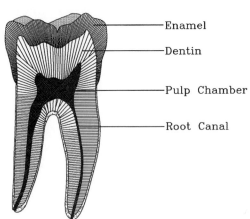

Enamel

Dentin

Pulp Chamber

Root Canal

The pulp cavity is divided into two major parts, the pulp chamber and the root canal. The pulp chamber occurs in the _____ portion of the tooth.

crown

Permanent
Mandibular
First Molar
MESIODISTAL
SECTION

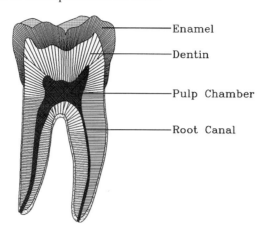

—Enamel

—Dentin

—Pulp Chamber

—Root Canal

The part of the pulp cavity occuring in the root is called the _____
_____ .

root canal

Permanent
Mandibular
1. First Molar
2. Canine
MESIODISTAL
SECTIONS

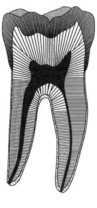

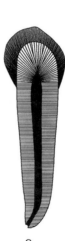

1   2

The two major portions of the pulp cavity are the pulp _____ and the
_____ _____ .

chamber, root canal

Permanent
Mandibular
Canine
MESIODISTAL
SECTION

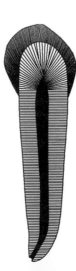

pulp cavity

The pulp chamber and root canal are the two parts of the _____ _____ .

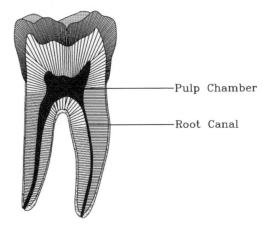

Permanent
Mandibular
First Molar
MESIODISTAL
SECTION

Pulp Chamber

Root Canal

roof

The occlusoapical extremes of the pulp cavity are the roof of the pulp chamber and one or more constricted openings over the apex called the apical foramen (plural: foramina). The dentin that forms the most occlusal (incisal) wall of the pulp cavity is called the _____ of the pulp chamber.

odontoblasts

The first layer of pulpal tissue within the walls of the pulp cavity is made up of dentin-producing cells called _____ .

foramen, foramina

The openings (one or more) near the apex of each root are called the apical _____ (plural: _____).

indistinct

The division between the pulp chamber and the root canals in teeth with more than one root canal is usually well defined. In teeth with a single root canal, the division between the pulp chamber and root canal is _____ (distinct/indistinct).

Permanent
Mandibular
1. Lateral Incisor
2. First Molar
MESIODISTAL
SECTIONS

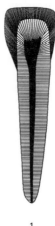

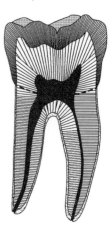

1   2

The division between the pulp chamber and root canal(s) lies at or apical to the division between the anatomical crown and root. In teeth with a more distinct division between the two parts of the pulp cavity, the dentin bounding the pulp chamber and lying somewhat parallel to the roof is called the floor of the pulp chamber. A chamber floor is present only when the pulp chamber gives rise to more than one _____ _____ .

Permanent
Mandibular
1. Lateral Incisor
2. First Molar
MESIODISTAL
SECTIONS

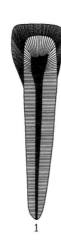
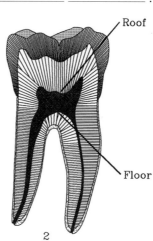

Roof

Floor

1

2

The occlusoapical level of the floor of the pulp chamber lies at or apical to the level of the _____ _____ .

Permanent
Mandibular
1. Lateral Incisor
2. First Molar
MESIODISTAL
SECTIONS

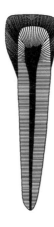
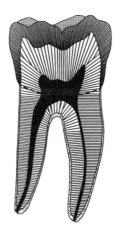

1

2

floor

Each of the openings leading from the pulp chamber to a root canal is called a root canal orifice. Therefore, a canal orifice is an opening in the _____ of the pulp chamber.

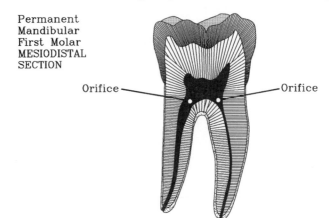

Permanent
Mandibular
First Molar
MESIODISTAL
SECTION

Orifice —   — Orifice

orifice

In teeth with a bifurcation of the pulp cavity at the floor of the chamber, each opening leading from the chamber to a root canal is called a root canal _____ .

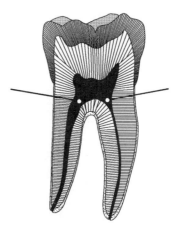

Permanent
Mandibular
First Molar
MESIODISTAL
SECTION

distal

The walls of the pulp cavity derive their names from the corresponding walls of the tooth surface. The name of pulp chamber wall A is the _____ wall.

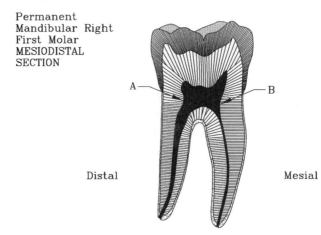

Permanent
Mandibular Right
First Molar
MESIODISTAL
SECTION

A —   — B

Distal   Mesial

Name the structures labeled A, B, and C.

A. _____

B. _____

C. _____

Permanent
Mandibular Right
First Molar
MESIODISTAL
SECTION

Distal   Mesial

A. Floor of the pulp
chamber; B. Mesial
wall of the pulp
chamber; C. Roof of
the pulp chamber.

The roof of the pulp chamber is frequently indented by small extensions called pulp horns, which generally occur directly beneath each cusp. Each horn is named for its corresponding cusp. Thus, pulp horn A is named the _____ pulp horn.

Permanent
Mandibular Right
First Molar
MESIODISTAL
SECTION

Mesiofacial Cusp

A

Distal   Mesial

mesial

The four-cusped mandibular second molar would have _____ (number) pulp horns, but the two-cusped maxillary first premolar would have only _____ (number) pulp horns.

Just as there are variations in the external shape of roots, the interior walls of the pulp chamber and root canals are irregular with many small concavities. The drawings in this program show the walls as very smooth, for simplicity, but the reader should think of them as irregular.

four, two

cervical

In single-rooted teeth, the root canal is continuous with the pulp chamber at approximately the _____ line.

Permanent
Mandibular
Canine
MESIODISTAL
SECTION

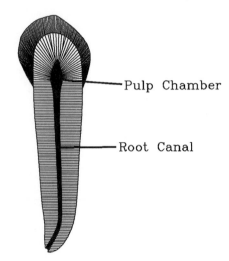

— Pulp Chamber

— Root Canal

pulp chamber

In multi-rooted teeth, the orifice of each root canal is located on the floor of the _____ _____ .

Permanent
Mandibular Right
First Molar
MESIODISTAL
SECTION

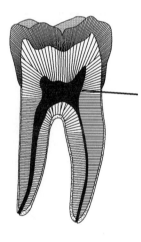

Each root canal terminates at one or more ＿＿＿＿＿ located near the ＿＿＿＿＿ of the root.

foramen (pl. foramina), apex

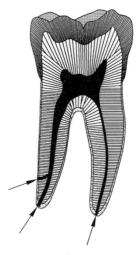

Permanent
Mandibular Right
First Molar
MESIODISTAL
SECTION

Accessory canals (small branches from the main root canal) usually occur in the ＿＿＿＿＿ third of the root, however, they can occur in the middle third of the root.

apical

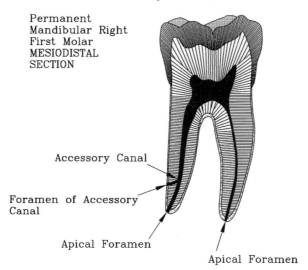

Permanent
Mandibular Right
First Molar
MESIODISTAL
SECTION

Accessory Canal

Foramen of Accessory
Canal

Apical Foramen

Apical Foramen

A, apical foramen;
B, accessory canal

The apical foramen is the opening at (or very near) the apex of the root as shown. A is an
_____ _____ ; B is an _____ _____ .

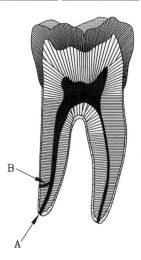

Permanent
Mandibular Right
First Molar
MESIODISTAL
SECTION

B

A

apical foramen

The blood vessels and nerves, nourishing and innervating the pulp, enter the pulp cavity
primarily through the _____ _____ . Accessory canals may also have
nerves and blood vessels.

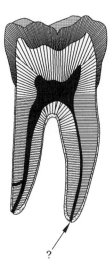

Permanent
Mandibular Right
First Molar
MESIODISTAL
SECTION

?

SUMMARY

A tooth is divided into a crown and a root, the crown being covered with enamel and the root with cementum. The cementum and enamel join to form the cementoenamel junction, also called the cervical line. Within this shell of enamel and cementum is the bulk of the tooth, the dentin. A cavity within the dentin is filled with pulpal tissues (odontoblasts, blood vessels, nerves, lymphatic vessels). The pulp cavity is divided into a pulp chamber and one or more root canals. Parts of the pulp cavity include the walls, floor, and roof of the pulp chamber, pulp horns, root canal orifices, accessory canals, and apical foramina. The walls of the pulp cavity are irregular with many small concavities. The drawing is a summarization of the structures learned in this section.

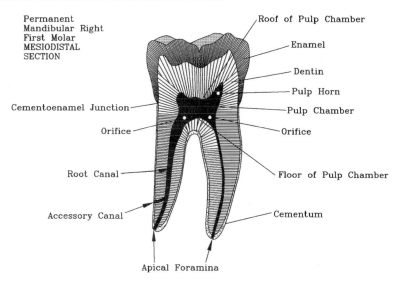

Permanent Mandibular Right First Molar MESIODISTAL SECTION

Roof of Pulp Chamber
Enamel
Dentin
Pulp Horn
Pulp Chamber
Orifice
Floor of Pulp Chamber
Cementum

Cementoenamel Junction
Orifice
Root Canal
Accessory Canal
Apical Foramina

TURN TO THE NEXT PAGE AND TAKE REVIEW TEST 1.4.

REVIEW TEST 1.4

Directions: Terms used in this section are listed in Group I (a-m). A set of definitions is given in Group II. In the blank to the right of each definition, write the letter (from Group I) of the term being defined.

GROUP I

a. enamel

b. accessory canal

c. cementum

d. dentin

e. floor

f. apical foramen

g. pulp horn

h. lymphatic vessels

i. orifice

j. pulp cavity

k. pulp chamber

l. roof

m. root canal

GROUP II

1. An outer opening at the apex of the root through which the blood and nerve supply of the pulp enter the tooth. _____

2. An accentuation of the roof of the pulp cavity corresponding to a cusp or lobe. _____

3. An opening in the floor of the pulp chamber leading to a root canal. _____

4. The central cavity within a tooth. _____

5. Lateral branches of the main root canal occurring in the apical third of the root. _____

6. One of the soft pulpal tissues. _____

7. Hard tooth tissue covering the anatomical root. _____

True/False

8. Tooth #8 (universal code) will have pulp horns.

9. Tooth #14 (universal code) will have a more distinct constriction of the pulp chamber at (or about) the cervical line than will tooth #9.

10. The part of the pulp cavity that occurs in the root is the pulp chamber.

CHECK YOUR ANSWERS IN APPENDIX A.

TOOTH TISSUES

1.5.0

Tooth tissues have been previously discussed in regard to anatomical definitions. The junction of the cementum and enamel (cementoenamel junction) forms the cervical line, separating the tooth into anatomical crown and root portions. The cementum and enamel together form the outer shell of the tooth. The dentin makes up the body or bulk of the tooth. The pulp contains nerve tissues and blood vessels to provide sensation and nutrition to the tooth. Of these four tissues, the first three—enamel, cementum, and dentin—are hard tissues; the fourth—pulp—is soft. These four tissues will be taken up in sequence with a more detailed explanation of their characteristics. The hard tissue that covers the anatomical crown of a tooth is known as _____ .

Permanent
Maxillary
Right Canine
FACIOLINGUAL
LONGITUDINAL
SECTION

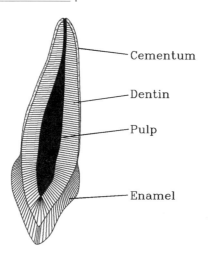

— Cementum

— Dentin

— Pulp

— Enamel

Beneath the enamel is another tissue, not quite as hard, called the _____ .

dentin

The hard outer shell of enamel serves to protect the tooth from wear and prolongs its working life. In fact, the hardest tissue in the body is _____ .

enamel

Enamel is translucent but has a bluish-white tint which contributes to the coloration of the tooth. Because of the translucency of the enamel, much of the tooth coloration is due to the _____ .

dentin

Question Frame

There will be two frames labeled Frame A and Frame B that will refer to this question frame.

Enamel is composed of microscopic rods called enamel rods. The rods are generally perpendicular to the dentin and are bound together by a cement substance. These rods can be cleaved with cutting instruments. The hardness of enamel makes it susceptible to fracture, especially where it is not supported by dentin. This may occur with dental caries (decay). Despite its hardness, enamel is subject to wear and, over a lifetime, a tooth may lose much of its incisal or occlusal enamel due to wear. The enamel is the only tissue completely formed before the tooth erupts, and once the enamel is laid down by the ameloblasts (enamel-producing cells), it does not have the ability of self repair. When enamel has been fractured, how is it mended?

By the enamel rods rebonding to each other . . . . GO TO FRAME A.
By artificial restoration methods . . . . GO TO FRAME B.

enamel rods rebond is
incorrect

>Frame A

You missed a small but very important concept. Enamel does not have the ability of self repair. After the enamel has initially been laid down, the process will not repeat itself for any type of enamel destruction, whether it is fractured or lost by normal abrasion. While the enamel rods are initially bonded together by a cement-like substance, this natural process cannot be repeated. Therefore, in tooth repair, artificial substances must be used; the correct choice of answers should have been "by artificial restoration methods."

RETURN TO THE QUESTION FRAME AND ANSWER AGAIN.

artificial restoration is
correct

wear

>Frame B

The study of artificial restoration methods would presumably lead to a study of operative or restorative dentistry, which will not be taken up now.

Enamel has at least three unique features: (1) it is complete by the time the tooth erupts; (2) the ameloblasts become inactive and the tissue ceases to form after the tooth has erupted; and (3) it is the hardest tissue in the human body. Despite its hardness, enamel is subject to considerable _____ during the life of the tooth.

Notice that the enamel layer is thickest on the _____ edge (surface) and tapers toward the _____ line.

Permanent
Maxillary
1. Canine
2. First Premolar
FACIOLINGUAL
SECTIONS

—Dentin—

—Pulp—

—Enamel—

1

2

Two types of cells that have a role in the formation of tooth tissue have been introduced. The names of these cells have the same suffix (ending). The first layer of pulp tissue that has a role in the formation of dentin is made up of cells called _____ . Enamel-producing cells are called _____ .

Enamel, the exterior tooth surface, covers the anatomical crown of the tooth. Cementum is another hard tooth tissue. It is also an exterior tooth tissue covering the anatomical root portion of the tooth. Cementoblasts, which lay down cementum, are very similar to the osteoblasts which form bone.

The similarity between cementum and bone is evident histologically, chemically, and in its physiologic behavior. Cementum is continually laid down during the life of the tooth in the areas of the apex and where multiple roots join. The basic difference between cementum and bone tissues is that bone undergoes resorption and formation in cycles. Cementum continues formation but normally does not resorb. Because of this process, pressure can be applied to a tooth with an orthodontic appliance ("braces"), and the resorption of the _____ _____ allows the tooth to be brought into proper alignment.

We can explain the process which permits orthodontic alignment to occur by studying, in more detail, the cementum and tooth attachment to the alveolar bone. A function of cementum is to attach the tooth root to a ligament called the periodontal ligament, which, in turn, attaches to the alveolar bone. A tooth is held in the alveolus by this attachment apparatus composed of three parts: the cementum, the periodontal ligament, and the alveolar bone. Orthodontic bands (or other sustained forces) produce pressure on areas of the periodontal ligament and alveolar bone, resulting in resorption of the bone in those areas. At the same time, tension is produced elsewhere on the periodontal ligament and alveolar bone, resulting in _____ (formation/resorption) of new bone tissue in the areas of tension.

dentin, enamel,
cementum

Both cementum and enamel are hard tooth tissues, enamel being the hardest tissue in the body. Cementum, a tooth tissue, is also termed a supporting structure, because it serves to attach the tooth to the alveolar bone. Together, enamel and cementum form the outer shell of the tooth.

Within this shell is the dentin, another hard tissue. Although measurements of the hardness of tooth tissues vary with the exact location on the tooth where the measurements are taken, on the average, dentin is found to be not as hard as enamel but harder than cementum. Thus, the order of hardness of the hard tooth tissues is enamel, dentin, and cementum.

Dentin forms the bulk of the tooth, both crown and root, and surrounds the pulp cavity. By making up the bulk of the tooth, dentin gives the tooth its general form and elastic strength. The hard enamel tissue which is laid directly upon the dentin depends upon this elastic strength for support. One can summarize the hard tissue makeup of the tooth as mostly _____ covered with _____ or _____ .

dentin, enamel,
(dentinoenamel)

The hard tissues of the tooth are the dentin, which is overlaid on the root with cementum and on the crown with enamel. Where the undersurface of the enamel joins the dentin, a junction is formed. The word that describes this junction, like many other dental terms, has been coined by using the letter "o" resulting in a name for the junction of the dentin and enamel. It is the _____o_____ junction, also called the D-E junction.

Permanent
Mandibular Right
First Molar
MESIODISTAL
SECTION

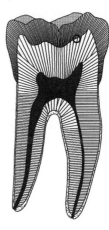

cementum

The dentin is thickest in the anatomic crown of a tooth, gradually tapering to thinner and thinner bulk as one approaches the root apex. You might remember that under the dentinoenamel junction (in the anatomical crown), the dentin is thicker than in the root. The root, of course, is not covered with enamel. It is covered with _____ .

Therefore, the dentinoenamel junction does not extend into the anatomical root. Instead, the dentin joins the cementum in this region. The same method for building a descriptive word for this junction holds true—the terms *dentin* and *cementum* are connected by an "o." At first everyone has difficulty remembering the correct sequence of words in building such terms. For instance, dentinoenamel junction is correct, but enamodental junction is incorrect. The proper order of connecting words is determined by convention and common usage within the dental profession.

What are two words that could be used to describe the junction of the dentin and the cementum? _____ and _____

The term that is commonly used is dentinocemental.

cementodentinal or
dentinocemental

To summarize, the hard tooth junctions are:

1. The C-E junction (the junction of the enamel and cementum) is also called the _____ junction, which also forms the _____ line.
2. The D-E junction (the junction of the enamel and dentin) is also called the _____ junction.
3. The D-C junction (the junction of the cementum and dentin) is also called the _____ junction.

1. cementoenamel;
   cervical;
2. dentinoenamel;
3. dentinocemental

Permanent
Mandibular Right
First Molar
MESIODISTAL
SECTION

Dentinoenamel

Cementoenamel

Dentinocemental

Because of the translucence of the enamel, the color of the dentin is one of the contributing factors of tooth color, varying from yellow to dark brown in color. Unlike enamel or cementum, dentin is sensitive to touch, thermal change, acids of foods, and the like. Dentin, like cementum, continues to form during the life of the tooth.

Does enamel also continue to form throughout the tooth's lifetime? (Yes or No) _____

no

Which tooth tissue is usually found to be harder—cementum or dentin? _____

dentin

odontoblasts

Enamel is the only tooth tissue which is completed upon eruption of the tooth. But, let's study the dentin. It isn't solid inorganic material, but has tube-like structures, called tubules, running through it from the pulp to the dentoenamel junction. These tubules contain extensions of the dentin-forming cells, the _____ .

primary

The structure of the tubules and the presence of living odontoblasts makes dentin a living tissue, permeable to fluids and sensitive to stimuli.

Dentin formation is active during the crown and root formation. We call this dentin the primary dentin. Dentin continues to form more slowly after the root is fully formed. This type of dentin differs in morphology from the primary dentin and is called secondary dentin.

When irritants act on the tooth, such as hot and cold temperatures, abrasion, dental caries, etc., the pulp and its odontoblasts are stimulated to form secondary dentin over the primary dentin in the pulp chamber and/or root canal to insulate the delicate pulp tissue from the irritation. The effect is to cause recession of the pulp into smaller and smaller confines. Such recession may, in some instances, obliterate the pulp cavity. Dentin also ages and aged dentin tubules may die, becoming dead tracts, or the tubules may calcify and become obliterated (sclerotic dentin). Sclerotic dentin is more highly mineralized, giving the dentin in the area a translucent appearance somewhat like an agate.

Considering only the dentin laid down along the D-E junction, which term properly identifies that dentin? _____ (primary/secondary).

Secondary dentin would be an incorrect answer to the previous question because the tooth forms its dentin from the dentinoenamel junction inward towards the pulp cavity. The dentin in the area adjacent to the D-E junction is primary dentin. Secondary dentin is laid down after the tooth is formed, well inwards from the D-E junction. Don't forget that dentin formation is a continual process as long as the pulp provides nutrients to the odontoblasts.

odontoblasts (in the dental pulp)

The fourth tooth tissue is dental pulp, which is a delicate, soft tissue organ. It is composed of odontoblasts to form dentin, blood vessels for nutrients, nerves for communication to the rest of the body, and connective tissues. The pulp is surrounded by the dentin and is the formative organ of the dentin. Among its functions are the formation of secondary dentin which is a defensive function to protect against irritants. Too much irritation can kill the pulp, ending its odontoblastic activity. Remember that the formation of secondary dentin causes the pulp cavity to become smaller as the tooth ages. What forms secondary dentin? _____

younger

Considering the changes in the pulp cavity that occur with age, which patients would generally have larger pulp cavities, younger or older patients? _____

SUPPORTING STRUCTURES
FOR THE TOOTH

1.5.1

The tooth-supporting structures, also four in number, are cementum, periodontal ligament, gingiva (JIN juh vuh), and alveolar bone.

Cementum, as previously noted, is a _____ (hard/soft) tooth tissue as well as being a supporting structure.

hard

Cementum is the hard tissue that bonds the tooth to the periodontal ligament, which is the soft tissue that surrounds the roots of the tooth and attaches to the alveolar bone. The periodontal ligament acts as a shock absorber, cushioning and stabilizing the tooth while transferring forces applied to the tooth into the bone. When severe forces are applied against the tooth, the periodontal ligament may become damaged and pain and inflammation may result. Other functions of the periodontal ligament include sensory and nutritive functions, which are fulfilled by nerves and blood vessels within the ligament. Also, located in the area of the periodontal ligament are cementum-forming cells, called _____ .

cementoblasts

— Cementum

— Periodontal Ligament

— Alveolar Bone

These items review the subject matter from the previous page. Refer back as necessary until the items are clear.

The tooth is attached to its socket by the _____ _____ .

periodontal ligament

The tooth tissue to which the fibers of the periodontal ligament are attached is called the

_____ .

cementum

The outer ends of these fibers are attached to the _____ bone.

alveolar

The periodontal ligament functions to protect against forces acting on the tooth by

_____ _____ .

absorbing shock (or synonym)

free

The outermost of the supporting tissues is the gingiva. Healthy gingiva, often incorrectly called "gums," is a firm, resilient, pink tissue which covers the alveolar bone and through which the tooth's clinical crown protrudes. The gingiva may be divided into attached gingiva and free gingiva. The gingiva directly adjacent to the alveolar bone is referred to as attached gingiva. Gingiva which extends coronally (toward the crown) from the attached gingiva is called _____ gingiva.

alveolar mucosa

The gingiva also attaches directly to the tooth. The attachment to the tooth is always slightly apical to the height of the visible tissue surrounding the tooth. There is, therefore, a space between the gingiva and the tooth, somewhat like a miniature trough, encircling the crown. We call this very narrow space the **gingival sulcus** (JIN juh vul SULL kuss). In healthy mouths, the gingival sulcus ranges from almost non-existence to 3 mm in depth.

The free gingival groove is a shallow indentation or groove found in some areas of the mouth, paralleling the margin of the free gingiva and roughly corresponding to the deepest point of the gingival sulcus.

Gingiva that extends apically (away from the crown) and located below the attached gingiva is called _____ _____ .

mucogingival junction

The attached gingiva is bound to bone and extends from the free gingival groove to the mucogingival junction. The gingiva extending apically from the mucogingival junction is the loosely attached alveolar mucosa. The alveloar mucosa is a thin, nonkeratinized darker pink tissue. The line of demarcation between the attached gingiva and the alveolar mucosa is the mucogingival junction. The alveolar mucosa extends apically from the _____ _____ .

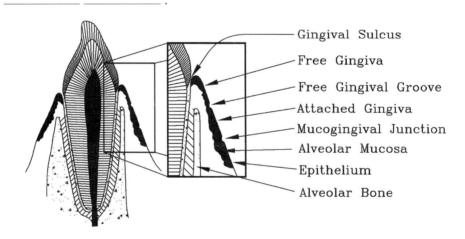

Gingival Sulcus
Free Gingiva
Free Gingival Groove
Attached Gingiva
Mucogingival Junction
Alveolar Mucosa
Epithelium
Alveolar Bone

does

The surface of gingival tissue is covered with a cell tissue that is common to protective surface tissue throughout the body and is called **epithelium** (e pith THEE lee um). The space located coronally from the connection of the epithelium to the tooth is called the gingival sulcus, which _____ (does/does not) completely surround each tooth.

The free gingiva is further subdivided as **papillary** (PAP ill larry) and marginal gingiva. The papillary gingiva occupies the space between the teeth. The marginal gingiva is free gingiva that is both facial and lingual to each tooth. Therefore, the free gingiva that forms the boundary of each clinical crown is both papillary and marginal gingiva.

Papillary gingiva is located _____ _____ .

between teeth

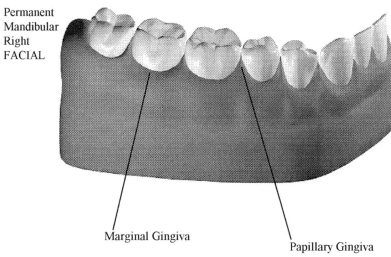

Permanent
Mandibular
Right
FACIAL

Marginal Gingiva

Papillary Gingiva

Papillary and marginal gingiva collectively form the free gingiva which extends coronally from the _____ _____ .

attached gingiva

The gingiva adjacent to the alveolar bone is called _____ gingiva.

attached

The free gingiva located facially and lingually to each tooth is called _____ gingiva.

marginal

papillary

Marginal gingiva is continuous with the free gingiva that extends into the spaces between the teeth, that is the _____ gingiva.

The illustration summarizes the classifications of gingiva.

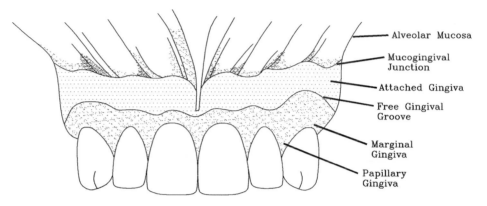

GO TO THE NEXT PAGE AND TAKE REVIEW TEST 1.5.

REVIEW TEST 1.5

1. Choose the *incorrect* statement.

   a. Cementum is classified as a supporting tissue.
   b. Papillary tissue is gingival tissue.
   c. The periodontal ligament is part of the marginal tissue.

2. Choose the *incorrect* statement.

   a. The dentinocemental junction is called the cervical line.
   b. The gingival sulcus is located between the tooth and the gingiva.
   c. Papillary gingiva occupies the space between the teeth.

3. Choose the *incorrect* statement.

   a. Pulpal stimulation causes the laying down of secondary dentin.
   b. Ameloblasts are bone-producing cells.
   c. The dentin constitutes the major portion of the tooth.

4. Select the *correct* term for each of the arrows to properly label each indicated structure.

   a. papillary gingiva
   b. marginal gingiva
   c. free gingival groove
   d. attached gingiva
   e. alveolar mucosa
   f. mucogingival junction

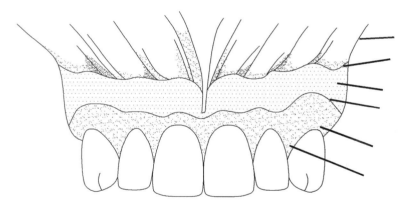

5. Select the *correct* term for each of the arrows to properly label each indicated structure.

    a. cementoenamel junction
    b. dentinoenamel junction
    c. dentinocemental junction

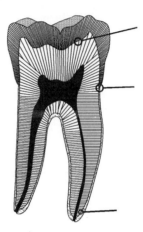

6. Label each arrow to indicate the name of the structure to which the arrow is pointing.

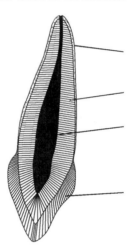

CHECK YOUR ANSWERS IN APPENDIX A.

LIFE HISTORY OF TEETH

All teeth initially develop from a tooth germ—a small clump of cells frequently called lobes, capable of differentiating into dental tissues. These tissues are the ameloblasts that form enamel, the odontoblasts that form dentin, and the other specialized cells necessary to produce the complex structure we call a tooth. Both primary and permanent teeth form in this way. The cells differentiated from the tooth germ form the organic structure which is subsequently calcified. Calcification is the process through which tooth tissues become hardened by deposits of mineral salts, including calcium salts. The tooth tissues that are hardened by calcification are enamel, dentin, and cementum. The cells that make the outer layer of the crown, or the enamel are called _____ .

ameloblasts

The first tooth germs of the primary dentition can be found approximately at 5 to 7 weeks of fetal development. The first tooth germs of the permanent dentition usually appear within 12 weeks after the first primary teeth begin to form—that is, they appear at approximately which point in fetal development? _____

a. at the first third
b. at the midpoint
c. at the last third

b. at the midpoint

Dentin forms inwardly from the dentinoenamel junction and enamel forms outwardly from the junction. The development and calcification of tooth tissue is paralleled by development of the alveolar bone which will support the tooth. The bone forms a crypt around the developing tooth. The process of tooth and bone formation and eruption is time consuming. Are any teeth normally visible in the mouth at birth? _____

No, not usually

The development of the hard tooth tissues in the crypt begins with the laying down of _____ , then enamel, and, finally, cementum.

dentin

Which type of dentin is laid down in the crypt, primary or secondary dentin? _____

primary

The first primary teeth begin to calcify at about the midpoint of fetal development and calcification of all primary teeth is normally completed at three to four years of age. For permanent teeth, calcification begins approximately at birth and is completed at eighteen to twenty-five years of age. The development of a tooth begins with the formation of the crown and continues apically until the apex is formed. We could describe the stage of development of permanent teeth in a 12-year-old child by saying:

"The hard tissues are not completely _____ , and the _____ portion of some teeth have not completely formed."

calcified, apical

1.6.1 GROWTH CENTERS AND LOBES

crown, root (apex)

Tooth development begins with increased cell activity in growth centers in the tooth germ. A growth center is an area of the tooth germ where the cells are particularly active. The active cells create projections or mounds. As the growth centers develop, they unite with one another. This union is called coalescence. The development of the tooth begins with the formation of the _____ (crown/root) and then continues in the direction of the _____ until the tooth is complete.

crypt

The initial formation of the crown is paralleled by growth of the alveolar bone, producing a _____ around the developing tooth.

four

In the illustration, you see the occlusal view of a mandibular second molar. The growth centers, called lobes, have been marked with circles to indicate the center from which the tooth was formed.

How many lobes make up the molar in this illustration? _____

Permanent
Mandibular
Right
Second Molar
OCCLUSAL

F

M

D

coalescence

Coalescence is a word you should know. It means "to fuse" or "to unite." Writing it once or twice may help you to remember it.

On the surface of crowns there may be grooves and/or cusps which mark significant anatomical divisions of the crown. These grooves and cusps are formed during _____ . Some developmental groves are deeper than others because they are not well coalesced.

On a newly erupted central incisor, the presence of three bulges on the incisal edge, called mamelons and two facial grooves appear to separate the facial and incisal portions of the incisor into three distinct areas. These three areas plus one area making up the lingual portion of the incisor crown, are called the _____ of the incisor.

lobes

Permanent
Maxillary
Right
Central Incisor
FACIAL

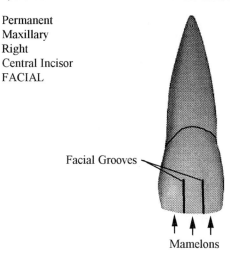

Facial Grooves

Mamelons

All anterior teeth show traces of four lobes, three facially and one lingually. The three facial lobes are visible as rounded eminences (mamelons) on newly erupted incisors. The facial surface of incisors, especially central incisors, often show traces of the fusion of three lobes. This evidence of lobes is in the form of lines called _____ grooves.

facial

	Number of Lobes	Number of Cusps
Molar	4 or 5	4 or 5
Pre-molar	4 or 5	2 or 3

Premolars usually have four lobes except for the mandibular second premolar, which frequently has five lobes (and two lingual cusps). Three lobes form the single facial cusp, and one or two lingually, depending upon the number of lingual cusps. Molars also have four or five lobes as a general rule. Each lobe of molar teeth is surmounted by a cusp. Fill in the table below by writing in the usual number of lobes and cusps for each tooth:

	Number of Lobes	Number of Cusps
Molar	_____ or _____	_____ or _____
Premolar	_____ or _____	_____ or _____

facial

The central lobe (No. 2) in each of the illustrations below is on which surface? _____

Permanent
Mandibular
Right
First Premolar
a. FACIAL
b. OCCLUSAL
c. LINGUAL

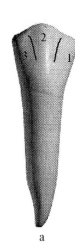
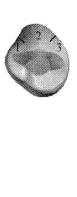
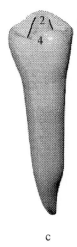

a   b   c

four

The incisors and canines are described as having how many lobes? _____

mamelons, lingual

The incisal edges of newly erupted incisors have three rounded bulges called _____ . They suggest the location of three lobes.

What would be the location of the fourth lobe of these incisors? _____ (facial/lingual).

NAMES OF LOBES AND TOOTH SURFACES

lingual

Knowing the correct technical term for each of the tooth surfaces will be very important throughout the remainder of this course. Names of surfaces, often in combined terms, are constantly used to locate various anatomical features. If you prefer to review these surface identifications, see section 1.2.2 on page 25.

All anteriors and premolars have three facial lobes and one lingual lobe with the exception of some mandibular second premolars which have two lingual lobes. All molars have two facial lobes and two lingual lobes with the exception of first molars which frequently have a fifth lobe.

For example, there are usually five lobes identified on the crown of the maxillary first molar: two to the facial, two to the lingual, and the fifth on the lingual side of the mesiolingual lobe. The facial lobes are known as the mesiofacial and distofacial lobes. The lingual lobes are known as the mesiolingual and distolingual lobes. The fifth lobe is a rudimentary lobe called the lobe of Carabelli, commonly called the cusp of Carabelli, deriving its name from the man who first described it. It is located _____ (facial/lingual/mesial/distal) to the mesiolingual lobe (see illustration).

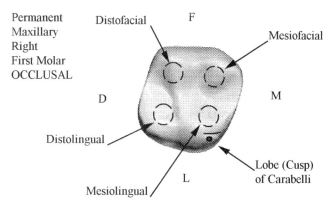

Permanent Maxillary Right First Molar OCCLUSAL — Distofacial — F — Mesiofacial — D — M — Distolingual — L — Mesiolingual — Lobe (Cusp) of Carabelli

The cusp of Carabelli is found on the _____ molar.

permanent maxillary first

Question Frame

The two frames following this question are labeled Frame A and Frame B for ease in location.

Is the cusp of Carabelli found toward the mesial or distal surface of the tooth? _____

mesial. . . . . GO TO FRAME B.
distal . . . . GO TO FRAME A.

Distal is incorrect

>**Frame A**

Distal is incorrect because the lobe of Carabelli is lingual to the mesiolingual lobe, placing it near the mesial and lingual surfaces.

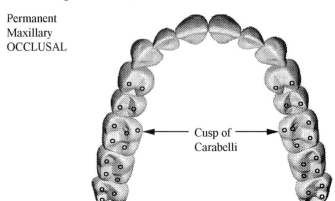

Permanent
Maxillary
OCCLUSAL

Cusp of Carabelli

Consider the illustration, then carefully picture in your mind the arrangement of these lobes.

RETURN TO THE QUESTION FRAME AND ANSWER AGAIN.

Mesial is correct

>**Frame B**

The mandibular first molar has five lobes also. The arrangement of the lobes differs from those of the maxillary first molar. There are two lingual lobes, mesiolingual and distolingual; and two facial lobes, mesiofacial and distofacial. The fifth lobe is positioned distal to the distofacial lobe and is known as the distal lobe (see diagram).

F

Permanent
Mandibular
Right
First Molar   M
OCCLUSAL

2

1   5

3   4

D

L

mamelons

The locations of three of the four lobes making up an incisor are seen from the bumps along the incisal edge of young children's incisors. These bumps are called _____.

Both the maxillary and mandibular second molars generally have four lobes, two to the facial and two to the lingual. Except for the fifth lobe on each of the first molars, the arrangement of the other four lobes is similar to the second molars, and the same terms apply.

The two facial lobes are the _____ and _____ lobes.
The two lingual lobes are the _____ and _____ lobes.

Permanent
1. Mandibular
   Right
   Second Molar
2. Maxillary
   Right
   Second Molar
   OCCLUSAL

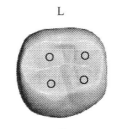

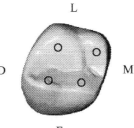

1

2

Many variations occur in the lobe arrangement of the third molars. Either four or five lobes may be present. At times only three lobes may be seen, and sometimes more than five. Because of the wide variation in the third molars, it is impractical to establish a standard for them.

The variations which occur throughout human dentition are also partially caused by the relationship of one lobe to another. Therefore, variations occur resulting from (1) the number of lobes, (2) the shape of the lobe, and (3) the arrangement of the lobes. These variables together affect the shape of any one particular tooth. A tooth is actually a _____ (fusion) of several lobes which has developed into a tooth.

DEVELOPMENT AND ERUPTION

The eruption of a tooth is most noticeable when it penetrates the **oral mucosa** (mew CO suh) and enters the oral cavity. At the time the tooth begins to erupt, the crown is fully developed, but the _____ is not.

4

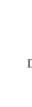

5

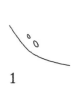

1

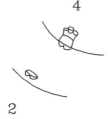

2

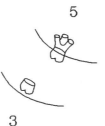

3

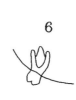

6

When the crown of the tooth is visible in the mouth, the process of enamel hardening, called _____ , has been completed.

the central incisors

The tooth usually continues to erupt until it meets its antagonist (opposing tooth) in the opposite jaw. This complex process is called active eruption and is the movement of teeth coronally through the oral mucosa. The active eruption of teeth in each dentition follows an eruption sequence, that is, an order of the progressive eruption of the teeth. The eruption sequence for the primary dentition is anterior to posterior except for the canines, which often lag behind the first molars. Which primary tooth can be expected to erupt first?

_____ _____ _____

B

Following is a graph showing the most frequent eruption sequence and the range of eruption dates for *primary* teeth. The sequence, central incisor, lateral incisor, first molar, canine, second molar, is found in the majority of cases, with the first molar and canine occasionally reversed. Study the graph carefully.

Which of the following series (A or B) of abbreviations represents the normal eruption sequence for primary teeth in each arch?

A: CI, LI, C, 1M, 2M
B: CI, LI, 1M, C, 2M

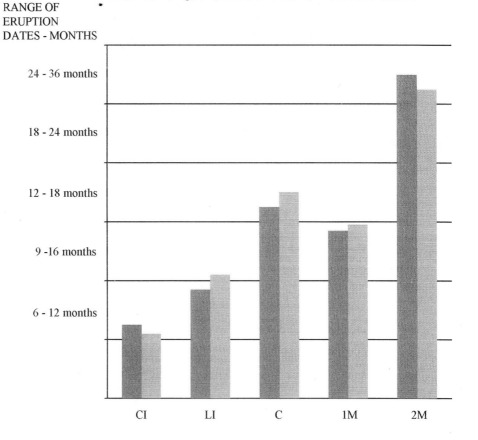

ERUPTION SEQUENCE AND DATES FOR PRIMARY TEETH

CI - Central Incisor
LI - Lateral Incisor
C - Canine
1M - First Molar
2M - Second Molar

Maxillary
Mandibular

Although there is a great variability in eruption sequence when we consider whether or not a particular mandibular tooth precedes a maxillary tooth, the aforementionued sequence seems to be an average eruption sequence for primary teeth. There may be a considerable difference between the mandibular and maxillary eruption dates for any one patient, however, in general, the tooth that can be expected to erupt first is the primary _____ (maxillary/mandibular) central incisor.

mandibular

Now, study the graph of eruption sequence and dates for *permanent* teeth. The eruption graph for permanent teeth shows a major difference in the eruption time of mandibular and maxillary canines. The mandibular canine usually erupts before the mandibular premolars. The maxillary canine usually erupts _____ (before/after) the maxillary premolars.

after

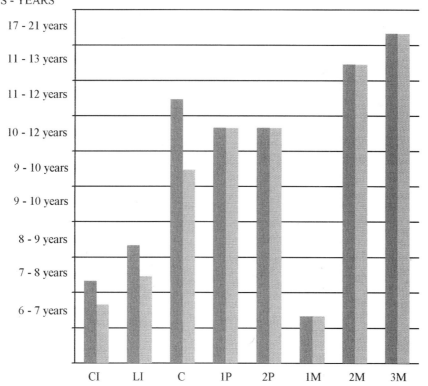

ERUPTION SEQUENCE AND DATES FOR PERMANENT TEETH

RANGE OF ERUPTION DATES - YEARS

17 - 21 years
11 - 13 years
11 - 12 years
10 - 12 years
9 - 10 years
9 - 10 years
8 - 9 years
7 - 8 years
6 - 7 years

CI   LI   C   1P   2P   1M   2M   3M

CI - Central Incisor
LI - Lateral Incisor
C - Canine
1P - First Premolar
2P - Second Premolar
1M - First Molar
2M - Second Molar
3M - Third Molar

☐ Maxillary
☐ Mandibular

before

Also, as shown in the eruption table, the permanent mandibular teeth usually erupt before the maxillary teeth except for the premolars and molars which have eruption dates very close together. For example, the mandibular central incisor usually erupts _____ (before/after) the maxillary central incisor.

nonsuccedaneous

An important difference between the eruption sequences for permanent and primary teeth is that the first molars erupt first in the permanent dentition. Recall that the permanent molars do not await the loss of any primary teeth in order to erupt—that is, the permanent molars are _____ .

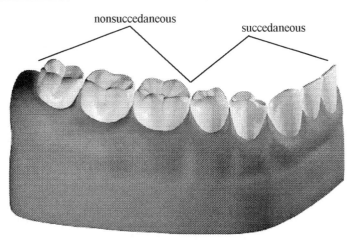

first molars, molars

The first permanent teeth to erupt are an exception to the general rule of an anterior to posterior eruption sequence. These are the _____ _____ , sometimes called the six-year _____ .

canines

The permanent maxillary canines also lag behind the first molars just as the primary _____ do.

first molars

We learned before that the primary canines normally lag behind the primary _____ _____ .

first molars

Also, that the first permanent teeth to erupt are the _____ _____ .

eruption

When a tooth meets its antagonist, further active _____ is restrained and continues only as necessary to compensate for wear on the functional surfaces.

After the primary tooth has met its antagonist through active eruption, it functions to hold space while the child grows, helps with mastication, swallowing, speech, etc., until the permanent tooth begins movement towards the oral cavity. A permanent tooth that moves into a position formerly occupied by a primary tooth is called a _____ tooth.

succedaneous

The succedaneous tooth continues its active eruption (root formation and movement) accompanied by the resorption of the roots of the primary tooth in its path.

Resorption of the primary tooth continues until the tooth has no root and no bone support and the epithelial attachment can no longer hold the tooth in place. The primary tooth then _____ _____ .

falls out (or any synonym)

Soon after the primary tooth falls out, the erupting permanent tooth is in place to pierce the mucosa and move into view in the mouth.

The natural process whereby the primary teeth are lost is known as exfoliation. Remember this term from the fact that primary teeth are also called deciduous and that a deciduous tree loses its leaves through exfoliation. Only the _____ dentition undergoes the process of exfoliation.

primary

The normal development of human dentition, therefore, consists of the active eruption, function, resorption of the root, and exfoliation of the primary teeth, followed by the appearance of the permanent teeth. The actual order of eruption for these teeth is known as the _____ _____ .

eruption sequence

Before a succedaneous permanent tooth can enter the oral cavity, first the _____ of the primary tooth root and finally the _____ of that tooth must take place.

resorption, exfoliation

As the tooth actively erupts, an increasingly larger segment of the tooth is visible. The free gingiva determines the boundary of this visible segment, called the _____ _____ .

clinical crown

active

The process of active eruption is basically completed when the tooth assumes its position in the mouth and the root is fully formed. Some active eruption related to additional growth of cementum and alveolar bone near the apex continues throughout life to compensate for the wear of occluding surfaces of teeth. A process called passive eruption may begin once the tooth enters the oral cavity. Passive eruption is the migration of the soft tissue attachment near the cementoenamel junction to a more apical attachment exposing more clinical crown. This recession of the supporting tissues may be a very slow process and of little significance, but can become a critical factor in pathological condition (e.g., periodontal disease) by weakening the tooth's support or actually causing loss of the tooth.

The laying down of additional bone at the base of the alveolus would be associated with _____ (active/passive) eruption.

enamel

One other factor in the history of a normal tooth is attrition, the wearing away of the incisal or occlusal surfaces. Attrition is initially the wearing away of what tooth tissue? _____

hardest

The enamel may show noticeable wear even though it is the _____ tissue in the body.

b. first molars

The most noticeable effect of attrition is the flattening of the occlusal cusp tips and incisal edges. It is not uncommon for the incisal edges to have worn to such an extent through attrition that the dentin is exposed.

Teeth cannot all be expected to wear at the same rate as a result of attrition. Differences in rate of wear are common. For example, it is possible that the first teeth to erupt may experience the most wear. Can you remember which of the permanent teeth erupt first?

a. The maxillary central incisors
b. The first molars

third molars

There is typically a lag of about six years between the eruption of the first and second molars and another six years between the second and third molars. The lag occurs because the maxilla and mandible have not completed their development, and there is insufficient space for the remaining nonsuccedaneous teeth. Normally, therefore, the last of the permanent teeth to erupt are the _____ _____.

The eruption sequence of the molars is important in considering attrition. Between the first and third permanent molars, there might be a considerable difference in wear from attrition because of a difference of how many years of use—6 years or 12 years? _____

The first molars erupt at approximately 6–7 years of age, as do the mandibular central incisors. The maxillary central incisors erupt at about age 7–8 years. The first, second, and third permanent molars are _____ and, therefore, do not follow any primary teeth.

All of the permanent molars cannot erupt early, however, for they must necessarily wait until the maxilla and mandible have reached the stage of development which allows enough room for them to erupt. Normally this means that the first permanent molars erupt about the sixth year, the second and third appearing later on at about six-year intervals.

The anterior teeth and premolars erupt at varying times within this interval of approximately twelve years. Therefore, we cannot expect these teeth to wear evenly.

Teeth, by meeting each of their antagonists through active eruption, form an imaginary occlusal plane along which each tooth makes contact with its antagonists. Is it correct to say that active eruption goes on throughout life, thereby maintaining the occlusal plane? _____

The life history of a tooth consists, therefore, of its development from one or more growth centers, coalescence when multiple centers exist, active eruption with root formation, continued active eruption to compensate for incisal/occlusal wear, and, in some cases, passive eruption through apical recession of the gingival attachment. The primary teeth usually have much less passive eruption than permanent teeth as they are not retained in the mouth for as many years, but they do, of course, undergo resorption of their roots and exfoliation.

NOW, TAKE REVIEW TEST 1.6 ON THE NEXT PAGE

REVIEW TEST 1.6

1. Choose the *incorrect* statement.

   a. Each tooth shows evidence of four or more lobes.
   b. Normally each tooth erupts after calcification of its crown is complete.
   c. Incisors develop from five growth centers.

2. Choose the *incorrect* statement.

   a. Grooves are visible lines which may separate the lobes.
   b. The fifth lobe normally found on the permanent mandibular first molars is known as the lobe of (cusp of) Carabelli.
   c. The lobe arrangement of most premolars is similar to that of the incisors.

3. Choose the *correct* statement. Normally, the first permanent teeth to erupt are

   a. the maxillary central incisors
   b. the canines
   c. the first premolars
   d. the first molars

4. Choose the *incorrect* statement.

   a. The development of permanent teeth is first evident in the crypt during the fifth to seventh week of fetal life.
   b. The primary eruption sequence is CI, LI, 1M, C, 2M.
   c. Active eruption of a tooth is completed when the tooth meets its antagonist.

5. Choose the *correct* statement.

   a. The third molars are generally lost through exfoliation.
   b. The roots of the primary teeth are resorbed before exfoliation.
   c. The molars are the succedaneous teeth.

CHECK YOUR ANSWERS IN APPENDIX A.

OCCLUSION

Occlusion refers to movements of the mandible and to the contacting of the maxillary and mandibular teeth resulting from those movements. Which arch is moveable?

mandible

Permanent
Maxillary
and
Mandibular

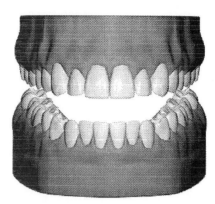

There is great variety in human occlusion. The study of occlusion is complex and demands far more attention than this volume could provide. We shall limit our discussion to some basic terminology and concepts.

lingual

Most commonly, the maxillary teeth overlap the mandibulars, and most teeth have two opposing teeth (antagonists). The maxillary anterior and posterior teeth are aligned towards the facial and therefore fit over the tops of the mandibular teeth. The mandibular teeth flare in towards the lingual. The maxillary teeth overlap the mandibular teeth when the teeth are in occlusion, or fitted together. Notice the illustration of the maxillary and mandibular arches from the back side. Which surface of the maxillary anterior teeth are touched by the mandibular anterior teeth—the incisal or lingual? _____

Permanent
Maxillary
and
Mandibular

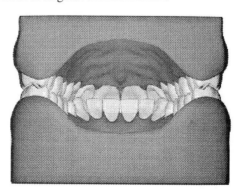

central incisors

Which mandibular teeth commonly have one antagonist? _____ _____

Schematic
Diagram of
Permanent
Maxillary
and
Mandibular
Left Quadrants

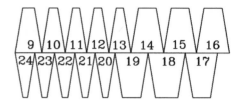

Permanent
Maxillary
and
Mandibular
Left Quadrants

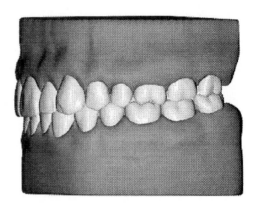

maxillary third

The maxillary teeth generally have two antagonists, except for the _____ _____ molars, which have one antagonist.

Schematic
Diagram of
Permanent
Maxillary
and
Mandibular
Left Quadrants

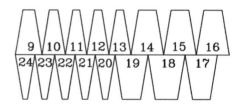

maxillary

Teeth are like stone blocks in a gothic arch. In the most frequent occlusion, which arch is larger—maxillary or mandibular? _____

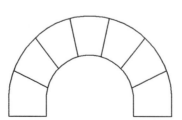
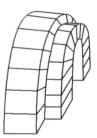

Tooth alignment usually involves a slight horizontal and vertical overlap. Overlap is a term used to describe the overlapping alignment seen when the two arches occlude. Horizontal overlap is also called overjet and vertical overlap is known as overbite. However, this text will use the simpler and more correct terms, horizontal overlap and vertical overlap. In Figure 2, identify the label (A or B) that represents horizontal overlap. _____

A

Permanent
Maxillary
Mandibular
1. Anteriors
   FACIAL (Occluded)
2. Central Incisors
   PROXIMAL (Occluded)

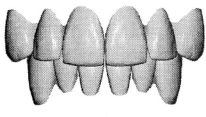

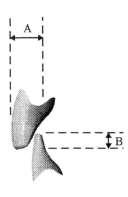

1   2

There are varying degrees of vertical overlap (overbite), which can be termed minimal, moderate, or severe as shown in the illustration. In Figure C, _____ overbite, it is apparent the maxillary teeth extend onto the facial surface of the mandibular teeth to the gingival margin of the mandibular anterior teeth.

severe

Permanent
Maxillary
Mandibular
Anteriors
FACIAL
Occluded
A. Minimal
B. Moderate
C. Severe

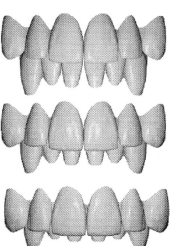

A. Minimal

B. Moderate

C. Severe

Figure A

The amount of horizontal overlap in an "ideal occlusion" should not be greater than 1 to 2 mm. Which figure (A or B) shows an ideal overjet? _____

Permanent
Maxillary
Mandibular
Left
Central
Incisors
PROXIMAL
Occluded

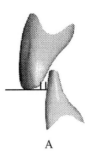 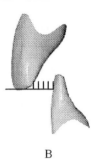

A   B

I

In 1899, Edward H. Angle developed a classification of human occlusion that is still basic and useful today. Angle described three classes of occlusion, Class I, Class II, and Class III. Class I is the most common, Class II less common, and Class III least common. Class I is the ideal. The associated skeletal type is called mesognathic or Class _____ skeletal type.

Mesognathic Facial Profile

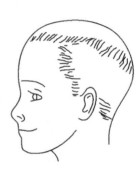

The classes can be defined in terms of the relationship between maxillary and mandibular first molars and canines as well as the skeletal type.

Angle felt, as many still do, that the first molars were good reference points because of their early eruption dates and significance in determining the space available for the succedaneous teeth. In Angle Class I occlusion, the mesiofacial cusp of the maxillary first molar lines up approximately with the facial groove of the mandibular first molar (see the illustration). The maxillary central incisors overlap the mandibulars with a slight vertical and horizontal overlap. Frequently the canine relationship is recorded. In the Class I relationship, the maxillary canine is a half tooth posterior to the mandibular canine. The associated skeletal type is called mesognathic or Class I skeletal type. The mesiofacial cusp of the maxillary first molar falls in the facial groove of the mandibular _____ _____ .

Permanent
Maxillary
Mandibular
Right Quadrants
FACIAL
Occluded

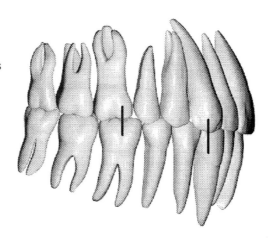

Class I Occlusion

In Angle Class II occlusion, the _____ cusp of the maxillary first molar falls approximately between the mandibular first molar and second premolar. The lower jaw and chin may also appear small and withdrawn, indicating the Class II skeletal type which is called retrognathic. The mandibular incisors occlude even more posterior to the maxillary incisors so that they may not touch at all. Compared to Class I, the maxillary incisors in Class II show more horizontal and sometimes more vertical overlap. The maxillary canine is a whole tooth anterior to the mandibular canine.

Permanent
Maxillary
Mandibular
Right Quadrants
FACIAL
Occluded

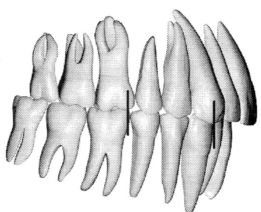

Class II Occlusion

retrognathic

The associated facial profile with the Class II distoclusion is _____ .

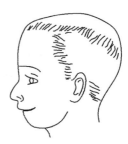

Retrognathic
Facial
Profile

Class II, distoclusion, is divided into two divisions. In Division 1 the mandible is retruded and all the maxillary incisors are protruded.

Permanent
Maxillary
Mandibular
Right Quadrants
FACIAL
Occluded

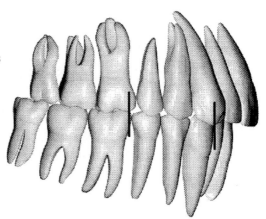

Class II. Division 1

In Class II, Division 2 the mandibular anteriors are retruded and one or more of the maxillary incisors are retruded.

Permanent
Maxillary
Mandibular
Right Quadrants
FACIAL
Occluded

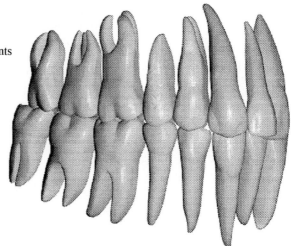

Class II, Division 2

Class II, _____, is divided into two divisions. In Division 2 one or more of the maxillary incisors are _____ .

distoclusion, retruded

In Angle's Class III occlusion, mesioclusion, the mandibular teeth are in a more anterior position than in Class I. The chin may also protrude like a bulldog's does. The associated skeletal type is called prognathic. The mandibular incisors overlap anterior to the maxillary incisors. The mesiofacial cusp of the maxillary first molar falls approximately between the mandibular first molar and the mandibular _____ . The maxillary canine falls posterior to the mandibular canine by a whole tooth width.

second molar

Permanent
Maxillary
Mandibular
Right Quadrants
FACIAL
Occluded

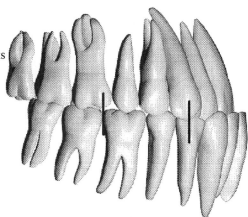

Class III Occlusion

The associated facial profile is prognathic.

Prognathic
Facial
Profile

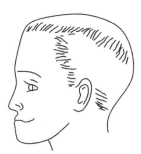

prognathic

In the Class III occlusion the mandibular anterior teeth are anterior to the maxillary anterior teeth. This relationship is often termed anterior crossbite. This is common with _____ facial profiles.

Permanent
Maxillary
Mandibular
Right Quadrants
FACIAL
Occluded

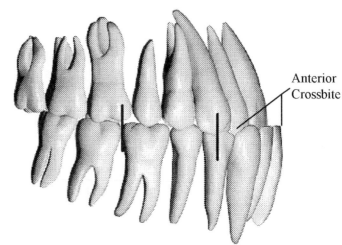

Anterior Crossbite

Class III Occlusion

mesiofacial

The cusp of the maxillary first molar that serves as a reference point in identifying Class I, II, and III occlusion is the _____ cusp.

Some of the different occlusal relationships that occur include an openbite in which the maxillary anterior teeth do not touch the mandibular anterior teeth.

Permanent
Maxillary
Mandibular
FACIAL

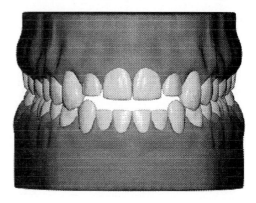

Anterior Openbite

Another frequently observed relationship is edge to edge in which the maxillary and mandibular anterior teeth are in occlusion on their edges as illustrated in this image of tooth number 8 and tooth number 25 (universal code) in edge to _____ occlusion.

Permanent
Maxillary
Mandibular
Right
Central
Incisors
MESIAL

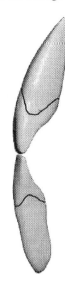

Edge to Edge Bite

When the posterior teeth occlude with their occlusal surfaces end to end it may look like this illustration of #3 and #30 (universal code) which are in end to _____ occlusion.

end

Permanent
Maxillary
Mandibular
Right
First Molars
FACIAL

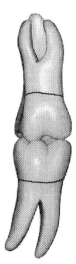

End to End Bite

a. central portion

Viewed from the distal, the premolars and molars normally occlude so that the mandibular facial cusps strike the central portion of the occlusal surface of their antagonists. Where would the lingual cusps of the maxillary posteriors strike their mandibular antagonists?

a. Central portion of the occlusal surface
b. Facial portion of the facial cusps

Permanent
Maxillary
Mandibular
Right
First Molars
DISTAL

L   F

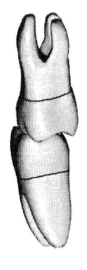

Centric Occlusion

facial

Human posterior teeth have double rows of cusps. As posterior teeth occlude, one set of cusps fits into fossae or marginal ridges and one set doesn't. Which cusp of the maxillary teeth is not occluding? (facial, lingual) _____

Permanent
Maxillary
Mandibular
Right
First Molars
DISTAL

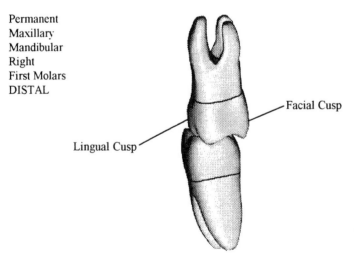

Facial Cusp

Lingual Cusp

Centric Occlusion

Cusps that do grinding work because they occlude in a fossa or marginal ridge are called working cusps. They are also sometimes called centric cusps because they hold the occlusion in a middle position where everything fits together called centric position of the teeth. Cusps that occlude are called _____ or _____ cusps.

The facial cusps of mandibular posteriors and the lingual cusps of the maxillary posterior teeth are called centric cusps, because they contact their antagonists and determine the position of the mandible in maximum opposing tooth contact called _____ occlusion.

Permanent
Maxillary
Mandibular
Right
Premolars
and
Molars
DISTOLINGUAL

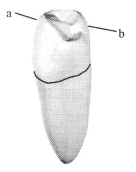

Lingual Cusps

Facial Cusps

Centric (working) Cusps

The form of teeth appears highly related to function in occlusion. For example, the centric cusps seem more bulky and rounded than noncentric cusps. Choose the letter (a or b) corresponding to the centric cusp shown in the illustration. _____

Permanent
Mandibular
Right
First Premolar
MESIAL

a

b

balancing

Cusps that do not occlude or fit into fossae or marginal ridge areas on the opposite arch are called balancing cusps or noncentric cusps. Though they are not used for grinding food, they still have an important job. They allow the dentition to move apart, out of occlusion. They allow the teeth to "unlock" and move back and forth and side to side. The working cusps occlude and the _____ cusps unlock the occlusion.

Permanent
Maxillary
Mandibular
Right
First Molars
DISTAL

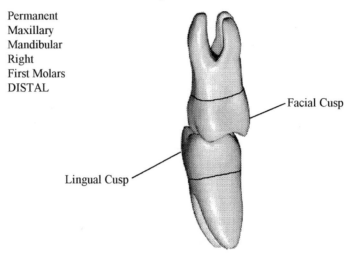

Facial Cusp

Lingual Cusp

Noncentric (balancing) Cusps

a, b

Balancing cusps, or noncentric cusps are on the opposite side as the working cusps. Working cusps are usually the larger, stronger, and rounder of the two types. Which of these cusps is a working cusp (also called centric cusp)? (a or b) _____ Which of the cusps is the more slender, weaker and more pointed? It is also called noncentric. (a or b)

_____

Permanent
Mandibular
Right
First Premolar
MESIAL

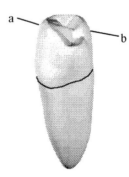

a

b

The maxillary posterior teeth have all their working cusps on the lingual side, while the balancing cusps are on the _____ .

facial

In some cases, you will see patients who have one or more posterior teeth or an entire quadrant that shows a crossbite. Study the illustration of the crossbite in Figure 1, and compare it to the illustration of a normal relationship in Figure 2.

facial

Permanent
Maxillary
Mandibular
Right Quadrants
1. Crossbite
2. Centric

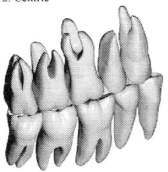
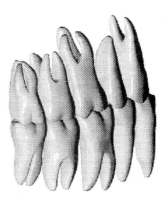

1   2

Which maxillary cusps, in crossbite, occlude in the central portion of the mandibular teeth? _____

lingual

The form of teeth is related to the way they occlude and function in the entire dentition. For example, the arch form of the upper and lower teeth determines to some extent the form of individual teeth.

Stone block arch

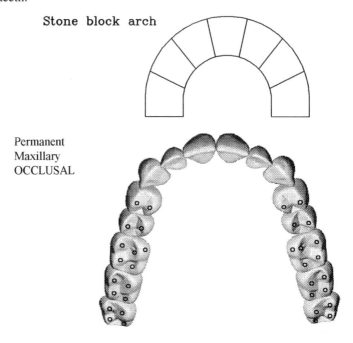

Permanent
Maxillary
OCCLUSAL

Stone blocks used to form an arch are wider at their outer surface than at their inner surface. When examining a dental arch, we can notice a similar relationship between the facial and lingual surfaces of the teeth, especially the anterior teeth. An incisal view of a maxillary central incisor demonstrates this concept.

Which surface of the incisor is narrower, the facial or lingual? _____

Permanent
Maxillary
Right
Central Incisor
INCISAL

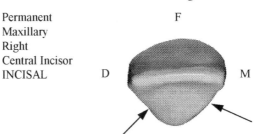

The study of the interrelationships of teeth in the arch should include an examination of the areas where adjacent teeth contact each other in the same arch. These proximal contact areas are described next.

PROXIMAL CONTACTS

1.7.1

···

mesial, distal

Each tooth contacts adjacent teeth on its proximal surfaces except the distal of third molars. The proximal surfaces are the _____ and _____ surfaces of a tooth.

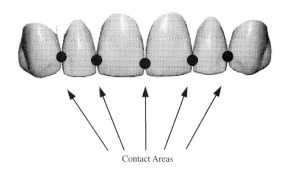

Permanent
Maxillary
Anterior
FACIAL

Contact Areas

···

···

facially

Proximal surfaces usually have contact areas rather than contact points. The contact areas are more _____ (facially/lingually) located.

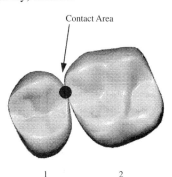

Permanent
Maxillary
Left
1. Second Premolar
2. First Molar
OCCLUSAL

Contact Area

1   2

···

···

faciolingual;
occlusocervical

The proximal contact area is located in (1) the incisocervical or occlusocervical dimension and (2) the faciolingual dimension. In the diagram below, dimension A is the _____ dimension, and B is the _____ dimension.

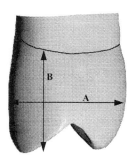

Permanent
Maxillary
Right
Second Premolar
MESIAL

B

A

cervical, middle, incisal (occlusal)

The contact location is determined by referring to thirds. Viewing the teeth from the facial aspect, the crowns are divided into three equal parts: the _____ , _____ , and _____ thirds.

Permanent
Mandibular
Right
Canine
FACIAL

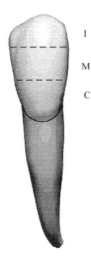

I

M

C

central incisors

Most proximal contacts involve a mesial and a distal surface. The proximal contact that involves the mesial surface of both teeth is between the two _____ _____ .

Permanent
Maxillary
Mandibular
INCISORS

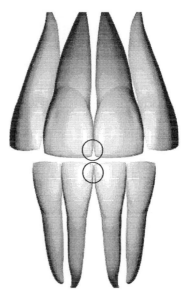

The remaining teeth contact mesial to distal except the third molars. The contact between the lateral incisor and canine involves the distal surface of the _____ _____ and the _____ surface of the canine.

Permanent
Maxillary
Right
1. Canine
2. Lateral Incisor

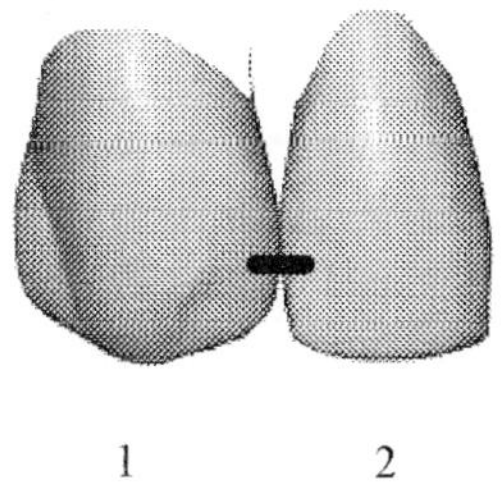

1   2

Each tooth is supported, in part, through contact with its neighboring teeth. In turn, a tooth lends support to the entire dental arch through its two proximal _____ _____ .

Permanent
Maxillary
OCCLUSALS

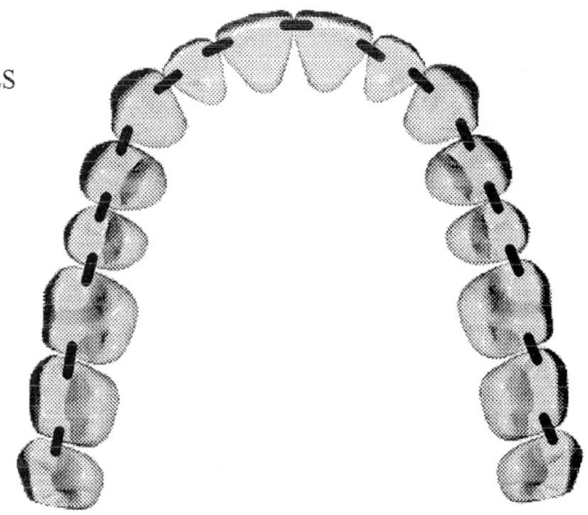

These proximal contact areas provide stability to the dental arch by helping support the individual tooth. The contact areas are located on the _____ and _____ surfaces, excepting the distal of the third molars.

junction of incisal and
middle thirds, middle
third

The permanent maxillary central incisor has a mesial contact in the incisal (I) third, and the distal contact at the junction (J) of the incisal and middle thirds. The lateral incisors have their contacts more apical than the centrals, with their mesial contact more incisal than their distal contact. Therefore, the permanent maxillary lateral incisor can be labeled J-M to indicate the location of its mesial contact (J—at the junction of the incisal and middle thirds) and distal contact (M—in the middle third). The maxillary canine can be labeled J-M also, which means that its mesial contact is at the _____ _____ _____ _____ _____ _____ and its distal contact is in the _____ _____ .

Permanent
Maxillary
Left
1. Central Incisor
2. Lateral Incisor
3. Canine
FACIAL

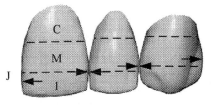

The contacts of the maxillary and mandibular anterior teeth are indicated in the illustrations as black dots. If you connect the black dots on the maxillary anterior teeth, they will make a gently curved line. This line is called the "smile line."

Permanent
Maxillary
Anterior
FACIAL

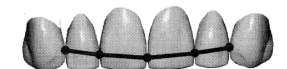

incisal

A straight line is formed upon connecting the dots on the mandibular anterior teeth. The contact on the mesial of the maxillary right central is located in the _____ third.

Permanent
Maxillary
Mandibular
Anterior
FACIALS

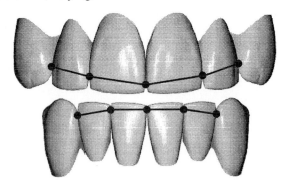

The contacts of the anterior teeth from the facial view can be summarized as follows:

Maxillary: IJ, JM, JM

Mandibular: II, II, IM

In this illustration of the posterior teeth, the contacts are marked with black dots. Again the location of the contacts can be indicated by naming which third or junction of thirds the contact falls. If you connect the contacts of the posterior teeth, it will also make a gently curving line. This gently curving upward line is called the curve of spee. The only tooth surface that does not make proximal contact is the _____ of _____ _____ .

(surface)   (teeth)

Permanent
Maxillary
Mandibular
Left
FACIALS

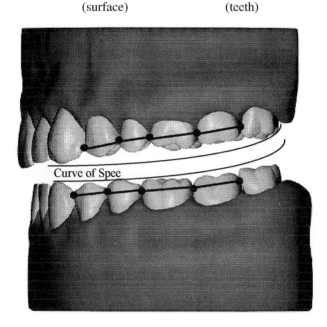

Curve of Spee

The *Curve of Wilson* is also associated with the way teeth curve. The lingual inclination of the mandibular molars and buccal inclination of the maxillary posterior teeth, indicate or follow a pathway commonly referred to as Curve of Wilson.

Permanent
Maxillary
Mandibular
First Molars
DISTAL

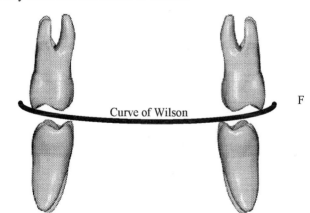

F   F

Curve of Wilson

The contacts of the posterior teeth can be summarized as follows:

Maxillary: MM, MM, MM, MM, M

Mandibular: MM, MM, MM, MM, M

incisal

In the incisocervical or occlusocervical dimension, if you examine the location of the proximal contact from the anterior teeth back to the posterior teeth, you will see that the contacts tend to be located in or near the incisal third between anteriors and in or near the middle third on the posteriors. This chart summarizes the contacts of all the teeth. Incisocervically, the central incisors of both arches have mesial contact areas well within the _____ thirds.

Maxillary: IJ, JM, JM, MM, MM, MM, MM, M

Mandibular: II, II, IM, MM, MM, MM, MM, M

It is possible to study the inciso/occlusocervical location of the proximal contact of individual teeth and to summarize the location of the contacts of all teeth with two rules that apply in every case:

1. The more anterior the tooth, the more incisal/occlusal are the location of the proximal contacts.
2. For any tooth, the mesial contact area is more toward the incisal/occlusal than is the distal contact area.

occlusal

All posterior teeth have proximal contacts in the middle third. The more posterior teeth—the molars—have contacts lower in the middle third than the premolars (Rule 1). Also, each posterior tooth has the mesial contact slightly more _____ (occlusal/apical) than the distal contact (Rule 2).

1.7.2 EMBRASURES

lingual

When viewing the arches from the occlusal, we see that the contacts are located towards the facial for all teeth. This happens because the crowns of all teeth have a shape that is tapered towards the lingual. It is said that the proximal sides of crowns of the teeth converge towards the lingual. Because teeth converge towards the lingual, and the contacts are located in the facial third, there are larger spaces between the teeth on the lingual than on the facial. These spaces are called embrasures. Which are greater—the facial embrasures or the lingual embrasures? _____ (In the illustration, the contacts are marked on the right side and the contacts and embrasures are marked on the left side.)

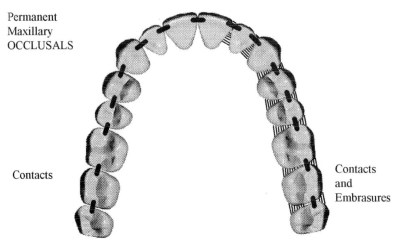

Permanent
Maxillary
OCCLUSALS

Contacts

Contacts
and
Embrasures

"Below" or cervical to each proximal contact and "between" adjacent teeth is the interdental area. The term that indicates the location "between" two teeth is _____ .

interdental

Occupying much of the interdental area is a projection of the free gingival tissue called "interdental papilla" or simply, papilla (puh PILL luh). Viewed facially, the interdental area and the interdental papilla are generally _____ in shape.

triangular

Permanent
Mandibular
Right
FACIAL

Interdental papilla

The interdental area is often called the interproximal area or interproximal space. It is not really a space because tissue fills much of the area. Since that tissue is interdental papilla, it is convenient to call the area the interdental area. Recall that the free gingiva lying between teeth was called _____ gingiva. Now, another term for that tissue is interdental _____ .

papillary, papilla

In healthy mouths, the tissue assumes much of the triangular shape of the interdental area from the facial view, but resembles a slightly sagging tent from the proximal view. The sagging area is the col (CALL) of the papillary gingiva and is apical to the _____ _____ area.

proximal contact

Permanent
Mandibular
Right
First Premolar
DISTAL

Contact Area

Col

The cervical third of the proximal surfaces of all teeth are relatively flat or even slightly concave in some areas, increasing the space for the free gingival tissue called the _____ .

papilla

embrasures

The curved tooth surfaces that sweep away from the proximal contact areas form open spaces: the interdental area (gingival to the contact) and embrasures (elsewhere around the contact). There are incisal or occlusal embrasures, lingual embrasures, and facial embrasures. Thus, the proximal contact is surrounded by the interdental area and the spaces are called _____ .

Permanent
Maxillary
Left
1. Second Premolar
2. Molar

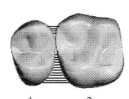

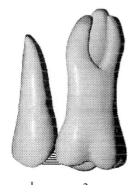

| 1. | 2. | 1. | 2. |

Occlusal   Facial

embrasures

These spaces allow chewed foods to escape from the occlusal surface. This self cleansing occurs when teeth are naturally cleared of food debris after chewing. The contacts provide a tight junction between teeth to prevent food from being impacted between them. The convex surfaces and the _____ provide natural spillways to lead food away from the surfaces of the teeth. Examples of the spillways are indicated in the drawing.

Permanent
Maxillary
OCCLUSALS

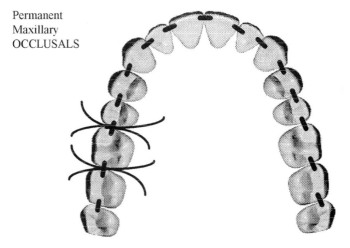

proximal surfaces

Embrasures make the natural hygienic factors in the mouth more effective by exposing tooth surfaces to oral fluids and the mechanical cleansing action of the tongue, lips, and cheeks. The curved surfaces discourage the impaction of food between the _____ _____ .

The embrasures also allow food to slide away from the chewing surfaces during mastication. This helps to protect the supporting structures from undue trauma by _____ (increasing/reducing) the forces exerted on the teeth during mastication.

reducing

The supporting structures are, therefore, protected from traumatic forces by the escape of food via the open _____ and by the transmission of occlusal forces to adjacent teeth through the solid _____ _____ _____ .

embrasures, proximal contact areas

Permanent
Maxillary
OCCLUSALS

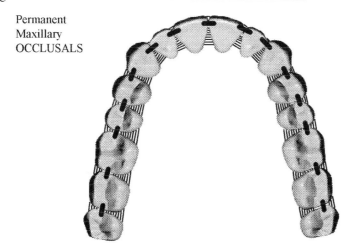

The embrasures are named according to their location in relation to the contact. The embrasures located incisally or occlusally to the contact are called the incisal or occlusal embrasures. The embrasures located facially are called facial embrasures, and those located lingually are called lingual embrasures.

occlusal

Facial and lingual embrasures are confluent with the interdental area; that is, their boundaries are indistinct and they blend together. The facial and lingual embrasures are also confluent with the space above the contact called the _____ embrasure.

Permanent
Maxillary
Left
1. Second Premolar
2. Molar

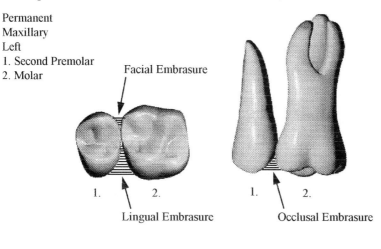

Facial Embrasure

Lingual Embrasure   Occlusal Embrasure

Occlusal   Facial

facial and lingual

Of the three embrasures created from the contact, which one(s) can be seen looking at the occlusal views: 1. facial embrasure, 2. lingual embrasure, or 3. incisal/occlusal embrasure? _____ _____ _____

Permanent
Maxillary
Left
1. Second Premolar
2. Molar

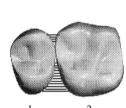
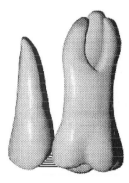

    1.   2.   1.   2.

      Occlusal   Facial

facially located

Study the illustration showing the contacts and embrasures from the occlusal and answer the following questions.

Permanent
Maxillary
OCCLUSALS

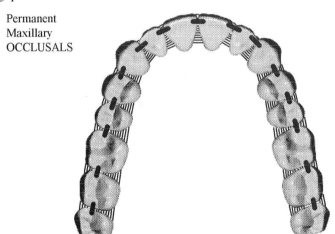

In the region of the anterior teeth, the facial and lingual embrasure have approximately equal depth. The proximal contacts between posterior teeth are _____ (centered/facially located) in the faciolingual dimension.

deeper

In the region of the posterior teeth, the lingual embrasures are _____(deeper/shallower) than the facial embrasures.

GO TO THE NEXT PAGE AND TAKE REVIEW TEST 1.7.

REVIEW TEST 1.7

For each question, choose the one *correct* answer.

1. Cervical to the proximal contact area is the:

   a. occlusal table
   b. interdental area
   c. distal embrasure

2. What surrounds the proximal contact areas in facial, occlusal, and lingual directions?

   a. papillary gingiva
   b. embrasures
   c. interdental area

3. What is located in the interdental area?

   a. alveolar bone
   b. attached gingiva
   c. interdental papilla

4. In the most common occlusion, which mandibular teeth have only one antagonist?

   a. third molars
   b. central incisors
   c. third molars and central incisors

5. In the most common occlusion, the facial cusp of a mandibular second premolar is a

   a. centric cusp
   b. non-centric cusp
   c. cusp in cross-bite position

6. In reference to the position of the central incisors in occlusion, match the following:

   a. mandibular incisors overlap anterior to maxillary incisors   I. Angle Class I occlusion
   b. normal maxillary horizontal and vertical overlap   II. Angle Class II occlusion
   c. extreme maxillary horizontal overlap   III. Angle Class III occlusion

7. In reference to the position of the mesiofacial cusp of tooth number 14 (universal code) in occlusion, match the following:

   Tends toward

   a. cusp aligned between 18 and 19   I. Angle Class I
   b. cusp aligned between 19 and 20   II. Angle Class II
   c. cusp aligned with facial groove of 19   III. Angle Class III

8. When the maxillary anterior teeth overlap the mandibular anterior exhibiting 5 to 7 mm of space between maxillary anterior and the mandibular anteriors, this is called

   a. horizontal overjet
   b. vertical overbite
   c. anterior crossbite

9. In Angle's Class II occlusion, the lower jaw and chin may appear withdrawn. The skeletal type is

   a. mesognathic
   b. retrognathic
   c. prognathic

TURN THE PAGE

10. Class II, distoclusion, is divided into two divisions. Identify the correct statement describing Division 1.

    a. The mandible is retruded and one or more maxillary incisors are retruded.
    b. The mandible is retruded and all the maxillary incisors are protruded.

11. In this canine relationship description, which occlusion classification is being described?"The maxillary canine falls posterior to the mandibular canine by a whole tooth width."

    a. Class I
    b. Class II
    c. Class III

12. When the mandibular anterior teeth are anterior to the maxillary anterior teeth, it is called

    a. posterior crossbite
    b. anterior crossbite
    c. vertical overlap

13. The facial cusps of the maxillary posterior teeth fall in the central groove of the mandibular posterior teeth. This is a description of

    a. centric occlusion
    b. crossbite
    c. noncentric cusps

14. The facial cusps of the mandibular posterior teeth are

    a. centric
    b. noncentric

15. The centric cusps are also

    a. balancing
    b. working

CHECK YOUR ANSWERS IN APPENDIX A.

CONTOURS OF TOOTH CROWNS

It is important to study the curved contours of crowns because there are many occasions for the dentist to operate on these contours in restoring or replacing crown surfaces. There is clinical evidence that smooth and properly contoured (not too convex) crown surfaces promote tooth cleaning and gingival health.

The curved contours of the crown are normally continuous with the gingiva, as shown in the drawing. This form seems to help make the _____ (cervical/occlusal) areas of the teeth cleanable.

Permanent
Mandibular
Right
First Premolar
DISTAL

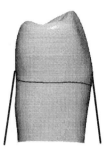

One of the best ways to study the contours of crowns is to focus on the height of contour.

The height of contour is an imaginary curved line encircling a tooth at its greatest bulge or circumference. One way to visualize this imaginary line is shown in the drawing, where a light source is depicted as being directed toward the incisal edge of an incisor. The height of contour encircles the entire crown and would be incisal or occlusal to a real line that encircles the tooth, the _____ line or cementoenamel junction.

Maxillary
Right
Central Incisor
DISTAL VIEW

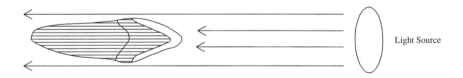

Light Source

One can also see the location of the height of contour by moving a pencil around the crown at its greatest bulge or circumference, and marking the height of contour.

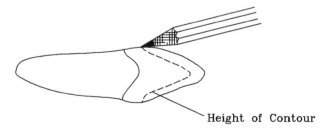

Height of Contour

along

The proximal contacts of a tooth lie _____ (along/above) the height of contour.

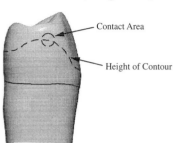

Permanent
Mandibular
Right
First Premolar
DISTAL

Contact Area

Height of Contour

proximal

The facial and lingual heights of contour are seen when a tooth is drawn from a _____ view.

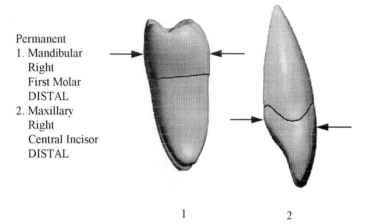

Permanent
1. Mandibular
   Right
   First Molar
   DISTAL
2. Maxillary
   Right
   Central Incisor
   DISTAL

1   2

anterior

Anterior teeth have facial or lingual heights of contour in the cervical third of the crown.

Examine the drawings for height of contour. The height of contour occurs in the cervical third on both the *facial* and *lingual* surfaces for all maxillary and mandibular _____ (anterior/posterior) teeth.

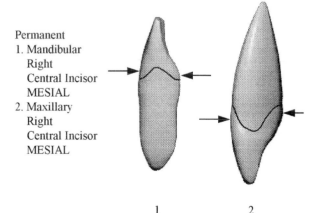

Permanent
1. Mandibular
   Right
   Central Incisor
   MESIAL
2. Maxillary
   Right
   Central Incisor
   MESIAL

1   2

All maxillary and mandibular posterior teeth have the height of contour in the middle third on the _____ surface.

lingual

Permanent
1. Maxillary
   Right
   First Molar
   MESIAL
2. Mandibular
   Right
   First Molar
   MESIAL

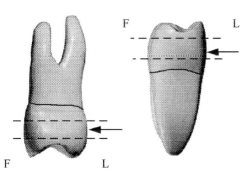

1   2

As with the maxillary incisors and canines, the mandibular anteriors have both the *facial* and *lingual* height of contour in the _____ third of the crown.

cervical

Permanent
Mandibular
1. Right Canine
2. Central Incisor
DISTAL

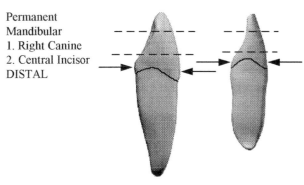

1   2

Both maxillary posterior teeth and mandibular posterior teeth have the height of contour on the *facial* surface in the _____ third and the *lingual* height of contour in the _____ third.

cervical, middle

Permanent
Mandibular
Right
First Premolar
DISTAL

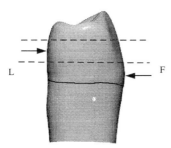

approximately 1/2 mm

In addition to knowing the location of the height of contour, you should know the amount of contour in a horizontal direction from the cervical line.

One way to measure the amount of contour of a tooth surface is to use a grid as shown here. If the grid has lines that are 1/2 mm apart, what is the amount of contour shown?

_____ _____ _____

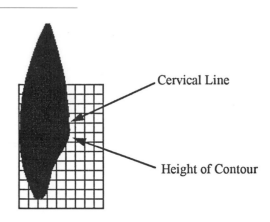

Permanent
Maxillary
Right
Central Incisor
MESIAL

Cervical Line

Height of Contour

cervical, 1/2,
middle, 1/2

All maxillary teeth exhibit *facial* and *lingual* contours that measure approximately 1/2 mm horizontally. The lingual surface of the maxillary right canine has the height of contour in the _____ third that measures _____ mm.

The lingual surface of the maxillary left first molar has the height of contour in the _____ third that measures _____ mm.

Permanent
Maxillary
Right
1. Canine
2. First Molar
DISTAL

L   F   L   F

1/2 mm   1/2 mm

1   2

In proximal view, maxillary teeth give the impression that the amount of contour is greater on the facial than on the lingual surface (especially true for anterior teeth). However, careful examination will show that the contour, both *facially* and *lingually,* for all maxillary teeth measures approximately _____ mm.

Permanent
Maxillary
Right
1. Canine
2. First Molar
DISTAL

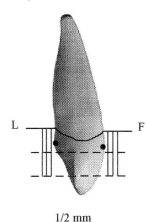

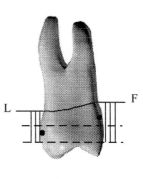

1/2 mm   1/2 mm

You should know that 1/2 mm is a very small amount of contour. For example, one-half millimeter is only as thick as four sheets of paper from this text held tightly between the fingers. It is approximately equal to the thickness of a human fingernail.

The facial and lingual amounts of contour of the mandibular anteriors are very slight. Mandibular incisors and canines have *facial* and *lingual* amounts of contour that measure

(each grid represents 1/2 mm)

A. more than 1/2 mm
B. 1/2 mm
C. less than 1/2 mm

Permanent
Mandibular
Right
1. Canine
2. Central Incisor
DISTAL

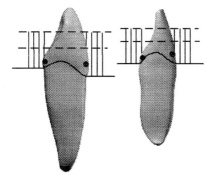

1   2

1/2

The amount of contour on the facial surfaces of mandibular posteriors are similar to those on the facial surfaces of the maxillary posterior teeth; that is, they measure approximately _____ mm.

Permanent
Mandibular
Right
1. Second Premolar
2. First Premolar
DISTAL

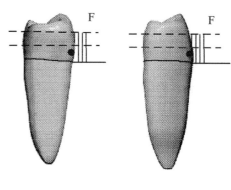

1/2 mm   1/2 mm

1

The mandibular posterior teeth have lingual curvatures that measure nearly double those of the maxillaries. The amount of contour on the *lingual* surface of mandibular posterior teeth approaches _____ mm in measurement.

Permanent
Mandibular
Right
First Molar
DISTAL

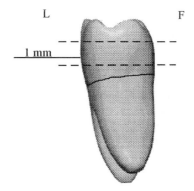

When examining teeth in the oral cavity, the location of the height of contour and the amount of contour may appear different than that of extracted teeth or drawings. The reason for this difference is shown in the accompanying drawing of a permanent mandibular molar. Because teeth are often inclined (toward the lingual in the case of the mandibular molars), the observed height of contour is noticeably different from the anatomical height of contour. The observed height of contour is closer to the occlusal surface and the amount of contour appears greater than the anatomical contour would suggest.

Permanent
Mandibular
Right
First Molar
MESIAL

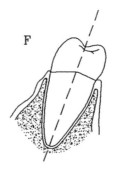

In preparation for the review test that follows, complete the following statements.

All permanent teeth have their height of contour in the cervical third on the _____ surface of the crown.

facial

The height of contour is located in the cervical third on the *lingual* surface of all maxillary and mandibular _____ (anterior/posterior) teeth.

anterior

Both maxillary and mandibular premolars and molars have heights of contour approximately in the middle third on the _____ surface of the crown.

lingual

Which tooth surfaces have curvatures that measure less than 1/2 mm? _____ _____ _____ _____ _____ (indicate whether maxillary or mandibular, anterior or posterior, facial or lingual)

mandibular anterior facial and lingual surfaces

Which tooth surfaces have curvatures that usually measure more than 1/2 mm? _____ _____ _____ _____ (indicate whether maxillary or mandibular, anterior or posterior, facial or lingual)

mandibular posterior lingual surfaces

In the discussion of facial and lingual contours, the average or most common tooth form was described. As with most anatomical features, individual deviations from the norm may occur on a specific tooth or a group of teeth. The model teeth used in the illustrations are not always anatomically correct, therefore, the height of contour is not properly represented making it very difficult to visualize.

Each of the following words is misspelled. Rewrite each word, spelling it correctly.

1. Ginegiva   _____
2. Facilingule   _____
3. Maxallary   _____
4. Procimal contracts _____
5. Cervacal   _____
6. Embrazures   _____

1. Gingiva;
2. Faciolingual;
3. Maxillary;
4. Proximal contacts;
5. Cervical;
6. Embrasures

TAKE REVIEW TEST 1.8 ON THE NEXT PAGE.

REVIEW TEST 1.8

For each question, choose the one *correct* answer.

1. In their position in the alveolar bone, the mandibular molars are
   a. tipped toward the facial
   b. in an upright, vertical position
   c. tipped toward the lingual

2. The proximal contact is usually located
   a. at the mesial or distal height of contour
   b. in the cervical third of the crown
   c. in the middle third of the crown

3. Indicate the incisocervical or occlusocervical location of the following proximal contact areas. Write the name of the third (incisal, middle, etc) and/or the junction of thirds where the area is located.
   a. mesial contact area of the maxillary central incisor _____
   b. distal contact area of the maxillary central incisor _____
   c. distal contact area of the maxillary lateral incisor _____
   d. mesial contact area of the mandibular central incisor _____
   e. distal contact area of the mandibular canine _____
   f. mesial contact area of the maxillary second premolar _____
   g. distal contact area of the mandibular second molar _____

4. In the region of the anterior teeth, the facial embrasures are approximately
   a. as deep as the lingual embrasures
   b. deeper than the lingual embrasures
   c. not as deep as the lingual embrasures

5. Choose the correct statement.
   a. Contact areas between posterior teeth are displaced lingually from the center of the faciolingual axis.
   b. Contact areas between posterior teeth are displaced facially from the center of the faciolingual axis.

CHECK YOUR ANSWERS IN APPENDIX A.

2

Permanent Anterior Teeth

REVIEW OF TOOTH SURFACES

2.1.0

wedge

The crowns of posterior teeth can be described as cube-shaped, and the crowns of anterior teeth can be described as _____-shaped.

Permanent
Mandibular Right
1. First Molar
2. Canine

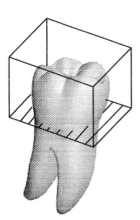

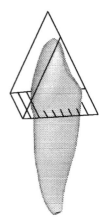

1
                           2

occlusal, incisal

One side of the cube or wedge used to describe tooth crowns is taken up by the root, and, consequently, it is not classified or named as a tooth surface. This leaves five tooth surfaces to be named on each tooth. The top or chewing surface of the posterior is larger than the top or biting surface of the anterior teeth. Remember that the biting surface of posterior teeth is called _____ and the biting surface of anterior teeth is called _____ .

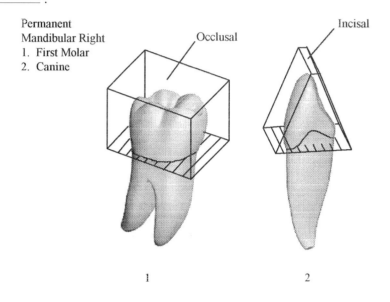

Permanent
Mandibular Right
1. First Molar
2. Canine

surface

Teeth are complex in shape with numerous surface refinements. Each edge or border must be studied as well as the area within these borders, called a tooth _____ .

cervical line (or CEJ)

Using the analogy of the cube or wedge and considering the "top" of the cube (or wedge) to be the occlusal surface (or incisal edge) and the outside the facial surface, the inside would then represent the lingual surface and the two sides would represent the mesial and distal surfaces. The border indicated with the question mark (?) in the illustration is the _____ _____ .

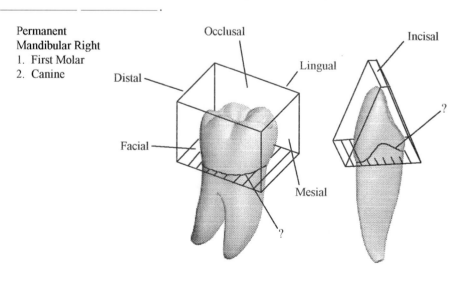

Permanent
Mandibular Right
1. First Molar
2. Canine

From the lingual aspect, four borders are seen. One border is cervical; the other three are the _____ , _____ , and the _____ borders.

Permanent
Maxillary
Right
Central Incisor
LINGUAL

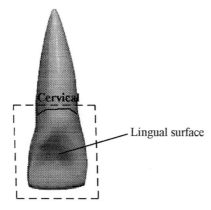

Cervical

Lingual surface

What surface on the posterior tooth in the illustration is designated with a question mark ?

_____

Permanent
Mandibular
Right
First Molar
MESIOFACIAL

?

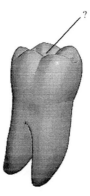

Three of the borders of the facial surface are also shared with other surfaces. For example, border (A) is a border of both the facial and the mesial surface. Often these borders are named by using a compound of two surfaces. In this case, the word would be

_____ .

Permanent
Mandibular
Right
First Molar
MESIOFACIAL

Facial

Mesial

A

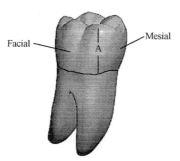

distofacial

When two surfaces meet and share a border, the border is often called a **line angle.** The border formed by the intersection of the mesial and facial surfaces would be called the mesiofacial line angle. In a similar manner, the distal border of the facial surface may also be called the _____ line angle.

incisal, distal

Each of the surfaces of anterior teeth can now be described. The biting edge of anterior teeth is called the _____ edge, and the four tooth surfaces labeled in the illustration are the: A. facial, B. lingual, C. mesial. The surface not seen in this mesiofacial view would be the _____ surface.

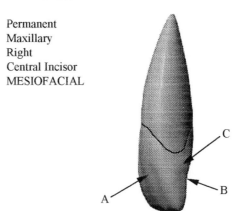

Permanent
Maxillary
Right
Central Incisor
MESIOFACIAL

five

The anatomical crown of each tooth will be explained from _____ (how many) views. The incisal or occlusal, mesial, distal, lingual, and facial.

Following the crown anatomy will be a brief discussion of the height of contour, contacts, embrasures, root anatomy, and pulp anatomy of each tooth.

2.1.1

MAXILLARY CENTRAL INCISOR: FACIAL VIEW

9, 8

The first tooth to be described, the permanent maxillary central incisor, is one of the most prominent teeth in the dental arch. The universal code number for this tooth in the left quadrant is _____ . The tooth number for this tooth in the right quadrant is _____ .

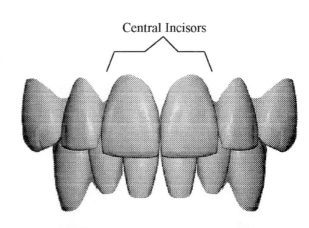

Permanent
Maxillary
Mandibular
Anteriors
FACIAL

Central Incisors

The maxillary central incisors contact one another across the midline on their _____ surfaces.

mesial

Permanent
Maxillary
Central Incisors
FACIAL

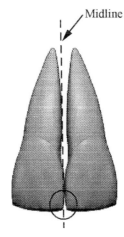

Midline

Viewed facially, the maxillary central incisor resembles a trapezoid. The four borders are called the _____ , _____ , _____ , and _____ borders.

incisal, mesial, distal, cervical

Permanent
Maxillary
Right
Central Incisor
FACIAL

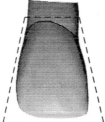

At eruption, the incisal surface has three mamelons which suggest three of the _____ (number) lobes of the central incisor.

four

Permanent
Maxillary
Right
Central Incisor
FACIAL

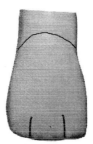

facial

Three of the four lobes are revealed by the grooves seen on the _____ surface of the crown.

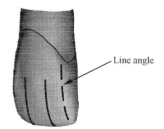

Permanent
Maxillary
Right
Central Incisor
FACIAL

Grooves

mesiofacial

The junction of the mesial and facial surface is called the _____ line angle.

Permanent
Maxillary
Right
Central Incisor
MESIOFACIAL

Line angle

distofacial

Similarly, the junction of the distal and facial surfaces would form the _____ line angle.

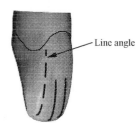

Permanent
Maxillary
Right
Central Incisor
DISTOFACIAL

Line angle

mesial

Of these two line angles or edges, the mesiofacial is slightly longer. Thus, the distance between the incisal edge of the tooth and the cervical line is greater at the _____ (mesial/ distal) border of the facial surface.

The facial surface of the central incisor is convex at both the mesial and distal borders. The mesiofacial line angle is said to be very slightly convex with the distofacial line angle somewhat _____ (more/less) convex.

The shorter line angle of the two is the _____ line angle.

Permanent
Maxillary
Right
Central Incisor
FACIAL

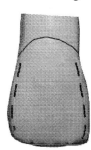

The angle formed at the intersection of the mesial and incisal surfaces is called the mesioincisal angle. As illustrated, the mesioincisal angle is an (obtuse, acute) _____ angle.

Permanent
Maxillary
Left
Central Incisor
FACIAL

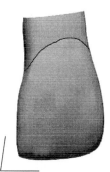

An obtuse angle is an angle that measures more than 90°. The illustration in this frame indicates an angle of less than 90°. The mesioincisal angle of a maxillary central incisor is less than 90° and, therefore, is an acute angle.

Permanent
Maxillary
Left
Central Incisor
FACIAL

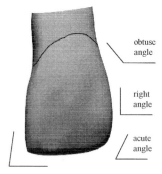

obtuse angle

right angle

acute angle

more

The distoincisal angle of the central incisor is _____ (more/less) rounded than the mesioincisal angle.

Permanent
Maxillary
Left
Central Incisor
FACIAL

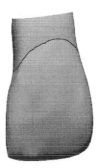

mesiofacial, distofacial

Of the two proximal line angles of the facial surface, the _____ is the longer, and the _____ is more curved.

Permanent
Maxillary
Right
Central Incisor
FACIAL

Line angle

Line angle

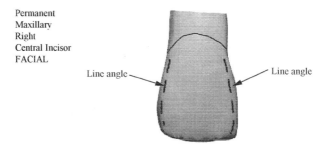

distal

The cervical line forms the fourth border of the facial or lingual surface, its curve blending into the mesial and distal borders. The illustration shows that the convexity is directed toward the root. The crest of convexity is slightly _____ (mesial/distal) to the longitudinal axis of the tooth as seen from a facial view.

Permanent
Maxillary
Left
Central Incisor
FACIAL

Longitudinal
axis

Crest of
convexity

Cervical
line

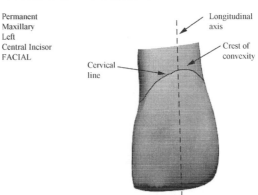

The curve of the cervical line is crested toward the root. In Figure 1 the crest of convexity is displaced slightly toward the distal. In Figure 2 the crest of convexity is also slightly displaced toward the _____ .

Permanent
Maxillary
1. Right Central Incisor
2. Left Central Incisor
FACIAL

1   2

distal

To which maxillary quadrant does this tooth belong? _____ (right/left)

Permanent
Maxillary
Central Incisor
FACIAL

right

Within its four borders, the facial surface of the maxillary central incisor is very slightly convex horizontally (from mesial edge to distal edge, or mesiodistally) and vertically (incisocervically). In other words, the facial surface is curved in _____ (one/two) dimensions.

Permanent
Maxillary
Right
Central Incisor
MESIOFACIAL

Mesiodistal
dimension

Incisocervical
dimension

two

Each of the following words is misspelled. Rewrite each, spelling it correctly.

distil   _____
oclusal   _____
labiul   _____
mesiel   _____
maxilarry   _____

distal, occlusal, labial, mesial, maxillary

2.1.2 MAXILLARY CENTRAL INCISOR: LINGUAL VIEW

true

The outline of a maxillary central incisor is the same when viewed from either the facial or lingual aspect. However, the lingual surface is slightly smaller than the facial surface. (true/false) _____

1. Stone Arch
2. Permanent
   Maxillary Arch
   OCCLUSAL

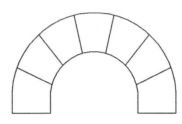

1

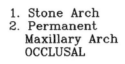

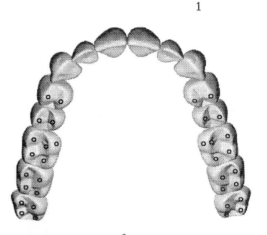

2

Recall that stone blocks used to form an arch are wider at their outer surface than at their inner surface. When examining a dental arch, we can notice a similar relationship between the facial and lingual surfaces of the teeth. The following three views of a maxillary central incisor demonstrate this concept.

Permanent
Maxillary
Central Incisor
3. INCISAL
4. LINGUAL
5. FACIAL

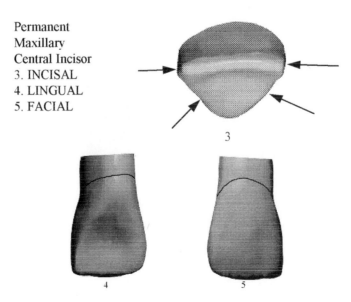

3

4   5

Similar to the facial surface, the lingual surface at the cervical line is convex toward the root and its crest of convexity is displaced toward the _____ (mesial/distal).

Permanent
Maxillary
Left
Central Incisor
LINGUAL

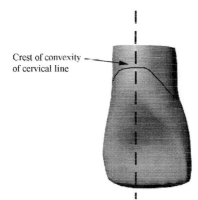

Crest of convexity
of cervical line

Along the mesial and distal margins are rounded ridges of enamel that are convex. The two lateral ridges are called the _____ marginal ridge and the _____ marginal ridge.

Permanent
Maxillary
Left
Central Incisor
LINGUAL

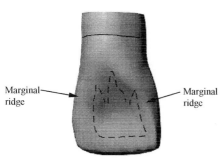

Marginal ridge

Marginal ridge

Identify the lettered areas using the correct nomenclature. A. _____ _____ _____ B. _____ _____ _____

Permanent
Maxillary
Left
Central Incisor
LINGUAL

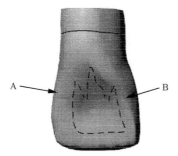

A

B

cervical

There is a pronounced convexity on the lingual surface representing the fourth or lingual lobe, which is referred to as the **cingulum** (SING gue lum). The cingulum is outlined with dashed lines in the illustration. It is located in the middle and _____ thirds.

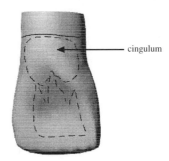

Permanent
Maxillary
Left
Central Incisor
LINGUAL

cingulum

lingual

In contrast to the convexity of the cingulum and marginal ridges, the remaining lingual surface is concave. This concavity, called a fossa, is named for the surface on which it occurs. It is, therefore, called the _____ fossa.

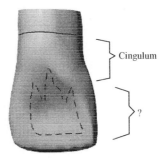

Permanent
Maxillary
Left
Central Incisor
LINGUAL

Cingulum

?

lingual

In some individuals there is a shallow pit called the *lingual pit*. This pit is in the cervical portion of the _____ fossa.

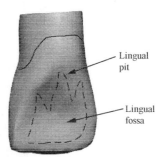

Permanent
Maxillary
Right
Central Incisor
LINGUAL

Lingual
pit

Lingual
fossa

The lingual fossa is concave in both dimensions and may have a small cervical extension called the _____ _____ .

Permanent
Maxillary
Right
Central Incisor
LINGUAL

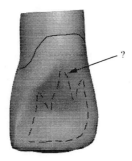

?

In contrast to the facial surface of this incisor tooth, which is slightly _____ (concave/convex), the lingual surface is both _____ and _____ when viewed from a proximal aspect.

Permanent
Maxillary
Right
Central Incisor
DISTAL

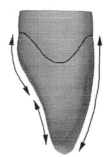

The three major ridges of the lingual surface are the _____ _____ _____ , the _____ _____ _____ , and the _____ .

Permanent
Maxillary
Right
Central Incisor
LINGUAL

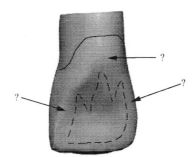

?

?

?

cingulum, lingual
fossa, lingual pit

The major convexity on the lingual surface in the cervical and middle thirds is the
_____ . The major concavity is the _____ _____ , which occasionally has a slight cervical extension called the _____ _____ .

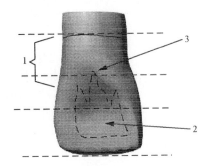

Permanent
Maxillary
Left
Central Incisor
LINGUAL

GO TO THE NEXT PAGE AND TAKE REVIEW TEST 2.1.

REVIEW TEST 2.1

1. The more convex line angle on the surface of the maxillary central incisor is the
   a. mesiofacial
   b. distofacial

2. The longer of the two line angles on the maxillary central incisor is the
   a. mesiofacial
   b. distofacial

3. The maxillary central incisor at eruption has how many mamelons?
   a. one
   b. three
   c. five
   d. four

4. The maxillary central incisor has how many lobes?
   a. three
   b. four
   c. five

5. Where are the following anatomical characteristics located on the lingual surface of the maxillary central incisor—in the cervical, middle, or incisal thirds? (Hint: Some of these are located in more than one of the thirds.) Draw a circle around the correct locations:
   a. cingulum: cervical   middle   incisal
   b. lingual pit   cervical   middle   incisal
   c. lingual fossa: cervical   middle   incisal

6. The more rounded incisal angle on the maxillary central incisor is the
   a. mesial
   b. distal

7. The convexities of enamel along the lateral borders of the lingual surface are
   a. lingual fossa
   b. mesial marginal ridge
   c. distal marginal ridge
   d. lingual pit
   e. cingulum

8. Which line angle of the maxillary central incisor is shorter in facial view?
   a. mesial
   b. distal

9. Which line angle of the maxillary central incisor is more nearly straight?
   a. mesial
   b. distal

10. The facial surface of the maxillary central incisor is
    a. both concave and convex
    b. slightly convex

CHECK YOUR ANSWERS IN APPENDIX A.

2.2.0

MAXILLARY CENTRAL INCISOR: PROXIMAL VIEW

incisal edge, cervical line

Viewing the maxillary central incisor from the mesial side reveals a triangular profile with the apex at the _____ _____ . The base corresponds roughly to the _____ _____ .

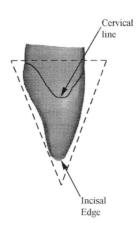

Permanent
Maxillary
Left
Central Incisor
MESIAL

Cervical line

Incisal Edge

cingulum

The most prominent feature of the lingual in proximal profile is the _____ .

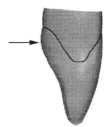

Permanent
Maxillary
Left
Central Incisor
MESIAL

convex, concave

In mesial profile, the cingulum appears _____ (convex/concave), but the remaining sweep of the lingual surface is gently _____ (convex/concave).

Permanent
Maxillary
Left
Central Incisor
MESIAL

Cingulum

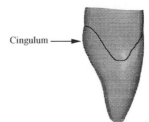

As shown, the cingulum occurs in both the _____ and _____ thirds of the anatomical crown.

Permanent
Maxillary
Left
Central Incisor
MESIAL

Examine the diagrams. The incisal edge occurs in the incisal third of the crown; the height of contour of the facial and lingual surfaces occurs in the _____ third, and the lingual fossa is in the _____ and _____ thirds.

Permanent
Maxillary
Right
Central Incisor
1. LINGUAL
2. DISTAL

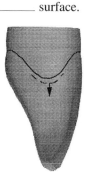

1   2

As seen in a proximal view, the cervical line appears as a rounded "U" shape with the "bottom" of the "U" projecting toward the _____ surface.

Permanent
Maxillary
Right
Central Incisor
DISTAL

cervical

From a proximal view of the maxillary central incisor, observe that the tooth axis that bisects the root apex and the incisal edge, also crosses through the crest of convexity of the _____ line.

Permanent
Maxillary
Right
Central Incisor
DISTAL

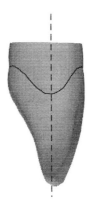

triangle

From a mesial view, the outline of the central incisor is roughly similar to what geometric shape? _____

Permanent
Maxillary
Right
Central Incisor
MESIAL

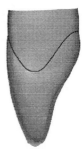

cingulum

The mesial view is very similar to the distal. Again, on the lingual surface one observes the large _____ (cingulum/lingual pit) occurring in the cervical and middle thirds.

Permanent
Maxillary
Right
Central Incisor
MESIAL

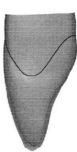

On the facial surface, the convexity is smooth with its height of contour occurring in the _____ third.

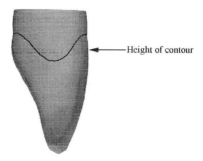

Permanent
Maxillary
Right
Central Incisor
DISTAL

Height of contour

To review briefly, on both facial and lingual aspects, these heights of contour occur in the _____ _____ of the crown.

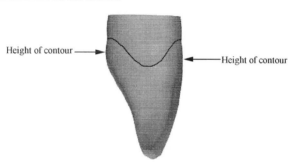

Permanent
Maxillary
Right
Central Incisor
DISTAL

Height of contour →

← Height of contour

The curvature of the cementoenamel junction (or cervical line) on the distal surface is similar to that of the mesial surface, the exception being the amount of curvature. For example, if the cervical line has a curvature that measures 3.5 mm on the mesial surface, the distal curvature will measure 2.5 mm. Although the amount of difference may vary, the amount of curvature of the cervical line on all teeth is greater on the _____ surface.

Permanent
Maxillary
Right
Central Incisor
1. MESIAL
2. DISTAL

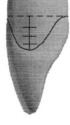

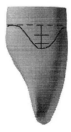

1

2

How many of the following terms are spelled correctly? _____
  mesial-distel
  cervikal
  lingual fose
  mesiodistally

2.2.1   MAXILLARY CENTRAL INCISOR: INCISAL VIEW

Figure 1 shows the central incisor as seen while turning to the incisal edge from the facial. Figure 2 shows the maxillary central as seen from an incisal view. Much of the facial surface can be seen. On the lingual surface, the most striking prominence is the large _____ .

cingulum

Permanent
Maxillary
Right Incisor
1. INCISOFACIAL
2. INCISAL

Facial

Incisal Edge

?

1   2

When examining a specimen tooth (maxillary central incisor) from an incisal view, how much of the root can be seen? _____

Incisal to the cingulum is the large lingual concavity, the _____ _____ .

lingual fossa

Permanent
Maxillary
Central Incisor
PROXIMAL

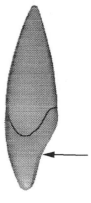

The incisal edge of a central incisor is centered over the root in the faciolingual direction. Thus, the plane that bisects the incisal edge and the cervical line on the proximal surfaces also bisects the _____ _____ .

Permanent
Maxillary
Central Incisor
PROXIMAL

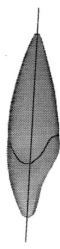

Examining a maxillary central incisor from the incisal view reveals three evident features of crown anatomy. First, the proximal surfaces taper in toward the cingulum. Second, very slight grooves are present on the facial surface. Third, the incisal view shows a geometric outline that is roughly triangular in shape. Fourth, the incisal edge appears long and _____ (narrow/wide).

narrow

Permanent
Maxillary
Right
Central Incisor
INCISAL

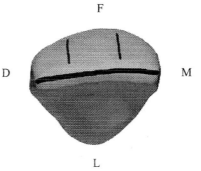

F

D

M

L

straight (or flat)

As we examine the facial surface progressively toward the incisal, the mesiodistal arc of convexity becomes less convex, until near the incisal border the curve of convexity is almost _____ .

Permanent
Maxillary
Right
Central Incisor
INCISOFACIAL

GO TO THE NEXT PAGE AND TAKE REVIEW TEST 2.2.

REVIEW TEST 2.2

1. The most prominent feature of the lingual surface of the maxillary central incisor from the proximal view is the _____ .

   a. cervical line
   b. cingulum
   c. lingual pit

2. The cingulum of the maxillary central incisor occurs in what thirds?

   a. incisal and middle
   b. cervical and middle

3. In a proximal view of the maxillary central incisor, the cervical line is a rounded "U" shape that is convex in the _____ direction.

   a. incisal
   b. apical

4. The height of contour on both the facial and lingual surfaces of the maxillary central incisor occurs in the _____ third.

   a. incisal
   b. middle
   c. cervical

5. The amount of curvature of the cervical line of the maxillary central incisor is greater on the _____ .

   a. mesial
   b. distal

6. Choose the correct statement about the maxillary central incisor.

   a. The lingual fossa is located incisally from the lingual pit.
   b. The cingulum is located incisally from the lingual pit.

7. Choose the incorrect statement.

   a. The distoincisal angle of the maxillary central incisor is more acute than the mesioincisal angle.
   b. The maxillary central incisor has a cingulum.

CHECK YOUR ANSWERS IN APPENDIX A.

2.3.0   HEIGHT OF CONTOUR, CONTACTS AND EMBRASURES OF MAXILLARY CENTRAL INCISORS

cervical

The permanent maxillary centrals have facial and lingual heights of contour in the _____ third of the crown.

Permanent
Maxillary
Central Incisor
MESIAL

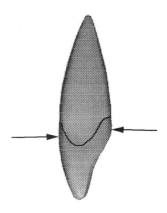

1/2

In proximal view, maxillary teeth give the impression that the amount of contour is greater on the facial than on the lingual surface (especially true for anterior teeth). However, careful examination will show that the contour, both facially and lingually, for all maxillary teeth measures approximately _____ mm.

Permanent
Maxillary
Central Incisor
MESIAL

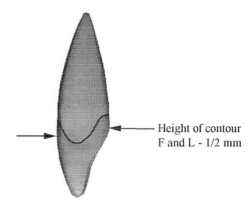

Height of contour
F and L - 1/2 mm

The incisocervical location of the proximal contact of the maxillary central incisors lies along the height of contour on the proximal surface. The contact area on the mesial of the central incisor is located in the _____ third.

incisal

Permanent
Maxillary
Incisors
1. FACIAL
2. INCISAL

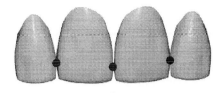

1

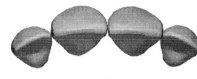

2

The contacts of the central incisor are centered in the faciolingual direction as seen in Figure 2 in the previous illustration. The _____ contact is located at the junction of the incisal and middle thirds. This is abbreviated _____ .

distal, J

Notice the small incisal embrasure between the two maxillary central incisors. This is because of the nearly right-angled mesioincisal angles of the incisors and the incisocervical location of their mesial contact areas in the _____ third of the crown.

incisal

Permanent
Maxillary
Incisors
FACIAL

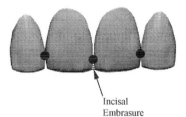

Incisal
Embrasure

The embrasures seen from the incisal view are the _____ and lingual.

labial

Permanent
Maxillary
Central Incisors
INCISAL

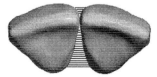

TURN TO THE NEXT PAGE AND TAKE REVIEW TEST 2.3.

REVIEW TEST 2.3

1. Which of the following descriptions of the maxillary central incisor is correct in all aspects?

   a. The height of contour on the facial and lingual surfaces occurs in the cervical third. On the proximal surface, the U-shaped contour of the cervical line projects apically. The cervical line has more curvature on the distal surface than on the mesial.

   b. The height of contour on the facial and lingual surfaces occurs in the cervical third. On the proximal surface, the U-shaped contour of the cervical line projects incisally. The cervical line has more curvature on the mesial surface than on the distal.

2. Choose the incorrect statement.

   a. The distoincisal angle of the maxillary central incisor is more acute than the mesioincisal angle.

   b. The maxillary central incisor has a cingulum.

3. The maxillary central incisors have facial and lingual heights of contour in the _____ third of the crown.

   a. incisal
   b. middle
   c. cervical

4. Choose the incorrect statement about the maxillary central incisors.

   a. The location of the mesial contact is along the height of contour.
   b. The distal contact is located in the incisal third.
   c. The mesial contact is in the incisal third.

5. The smallest embrasure of the maxillary central incisor is the

   a. facial
   b. lingual
   c. incisal

CHECK YOUR ANSWERS IN APPENDIX A.

ROOTS OF MAXILLARY CENTRAL INCISORS

The root of the maxillary central incisor is roughly cone-shaped. A cross section of the root is sometimes described as having a triangular form with rounded edges but the exact shape varies depending on the part of the root from which the cross section is drawn. Similar to the crown, the mesial and distal root surfaces converge toward the lingual, slightly distorting the conical form. The lingual convergence reduces the lingual measurement of the root in the _____ (mesiodistal/faciolingual) direction.

Permanent
Maxillary
Right
Central Incisor
1. LINGUAL
2. CROSS SECTION

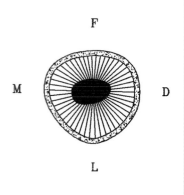

1

2

An illustration of the facial and lingual surfaces as seen from the apicoincisal view, reveals the lingual convergence of the root. Notice in Figure 1 the flatter convex surface on the facial and compare it with the even more convex lingual surface in Figure 2.

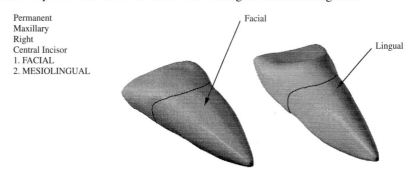

Permanent
Maxillary
Right
Central Incisor
1. FACIAL
2. MESIOLINGUAL

Facial

Lingual

1   2

The roots of all single-rooted teeth (incisors, canines, and most premolars) show a lingual convergence similar to the maxillary central incisor. As illustrated by this mesiolingual view of the maxillary right central incisor, the convergence of the root to the lingual is apparent. Which root surface is the narrowest? _____

Permanent
Maxillary
Right
Central Incisor
MESIOLINGUAL

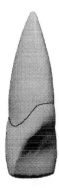

The definition of *cervix* is "the neck" or "any constricted part." Barring extreme variations, every tooth is constricted in the region of the cementoenamel junction or cervical line. This constriction occurs at the junction of the crown and root of the tooth where the enamel and cementum meet. A very distinct _____ (concave/convex) region can be determined at the cervical line.

Permanent
Maxillary
Right
Central Incisor
LINGUAL

M   D

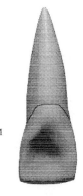

Because of the higher degree of variability in form at the apical portion of a root, our discussion of root anatomy will concentrate on the more consistent form exhibited by the _____ portion of the root.

Permanent
Maxillary
Left Incisors
FACIAL

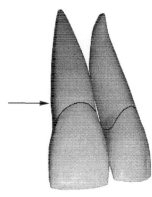

Viewed from the mesial, which root surface of the maxillary central incisor is more convex in the longitudinal direction? _____ (facial/lingual)

Permanent
Maxillary
Central Incisor
MESIAL

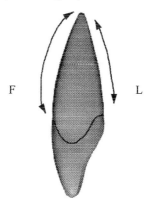

As seen in the cross section (Fig. 2), the faciolingual curvature of the mesial root surface of the maxillary central incisor has a convex portion and a portion that tends to be straight or flat. The convex portion is toward the _____ (facial/lingual), the straight portion toward the _____ (facial/lingual).

Permanent
Maxillary
Right
Central Incisor
1. LINGUAL
2. CROSS SECTION

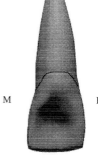

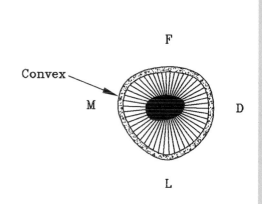

Convex

1

2

The faciolingual curvature of the distal surface is entirely _____ .

Permanent
Maxillary
Right
Central Incisor
1. LINGUAL
2. CROSS SECTION

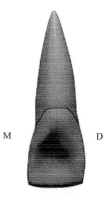

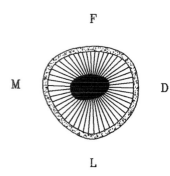

1

2

cervical

Some maxillary central incisors will have a mesial and/or distal convexity at the _____ third, although it is the least likely tooth to have a root depression on a proximal surface.

2.4.1 PULP ANATOMY OF MAXILLARY CENTRAL INCISORS

dentin

The description of the pulp cavity of a permanent tooth described in this chapter will be indicative of the average form after the root is formed. If the root of a tooth in the mouth of a young person is not completely formed, the average description will not be applicable.

In older people, secondary dentin may occupy part of the original pulp cavity. The progressive change in the pulp cavity that begins with the early formation of a tooth in the crypt takes place as the pulp performs its primary function of laying down _____ .

mesiodistal

The maxillary central incisor has a large, simple pulp cavity. Near the roof, the pulp chamber is widest in the _____ direction.

Permanent
Maxillary
Right
Central Incisor
1. MESIAL FACIOLINGUAL
LONGITUDINAL SECTION
2. LINGUAL MESIODISTAL
LONGITUDINAL SECTION

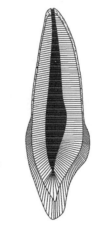
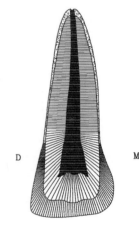

F   L   D   M

1   2

lobes

In a mesiodistal longitudinal section, three pulp horns may be seen at the roof of the pulp chamber. These horns roughly correspond to the three facial _____ .

Permanent
Maxillary
Right
Central Incisor
MESIODISTAL
LONGITUDINAL SECTION
LINGUAL

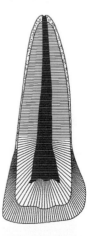

A faciolingual longitudinal section of the maxillary central incisor shows the pulp cavity tapering toward the incisal and apical. The gradual taper of the pulp cavity is interrupted by a slight faciolingual constriction at the level of the _____ _____ .

Permanent
Maxillary
Right
Central Incisor
FACIOLINGUAL
LONGITUDINAL SECTION
MESIAL

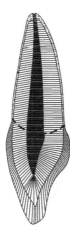

A series of cross sections show that the pulp cavity of the maxillary central incisor gradually changes from an elliptical to a circular shape. Near the roof of the pulp chamber, the shape is elliptical. This elliptical form is widest in the _____ direction.

Permanent
Maxillary
Right Central Incisor
1. LINGUAL MESIODISTAL
   LONGITUDINAL SECTION
2. CROSS SECTIONS

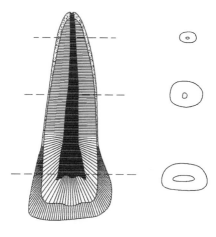

1   2

cervical line

mesiodistal

SUMMARY OF PERMANENT MAXILLARY CENTRAL INCISORS

These illustrations summarize the information presented about the crown of the permanent maxillary central incisor.

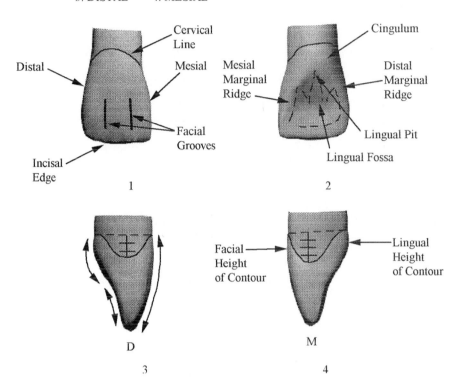

Permanent Maxillary Right Central Incisor - Summary
1. FACIAL   2. LINGUAL
3. DISTAL   4. MESIAL

The information concerning anatomical landmarks, contacts, embrasures, and universal code numbers for the permanent maxillary central incisors is summarized in these illustrations.

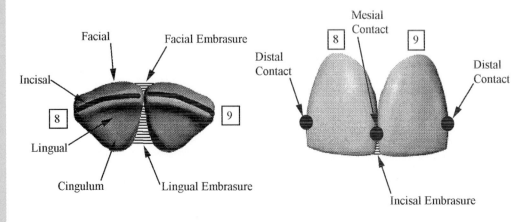

Permanent Maxillary Central Incisors - Summary
1. INCISAL   2. FACIAL

The illustrations in this frame summarize root anatomy and pulp anatomy. Notice the lingual convergence of the root in Figure 2, and the convexity of the lingual root surface in a longitudinal direction.

Permanent Maxillary Right Central Incisor - Summary
1. MESIAL   2. MESIOLINGUAL

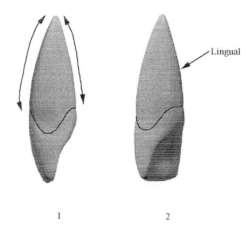

Lingual

1   2

In Figure 2, the mesiodistal section, remember the number of pulp horns is _____. In which direction is the pulp chamber widest? _____

two, mesiodistal

Notice the constriction of the pulp at the level of the CEJ.

Permanent Maxillary Right Central Incisor Longitudinal Sections – Summary
1. FACIOLINGUAL   2. MESIODISTAL

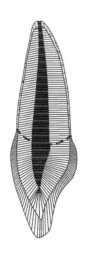
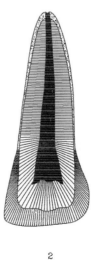

1   2

TURN TO THE NEXT PAGE AND TAKE REVIEW TEST 2.4.

REVIEW TEST 2.4

1. Label the indicated items (a through e) on the illustration.

   a.
   b.
   c.
   d.
   e.

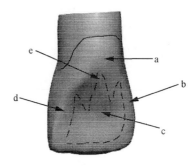

2. The pulp of the maxillary central incisor has

   a. one pulp horn
   b. two pulp horns
   c. three pulp horns

3. The apex of the maxillary central incisor is

   a. pointed
   b. blunted

4. The pulp of the maxillary central incisor is wider in the

   a. faciolingual
   b. mesiodistal

5. The proximal contact of tooth number 8 is located in the incisal third on the

   a. mesial
   b. distal

6. The facial and lingual heights of contour on tooth number 9 are located in the

   a. cervical third
   b. middle third
   c. incisal third

CHECK YOUR ANSWERS IN APPENDIX A.

MAXILLARY LATERAL INCISOR

2.5.0

The maxillary lateral incisor closely resembles its neighbor, the central incisor. Facially, the geometric shape of the lateral incisor is the same; that is, _____ in shape.

trapezoidal (or quadrilateral)

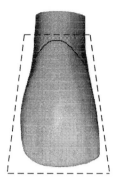

Permanent
Maxillary
Right
Lateral Incisor
FACIAL

This is an illustration of the permanent maxillary right and left lateral incisors. The universal code for the permanent maxillary right lateral incisor in Figure 1 is _____ . The code for the lateral in Figure 2 is _____ .

7, 10

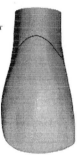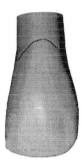

Permanent
Maxillary
1. Right Lateral Incisor
2. Left Lateral Incisor
FACIAL

1   2

The lateral incisor is smaller than the central incisor in all dimensions. Mesiodistally (horizontally), it is _____ (narrower/wider); incisocervically (vertically), it is _____ (longer/shorter).

narrower, shorter

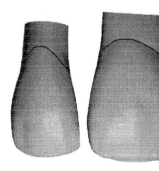

Permanent
Maxillary
Right
1. Lateral Incisor
2. Central Incisor
FACIAL

1   2

distal

A maxillary lateral incisor is more rounded from a facial view than its adjacent central incisor. The angles formed by the intersection of the incisal with the two proximal surfaces are definitely rounded. Of the two incisal angles, the more rounded is the _____ angle.

Permanent
Maxillary
Right
Lateral Incisor
FACIAL

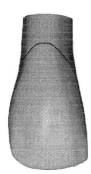

lateral incisor

Keeping in mind the overall comparison in curvature between a maxillary lateral and central incisor, which tooth has the more rounded distofacial line angle? _____ _____ .

Permanent
Maxillary
Right
1. Lateral Incisor
2. Central Incisor
FACIAL

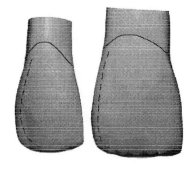

1   2

straighter

Although the lateral incisor is more curved than the central incisor, there is one feature that is an exception. The mesiofacial line angles of the two maxillary incisors closely resemble each other. The maxillary lateral incisors will deviate from the norm more often than any other tooth, with the exception of the third molars. At times, the general trend of a more rounded form for the lateral incisor is reversed, so that the mesial border of a lateral incisor appears to be _____ than that of the central incisor.

Permanent
Maxillary
Right
1. Lateral Incisor
2. Central Incisor
FACIAL

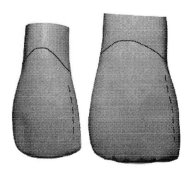

1   2

Lingually, the features of a maxillary lateral incisor are more prominent than those of a central incisor. Each of the four convexities that form the borders of the lingual surface is well developed. By comparison to the central incisor, these well-developed ridges create a lingual fossa that is slightly _____ (deeper/shallower).

deeper

Permanent
Maxillary
Right
1. Central Incisor
2. Lateral Incisor
LINGUAL

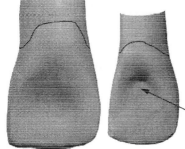

Lingual
Fossa

1   2

The mesial and distal marginal ridges unite, cervically, with the major lingual convexity, the _____ .

cingulum

Permanent
Maxillary
Right
Lateral Incisor
LINGUAL

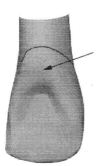

Incisally, a well-developed linguoincisal ridge completes the marginal convexity of the lingual surface. Which of the following statements describes the effect the well-developed linguoincisal ridge has on the incisal surface of the lateral incisor?

Proportionately, the faciolingual measurement of the incisal edge of the maxillary central and maxillary lateral incisor would be

a. the same on both incisors
b. relatively thicker on the lateral incisor

b. relatively thicker on the lateral incisor

Permanent
Maxillary
Right
1. Lateral Incisor
2. Central Incisor
INCISAL

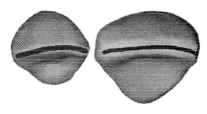

1   2

A maxillary central incisor is larger than a maxillary lateral incisor, but the well-developed linguoincisal ridge on a lateral incisor gives the lateral incisor added thickness at the incisal.

The lingual surface of a maxillary lateral incisor has mesial and distal marginal ridges that are _____ (more/less) prominent than a maxillary central incisor.

The term used to identify area A is _____ _____ _____ .

Permanent
Maxillary
Right
Lateral Incisor
LINGUAL

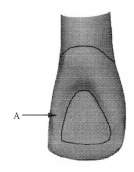

A ——▶

The term used to identify area B is _____ ridge.

Permanent
Maxillary
Right
Lateral Incisor
LINGUAL

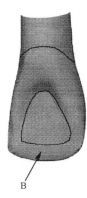

B

The area marked B is called _____ _____ (lingual fossa/lingual pit).

Permanent
Maxillary
Right
Lateral Incisor
LINGUAL

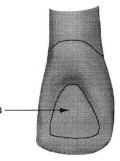

B ——▶

more

mesial marginal ridge

linguoincisal

lingual fossa

The cingulum is indicated by arrow A, B, or C. _____

A is correct; B is the
lingual fossa; C is the
distal marginal ridge

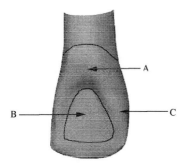

Permanent
Maxillary
Right
Lateral Incisor
LINGUAL

From a facial view, which tooth is larger: a maxillary central incisor or a maxillary lateral incisor? _____ _____ _____

maxillary central
incisor

From a proximal view, which tooth appears relatively thicker at the incisal: a maxillary central incisor or a maxillary lateral incisor? _____ _____
_____

maxillary lateral incisor

Both proximal surfaces of a maxillary lateral incisor are generally similar to the proximal surfaces of a central incisor. The actual amount of curvature of the cervical line is slightly less on the proximal surfaces of a _____ incisor.

lateral

Permanent
Maxillary
Right
1. Central Incisor
2. Lateral Incisor
MESIAL

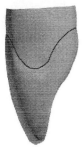   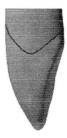

1   2

As on a maxillary central incisor, the cervical line on the proximal surface of a maxillary lateral incisor appears as a rounded "U" shape. The cervical line is convex toward the _____ edge.

incisal

Permanent
Maxillary
Right
Lateral Incisor
MESIAL

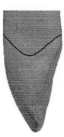

interdental papilla

As with all teeth, the lateral incisors are relatively flat on the proximal surfaces, gingival to the interproximal contact area. This relatively flat contour allows room for the gingival tissue called the _____ _____ .

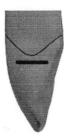

Permanent
Maxillary
Right
Lateral Incisor
MESIAL

mesial

On which proximal surface of any given tooth does the cervical line have the greater amount of curvature? _____

Figure 1

Although a maxillary central incisor is larger than a lateral incisor, the lateral incisor appears to be more rounded from an incisal view. Because a lateral incisor is narrower mesiodistally, the curvature on the facial surface is proportionately greater than that of a central incisor. Lingually, the major convexities (the mesial and distal marginal ridges, the linguoincisal ridge, and cingulum) are more fully developed on a lateral incisor.

Of the two figures, which is the lateral incisor (incisal view), Figure 1 or Figure 2? _____

Permanent
Maxillary
Right
1. Lateral Incisor
2. Central Incisor
INCISAL

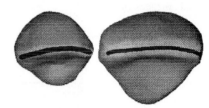

1   2

B

Maxillary laterals will deviate from the normal description more than any other tooth except maybe the third molars. The laterals will sometimes have a pointed crown commonly referred to as "peg lateral." In the illustration shown, _____ is an example of a "peg lateral."

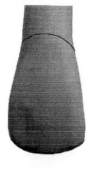
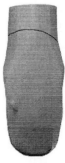

A   B

Another common deviation of maxillary laterals is congenitally missing laterals. Congenital means the condition at birth. So congenitally missing would mean _____ _____ _____ .

Some other malformations may include
1. a large pointed tubercle as part of the cingulum
2. deep developmental groove extending from the cingulum on the lingual down the lingual root

Identify each of the four teeth by arch (maxillary/mandibular), quadrant (right/left), and tooth name.

A. Permanent _____ _____ _____ _____
B. Permanent _____ _____ _____ _____
C. Permanent _____ _____ _____ _____
D. Permanent _____ _____ _____ _____

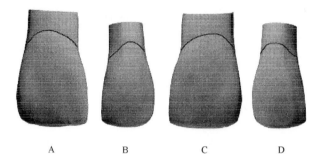

A   B   C   D

Identify each of the anatomical landmarks in the illustration of the permanent maxillary right lateral incisor.

The term used to identify area A is _____ _____ _____ .
The term used to identify area B is _____ ridge.
Area C is called _____ _____ _____ .
Area D is called _____ _____ .
Area E is called _____ .

Permanent
Maxillary
Right
Lateral Incisor
LINGUAL

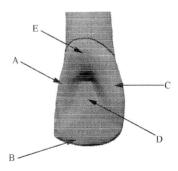

cervical, fossa,
concave, mesiodistal

Each of the following terms is spelled incorrectly. Revise each.

1. cervecol   1. _____
2. fosse   2. _____
3. conkave   3. _____
4. meseodistol   4. _____

2.5.1 HEIGHT OF CONTOUR, CONTACTS AND EMBRASURES OF MAXILLARY LATERAL INCISORS

lateral

The arrows indicate the height of contour. The height of contour occurs in the cervical third on both the facial and lingual surfaces of maxillary _____ incisors.

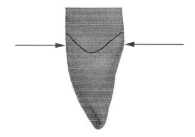

Permanent
Maxillary
Right
Lateral Incisor
MESIAL

at the junction of the
incisal and middle
thirds (J)

The incisocervical location of the proximal contact of the maxillary lateral incisors lies along the height of contour on the proximal surface. The contact areas of the lateral incisors are marked in the illustration. The mesial contact of tooth numbers 7 and 10 is located _____ .

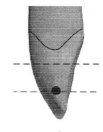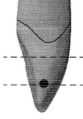

Permanent
Maxillary
1. Right Lateral Incisor
2. Left Lateral Incisor
MESIAL

1   2

middle

The contact in the incisocervical direction of the distal of the maxillary lateral incisors is located in the _____ third of the crown.

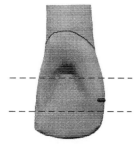

Permanent
Maxillary
Right
Lateral Incisor
LINGUAL

Incisocervically, the contact between a maxillary central and lateral incisor occurs approximately at the junction of the incisal and middle thirds. Therefore, "the junction of the incisal and middle third," or simply "J," describes the location of the distal contact of the _____ incisor and the mesial contact area for a maxillary _____ incisor. The distal contact of the maxillary lateral incisor is located in the _____ third.

Permanent
Maxillary
Right
Central Incisor

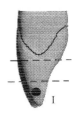

I

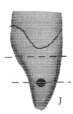

J

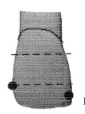

I J

Permanent
Maxillary
Right
Lateral Incisor

J

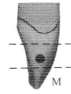

M

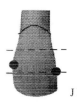

J M

Study the illustration of the maxillary incisors and note the location and depth of the embrasures. The largest embrasures are located on the _____ , while the smallest embrasures are on the _____ .

Permanent
Maxillary
Incisors
1. Facial
2. Incisal

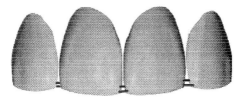

1

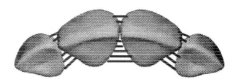

2

2.5.2   ROOTS OF MAXILLARY LATERAL INCISORS

longer

The root form of the maxillary lateral incisor is highly variable. Typically, it is different from that of the central incisor. The roots of the two incisors are nearly equal in length; but in proportion to crown length, the maxillary lateral incisor has a root that is proportionally _____ (shorter/longer) than the central incisor.

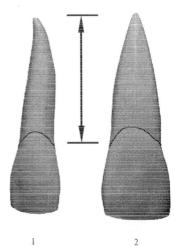

Permanent
Maxillary
Right
1. Lateral Incisor
2. Central Incisor
FACIAL

1   2

central incisor

In the mesiodistal direction, which maxillary incisor has a thicker root? _____

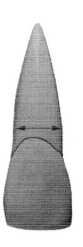

Permanent
Maxillary
Right
1. Lateral Incisor
2. Central Incisor
FACIAL

D   M

1   2

Which maxillary incisor has the thicker root in the faciolingual direction? _____
_____

Permanent
Maxillary
Right
1. Lateral Incisor
2. Central Incisor
MESIAL

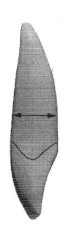 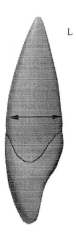

F   L

1   2

The mesial and distal surfaces of the maxillary lateral incisor sometimes have a broad groove running in the longitudinal direction. Named for the direction they run, these grooves are called _____ grooves.

Permanent
Maxillary
Right
Lateral Incisor
1. Mesial
2. Distal

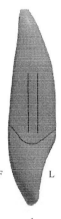 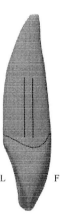

F   L   L   F

1   2

When present, a longitudinal groove is sometimes distinct, sometimes faint. The presence of a longitudinal groove causes the mesial and distal root surfaces to have a faciolingual curvature that varies from nearly flat to _____ (concave/convex).

Permanent
Maxillary
Right
Lateral Incisor
MID—ROOT
CROSS SECTIONS

F   F

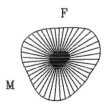 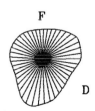

M   D

distal

Because the root form of the lateral incisor is highly variable, the shape of the horizontal section varies. Longitudinal grooves may or may not be present on the mesial and distal root surfaces of the maxillary lateral incisor. On which of these two root surfaces does a longitudinal groove appear more often? _____

Permanent
Maxillary
Right
Lateral Incisors
MID–ROOT
CROSS SECTIONS

F

F

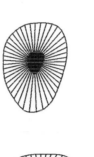

M

D

pointed (or narrower)

Of the two maxillary incisors, one has a blunt apex, the other a pointed one. The apex of the maxillary lateral incisor is _____ .

Permanent
Maxillary
Right
1. Lateral Incisor
2. Central Incisor
FACIAL

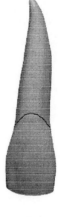

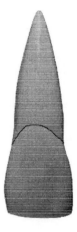

1

2

The apical portion of the root of different specimens of maxillary lateral incisors may be found to show deflections or deviations in any direction. Notice the root deviations in the illustration of the maxillary lateral incisor. The facial view shows a deviation toward the _____ (mesial/distal) and the proximal view shows deviation toward the _____ (facial/lingual).

distal, facial

Permanent
Maxillary
Right
Lateral Incisor
1. FACIAL
2. MESIAL

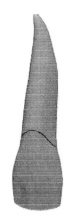 

1   2

PULP ANATOMY OF MAXILLARY LATERAL INCISORS

2.5.3

The pulp cavity of the maxillary lateral incisor is similar in shape to that of the maxillary central incisor except that the lateral usually has _____ (two/three) pulp horns. Because of the relative sizes of the two teeth, the measurements of the pulp cavity of the lateral incisor are slightly _____ (larger/smaller) than those of the maxillary central incisor.

two, smaller

Permanent
Maxillary
Right
1. Lateral Incisor
2. Central Incisor
MESIODISTAL
LONGITUDINAL SECTIONS
LINGUAL

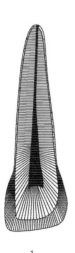 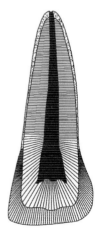

1   2

lateral incisor

The pulp cavity of either maxillary incisor may have fine, irregular constrictions along the incisoapical path and accessory canals. Which maxillary incisor is more likely to have accessory canals? _____ _____

Permanent
Maxillary
Right
1. Lateral Incisor
2. Central Incisor
MESIODISTAL
LONGITUDINAL SECTIONS
LINGUAL

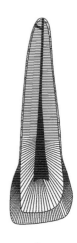
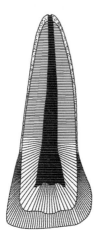

1   2

mesiodistal

Like the maxillary central incisor, the maxillary lateral incisor shows the pulp chamber to be widest in the _____ direction at the level of the crown.

Permanent
Maxillary
Right
Lateral Incisor
1. Mesiodistal Longitudinal
   Section
2. Faciolingual Longitudinal
   Section

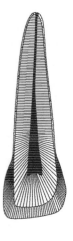
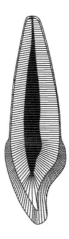

1   2

SUMMARY OF PERMANENT MAXILLARY LATERAL INCISORS

Permanent Maxillary Lateral Incisors - Summary

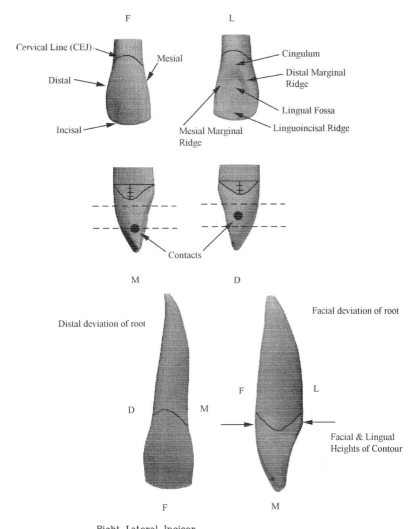

F   L

Cervical Line (CEJ)   Mesial

Distal

Incisal

Cingulum

Distal Marginal Ridge

Lingual Fossa

Linguoincisal Ridge

Mesial Marginal Ridge

Contacts

M   D

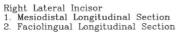

Distal deviation of root

Facial deviation of root

D   M

F   L

Facial & Lingual Heights of Contour

F   M

Right Lateral Incisor
1. Mesiodistal Longitudinal Section
2. Faciolingual Longitudinal Section

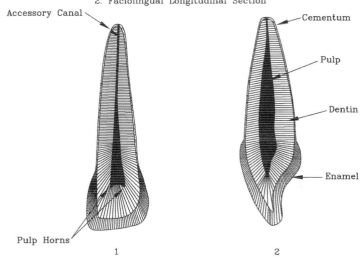

Accessory Canal

Cementum

Pulp

Dentin

Enamel

Pulp Horns

1   2

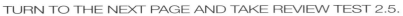

TURN TO THE NEXT PAGE AND TAKE REVIEW TEST 2.5.

REVIEW TEST 2.5

1. Choose the *correct* statement.

   a. The lateral incisor usually has a straighter distofacial line angle than the central incisor.
   b. The lateral incisor has a more rounded distofacial line angle than the central incisor.

2. Choose the *correct* statement.

   a. The lateral incisor has more curvature to the cervical line on the mesial and distal surfaces than does the central incisor.
   b. The cervical line of the lateral incisor has less curvature on the mesial and distal surfaces than does the cervical line on the corresponding surfaces of the central incisor.

3. If someone said, "The maxillary incisors are relatively flat on their proximal surfaces, gingival to the proximal contact areas," which of the following responses would be the most complete and accurate reply?

   a. "This is false, because they are convex."
   b. "This is false, because the line angles of these teeth are curved."
   c. "That is true, because the enamel is thin."
   d. "That is true, because this flatness provides space for the interdental papilla."

4. Choose the *incorrect* statement.

   a. The distoincisal angle of the maxillary lateral incisor is more rounded than the mesioincisal angle.
   b. The maxillary central incisor has more distinct mesial and distal marginal ridges than the maxillary lateral incisor.

5. The mesial contact of the maxillary lateral is located

   a. in the incisal third
   b. at the junction of the incisal and middle thirds
   c. in the middle third

6. The apex of the lateral incisor is

   a. pointed
   b. blunted

7. Choose the *correct* statement.

   a. The root of the maxillary lateral incisor is wider than the root of the maxillary central incisor.
   b. The root of tooth number 9 (universal code number) is wider than the root of number 10.

8. The pulp anatomy with three pulp horns is found in which incisor?

   a. tooth number 7
   b. tooth number 8

9. The root of which maxillary incisor could be deviated to the distal?

    a. central incisor

    b. lateral incisor

10. Which incisor would be more likely to have accessory canals?

    a. lateral incisor

    b. central incisor

CHECK YOUR ANSWERS IN APPENDIX A.

2.6.0   MANDIBULAR CENTRAL INCISORS

The mandibular incisors are the smallest teeth of the human dentition. In normal occlusion, the maxillary central incisor occludes with the central and lateral incisors of the mandibular arch. Which incisor normally has only one antagonist? _____ _____
_____

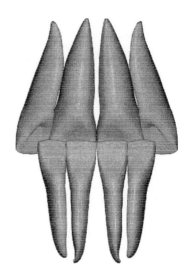

Permanent
Maxillary and
Mandibular
Incisors
LINGUAL

wedge

The form of a mandibular incisor is distinctly different from that of a maxillary incisor. Despite the differences in tooth form, the maxillary and mandibular incisors have general similarities that place them in the classification of incisors. Each of the crowns of the incisors has a _____ shape.

four

As with maxillary anteriors, the mandibular incisors have _____ (number) lobes.

mamelons

Similar to maxillary incisors, the incisal edges of newly erupted mandibular incisors have three rounded bumps. These bumps, which suggest three of the four lobes, are called _____ .

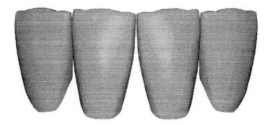

Permanent
Mandibular
Incisors
FACIAL

mesiofacial, central-
facial, distofacial

The four lobes are called the distofacial, central-facial, mesiofacial, and lingual lobes. Which three lobes represent that part of the tooth seen in a facial view? _____ ,
_____ , _____ .

The fourth lobe is represented on the lingual surface of the crown by the prominent convexity called the _____ .

Permanent
Mandibular
Right
Central Incisor
DISTAL

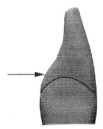

As seen from a facial view, the geometric outline of a mandibular incisor is roughly quadrilateral. From a proximal view, each of the eight incisors has a geometric outline that is roughly _____ .

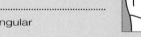

Permanent
Maxillary
Right
Central Incisor
1. FACIAL
2. DISTAL
Permanent
Mandibular
Right
Central Incisor
3. FACIAL
4. DISTAL

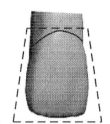

1

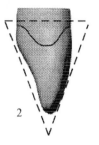

2

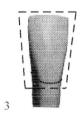

3

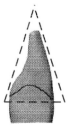

4

The nomenclature established for the maxillary incisors applies to the corresponding features of mandibular incisors. The prominent features are located in similar positions on the crowns of all eight incisors.

For example, the intersection of the facial and mesial surfaces forms the mesiofacial line angle, and the concavity of the lingual surface is termed the lingual _____ .

Permanent
Mandibular
Right
Central Incisor
1. MESIOFACIAL
2. LINGUAL

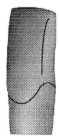

1

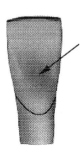

2

convex

The facial surface of a mandibular central incisor is curved in the incisocervical and mesiodistal dimensions. In both dimensions, the facial surface is slightly _____ (convex/concave). The facial of this tooth is smooth with few ridges and valleys, making it a very symmetrical tooth.

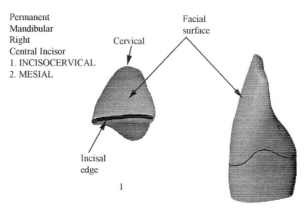

Permanent
Mandibular
Right
Central Incisor
1. INCISOCERVICAL
2. MESIAL

Cervical

Facial
surface

Incisal
edge

1

2

incisal

Facially, the mandibular central incisor is very smooth with a slight convexity at the cervical third of the crown. The degree of convexity of the facial surface decreases progressively from the narrow cervical third toward the wider, nearly flat _____ edge.

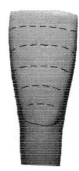

Permanent
Mandibular
Right
Central Incisor
FACIAL

incisal edge

As the facial surface becomes less convex, it becomes wider, so the broadest portion of a mandibular central incisor is found near the _____ _____ .

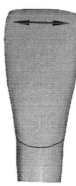

Permanent
Mandibular
Right
Central Incisor
FACIAL

When one examines a mandibular central incisor from a facial view, it is difficult to identify characteristics that distinguish the mesial from the distal surface. The distinguishing features are very slight.

From the facial view,

1. the distofacial line angle is slightly more convex.
2. the cervical line has its crest slightly toward the distal.
3. the straight line distance between the end-points of the distofacial line angle is slightly less than the straight-line distance between the end-points of the mesiofacial line angle. That is, the incisal edge is inclined slightly toward the gingival at the distal.
4. the distoinciscal angle is slightly greater than the mesioincisal angle.

Permanent
Mandibular
Right
Central Incisor
FACIAL

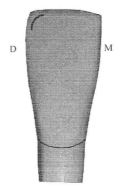

The illustrations represent three mandibular central incisors. In each tooth, which letter (A or B) is toward the distal?

A, B, B

_____ _____ _____

(Figure 1)   (Figure 2)   (Figure 3)

Permanent
Mandibular
Central Incisors
FACIAL

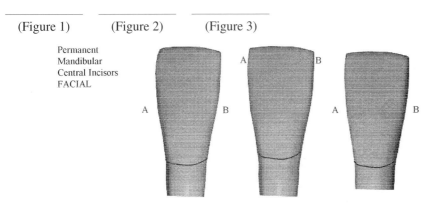

Both the mesioincisal and the distoincisal angles of a mandibular central incisor are acute. Of the two angles, which is more acute? _____

mesioincisal

root, distal

From a facial view, the cervical line is convex toward the _____ of the tooth. The crest of this convexity is slightly _____ (distal/mesial) to the midline of the facial surface.

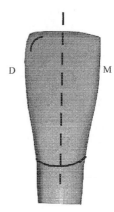

Permanent
Mandibular
Right
Central Incisor
FACIAL

D   M

A, C

Let the geometric shape shown represent the outline of the facial surface on a model of a mandibular central incisor that has been dropped on a tray. Which of the line segments (A, B, C, D) represents the incisal and cervical borders? Incisal _____ , cervical _____ .

A
B
C
D

smooth

The faint facial grooves seen on the facial surfaces of the maxillary incisors are absent on the mandibular central incisors except when they are newly erupted. Compared to maxillary centrals, the mandibular centrals have a facial surface that is quite _____ and straight.

four

The geometric outlines of the facial and lingual surfaces of the mandibular central incisor are similar. How many borders or edges does the outline have? _____

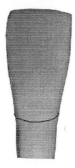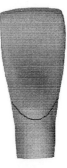

Permanent
Mandibular
Right
Central Incisor
1. FACIAL
2. LINGUAL

1   2

As with maxillary incisors, the lingual surface is somewhat _____ (smaller/larger) than the area within the facial surface.

As seen from an incisal view, the smaller lingual outline is a result of the convergence toward the _____ surface.

Permanent
Mandibular
Right
Central Incisor
INCISAL

F

M   D

L

In contrast to what is observed on the maxillary incisors, the mesial and distal marginal ridges of the mandibular central incisor are quite _____ (size).

Permanent
Mandibular
Left
Central Incisor
LINGUAL

Mesial Marginal Ridge

Distal Marginal Ridge

Comparing the lingual convexity of the maxillary and mandibular central incisors, the cingulum on the lingual surface of a mandibular central incisor is _____ (less/more) pronounced.

Permanent
Right
Central Incisors
1. Maxillary
2. Mandibular
MESIOLINGUAL

Cingulum

1

Cingulum

2

fossa

The lingual surface of a mandibular central incisor is concave in both the incisocervical and mesiodistal dimensions. The small cingulum and indistinct marginal ridges result in a shallow and generally less distinct lingual _____ .

pit

The resulting lingual surface of a mandibular central incisor forms a smooth area that flows in a concave, then convex curve from the incisal edge to the cervical line. The less pronounced lingual anatomy results in the absence of small extensions of the fossa into the cingulum. A mandibular central incisor, therefore, has no lingual _____ .

Permanent
Mandibular
Right
Central Incisor
1. MESIAL
2. LINGUAL
3. INCISAL

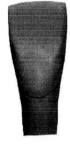 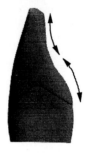

1   2   3

mesiodistal

Although the lingual fossa of a mandibular central incisor is small or less distinct, the lingual surface is concave in two dimensions: the incisocervical dimension as well as very slightly concave in the _____ dimension.

pit

Contributing to the smooth lingual surface of a mandibular central incisor are the reduced marginal ridges and cingulum and the absence of a lingual _____ (pit/fossa).

Permanent
Mandibular
Right
Central Incisor
MESIOLINGUAL

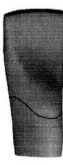

Like the crowns of the maxillary incisors, the mandibular central incisor crown (mesial view) is approximately _____ in shape.

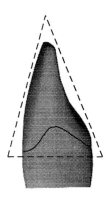

Permanent
Mandibular
Right
Central Incisor
MESIAL

The apex of this triangle represents the _____ edge of the tooth; the base of the triangle corresponds roughly to the _____ _____ .

The vertical axis of the tooth that bisects the cervical line on the mesial surface shows the incisal edge displaced slightly toward the _____ surface.

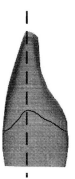

Permanent
Mandibular
Right
Central Incisor
MESIAL

As seen from a mesial view, the facial surface of a mandibular central incisor is _____ (convex/concave).

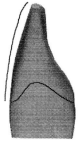

Permanent
Mandibular
Right
Central Incisor
MESIAL

The bulk of the convexity of the lingual surface occurs in the _____ third of the crown and forms the _____ .

Permanent
Mandibular
Right
Central Incisor
MESIAL

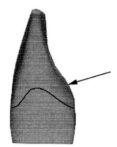

The mesial view also shows a concavity of the lingual surface from the small _____ to the _____ edge.

Permanent
Mandibular
Right
Central Incisor
MESIAL

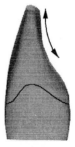

Identify the lettered areas on the illustration.

A. _____

B. _____

C. _____

Permanent
Mandibular
Right
Central Incisor
MESIOLINGUAL

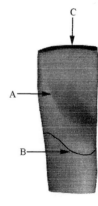

There is a difference in the amount of curvature of the cervical line on the two proximal surfaces. The cementoenamel junction curves slightly more toward the incisal on the mesial. On which of the two proximal surfaces is the cervical line less convex toward the incisal? _____

Permanent
Mandibualr
Right
Central Incisor
1. MESIAL
2. DISTAL

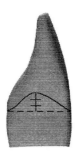

1   2

The crest of convexity of the cervical line is more incisally located on the _____ (mesial/distal) surface (Fig. 1 and Fig. 3).

The incisal edge slopes slightly downward (Fig. 2) toward the distal surface and the disto-facial line angle is slightly _____ (shorter/longer) than the mesiofacial.

Permanent
Mandibular
Right
Central Incisor
1. DISTAL
2. FACIAL
3. MESIAL

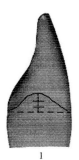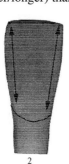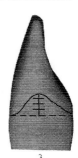

1   2   3

The mesial surface is slightly _____ (longer/shorter) than the distal, and the incisal edge slopes down toward the _____ .

Permanent
Mandibular
Right
Central Incisor
FACIAL

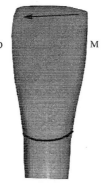

D   M

lingual

From the incisal view, we see the proximal surfaces taper in toward the _____ (facial/lingual) surface.

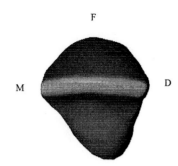

Permanent
Mandibular
Right
Central Incisor
INCISAL

F

M

D

Question Frame

With normal occlusion, the mamelons on mandibular incisors are eventually worn away. Maxillary and mandibular incisors do not usually occlude end to end, but occlude so that the mandibular incisors strike the incisolingual surfaces of the maxillary incisors (Fig. 2). Under normal conditions, which portion of the incisal edge on a mandibular incisor receives more wear?

linguoincisal . . . . GO TO FRAME A.
facioincisal. . . . . GO TO FRAME B.

Permanent
Maxillary and
Mandibular
Incisors
1. LINGUAL
2. DISTAL

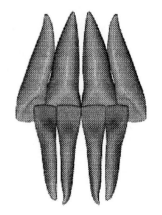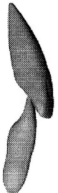

1   2

linguoincisal is
incorrect

facial

>Frame A

Try the following experiment. Slide your lower jaw back and forth in a faciolingual direction. You, like most people, will probably feel the mandibular incisors slide over the lingual surface of the maxillary incisors. Does the abrasion on the mandibular incisors involve a portion more toward the facial or the lingual? _____

RETURN TO THE QUESTION FRAME AND ANSWER AGAIN.

>**Frame B**

With increased wear at the facioincisal, the incisal edge tends to incline. In some individuals, the incisal edge of a mandibular incisor has an obvious slope downward toward the _____ (facial/lingual) surface.

facioincisal is
correct

facial

Permanent
Maxillary and
Mandibular
Right
Central Incisors
DISTAL

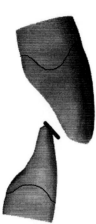

Attrition also influences the incisal edge of maxillary incisors. On a maxillary incisor, which area (facioincisal/linguoincisal) receives more wear? _____

linguoincisal

Permanent
Maxillary and
Mandibular
Right
Central Incisors
DISTAL

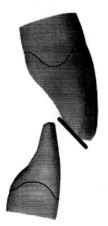

The slope of the arrow represents the incline of the worn incisal edges of both maxillary and mandibular incisors. The slope is upward toward the lingual and downward toward the facial. With wear, the incisal edges of maxillary and mandibular incisors tend to become parallel surfaces.

Permanent
Maxillary and
Mandibular
Right
Central Incisors
DISTAL

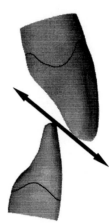

facial

When describing the slope of worn incisal edges of the maxillary and mandibular incisors, we say that the incisal edge of a maxillary incisor is inclined toward the lingual, and the incisal edge of a mandibular incisor is inclined toward the _____ surface.

Permanent
Right
Central Incisors
1. Mandibular
2. Maxillary
DISTAL

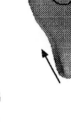

1   2

GO TO THE NEXT PAGE AND TAKE REVIEW TEST 2.6.

REVIEW TEST 2.6

1. Which border of the mandibular central incisor is longer?

   a. mesial
   b. distal

2. Which border of the mandibular central incisor is broadest in the facial view?

   a. incisal
   b. cervical

3. Which incisal angle of number 24 is more acute?

   a. mesial
   b. distal

4. Which border of number 25 is longer in the facial view?

   a. mesial
   b. distal

5. The convexity of the cervical line of number 24 is more incisally located toward the _____ surface.

   a. mesial
   b. distal

6. Choose the *correct* statement.

   a. The mandibular central incisor has a less prominent lingual fossa than the maxillary central incisor and the marginal ridges are less distinct.
   b. A lingual pit is occasionally found on the mandibular central incisor.

7. What is the word that describes the process that causes adult mandibular incisors to show no signs of the mamelons that were present at eruption (in the most common type of occlusion)? _____

8. Which one of the following teeth has only one antagonist in the normal (most frequent) occlusion?

   a. maxillary central incisor
   b. maxillary lateral incisor
   c. mandibular central incisor

9. The cervical line on the facial of the mandibular central incisor is convex in which direction?

   a. apical
   b. incisal

10. On which surface is the cervical line of the mandibular central incisor more convex?

    a. mesial
    b. distal

CHECK YOUR ANSWERS IN APPENDIX A.

2.7.0

HEIGHT OF CONTOUR, CONTACTS AND EMBRASURES OF MANDIBULAR CENTRAL INCISORS

height of contour

Incisocervically, the imaginary line encircling the tooth and defining the peak or height of curvature is called the _____ _____ _____ .

Permanent
Mandibular
Right
Central Incisor
MESIOLINGUAL

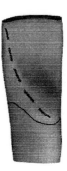

cervical

The height of contour is an imaginary curved line that completely surrounds the crown. The height of contour is marked on the facial, mesial, and lingual of tooth number 25 in the illustration. On the facial and lingual surfaces of a mandibular incisor, the height of contour occurs in the _____ third of the crown.

Permanent
Mandibular
Right
Central Incisor
MESIOFACIAL

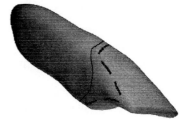

Recall that the amount of contour is a horizontal measurement. On the facial and lingual surfaces of a mandibular incisor, the amount of contour is _____ . The dot on the mandibular right central incisor in the illustration indicates the lingual height of contour.

Permanent
Mandibular
Right
Central Incisor
DISTAL

1 mm Grid

F

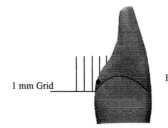

more than 1/2 mm . . . . GO TO FRAME A.
less than 1/2 mm . . . . GO TO FRAME B.

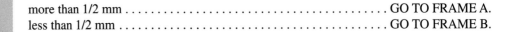

> ## >Frame A

Let us review some material presented earlier. For the majority of the teeth in the human dentition, the facial and lingual amount of contour measures approximately 1/2 mm. There are, however, several exceptions, the mandibular incisors being one. The amount of contour on the mandibular incisors is very slight, at times nearly indistinguishable. Therefore, on mandibular incisors, the facial and lingual amount of contour measures less than 1/2 mm.

RETURN TO THE QUESTION FRAME AND ANSWER AGAIN.

more than 1/2 mm is incorrect

less than 1/2 mm is correct

incisal

> ## >Frame B

The contact areas are located on the height of contour on the mesial and distal surfaces. The mandibular central incisors have contact areas located in the _____ third, indicated by the dot on the centrals. The location of the contact and the acute angle of the central incisors forms a small incisal embrasure.

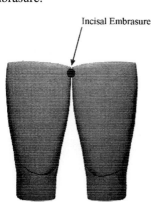

Permanent
Mandibular
Central Incisors
FACIAL

Incisal Embrasure

This incisal embrasure may be obliterated by wear of the incisal edges. No embrasure means that the contact area extends *up* to the _____ _____ .

incisal edge

The contacts of the mandibular central incisors are located along the height of contour near the incisal third of the crown leaving a very small incisal embrasure. Because the contacts are located near the incisal, they are said to be incisally located. The location of the contact area for both the mesial and distal is the _____ third of the crown.

incisal

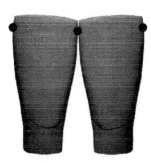

Permanent
Mandibular
Central Incisors
FACIAL

Viewing the mandibular central incisors from the incisal, one can see the facial and lingual embrasures as indicated in the illustration. The slightest or sometimes absent embrasure is the _____ embrasure.

Permanent
Mandibular
Central Incisors
1. FACIAL
2. INCISAL

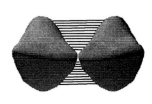
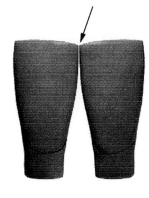

1   2

The illustrations in this frame are a summary of heights of contour, contacts and embrasures. The contacts and incisal embrasure are marked in Figure 1. The labial and lingual embrasures are indicated in Figure 2. The model teeth are not necessarily indicative of all mandibular central incisors as they appear to be tipped toward each other at the incisal edge, thus creating excessively large labial and lingual embrasures.

Permanent
Mandibular
Central Incisors
1. FACIAL
2. INCISAL

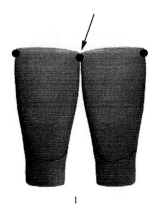
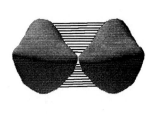

1   2

In this illustration, the mesiolingual height of contour is indicated with a dashed line.

Permanent
Mandibular
Right
Central Incisor
MESIOLINGUAL

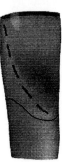

ROOTS OF MANDIBULAR CENTRAL INCISORS

The roots of the mandibular incisors are flattened or pinched from the mesial and distal directions. In which direction does the root of the mandibular central incisor have a greater measure? _____

Permanent
Mandibular
Right
Central Incisor
1. FACIAL
2. MESIAL

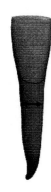
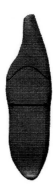

1   2

Viewed from the facial, the root of the mandibular central incisor is symmetrical and straight; that is, the mesial and distal surfaces tend to be relatively straight in the _____ direction.

Permanent
Mandibular
Right
Central Incisor
FACIAL

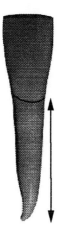

distal

The apical portion of the root on the mandibular central incisor may deviate toward the
_____ .

Permanent
Mandibular
Right
Central Incisor
FACIAL

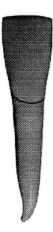

---

proximal

Longitudinal grooves may or may not be present on the mesial and distal root surfaces of
the mandibular central incisor. When present, these grooves are broad and run most of the
root length, causing a concavity on the _____ surface.

Permanent
Mandibular
Right
Central Incisor
MESIOLINGUAL

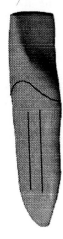

---

maxillary central
incisor

Of the maxillary and mandibular incisors, which one is least likely to have longitudinal
grooves on the mesial and distal root surfaces?

_____   _____   _____
  (arch)   (tooth)   (name)

Study the drawings in this frame. All the teeth have been inserted with their crowns toward the top of the page even though they may be maxillary. Identify each of the incisors shown by writing their names below.

A. _____

B. _____

C. _____

D. _____

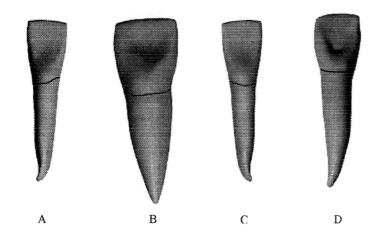

A   B   C   D

A, mandibular left central incisor:
B, maxillary right central incisor;
C. mandibular right central incisor;
D, maxillary right lateral incisor

PULP ANATOMY OF MANDIBULAR CENTRAL INCISORS

2.7.2

In the mandibular arch, the pulp canals of the two incisors are similar. For most of its incisoapical length, the pulp cavity of a mandibular incisor is wider in the _____ direction.

faciolingual

Permanent
Mandibular
Right
Central Incisor
1. FACIOLINGUAL
2. MESIODISTAL

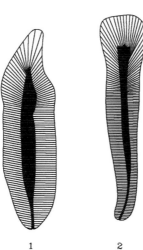

1   2

mesiodistal

Examine the series of cross sections. Near the roof of the pulp chamber, the elliptical form of the pulp cavity is widest in the _____ direction.

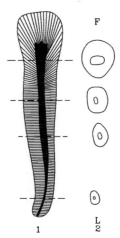

Permanent
Mandibular
Right
Central Incisor
1. MESIODISTAL
2. CROSS SECTIONS

faciolingual

Near mid-root of a mandibular incisor, the elliptical form is widest in the _____ direction.

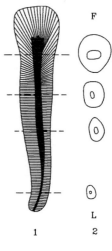

Permanent
Mandibular
Right
Central Incisor
1. MESIODISTAL
2. CROSS SECTIONS

Near the apex of a mandibular incisor, the cross section form of the pulp cavity is
_____ .

Permanent
Mandibular
Right
Central Incisor
1. MESIODISTAL
2. CROSS SECTIONS

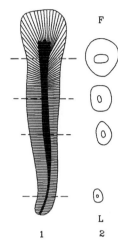

Sometimes, a thin wall of dentin divides the flattened root canal of the mandibular incisor.
These two root canals are called the _____ and _____ root canals.

Permanent
Mandibular
Right
Central Incisor
FACIOLINGUAL
Longitudinal Sections

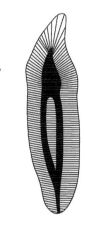
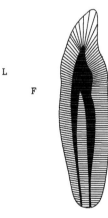

If two root canals are present, they either have separate apical foramina or converge apically to form a single canal. Mandibular incisors have few accessory canals, relative to
maxillary incisors. The incisor with the most variable root and most frequent accessory
canals is the _____ _____ _____ .

Permanent
Mandibular
Right
Central Incisor
FACIOLINGUAL
Longitudinal Sections

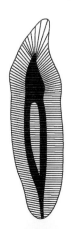
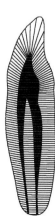

Study the summaries and review the information previously presented if necessary.

Permanent Mandibular Right Central Incisor - Summary

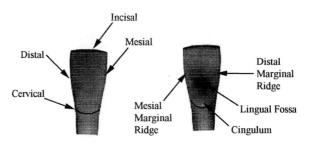

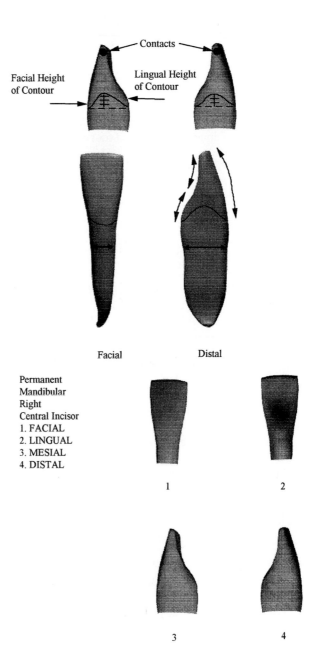

Facial   Distal

Permanent
Mandibular
Right
Central Incisor
1. FACIAL
2. LINGUAL
3. MESIAL
4. DISTAL

1   2

3   4

GO TO THE NEXT PAGE AND TAKE REVIEW TEST 2.7.

REVIEW TEST 2.7

1. Choose the *correct* statement.

   a. The mandibular central incisor has a less prominent lingual fossa than the maxillary central incisor and the marginal ridges are less distinct.

   b. A lingual pit is occasionally found on the mandibular central incisor.

2. Mandibular incisors have an amount of contour on the facial and lingual surfaces that measures

   a. between 1 mm and 1/2 mm

   b. approximately 1/2 mm

   c. less than 1/2 mm

3. What is the word that describes the process that causes adult mandibular incisors to show no signs of the mamelons that were present at eruption (in cases where the adult has had the most common type of occlusion)? _____

4. Which one of the following teeth has only one antagonist in the normal (most frequent) occlusion?

   a. maxillary central incisor

   b. maxillary lateral incisor

   c. mandibular central incisor

   d. mandibular lateral incisor

5. Incisal wear will cause the _____ embrasure of the mandibular centrals to become very small or nonexistent.

   a. facial

   b. incisal

   c. lingual

6. The pulp of the mandibular central incisor is widest in the _____ direction.

   a. faciolingual

   b. mesiodistal

7. When the root canal is divided in the mandibular central incisor, the names of the two roots are (choose two selections)

   a. mesial

   b. distal

   c. facial

   d. lingual

CHECK YOUR ANSWERS IN APPENDIX A.

2.8.0

MANDIBULAR LATERAL INCISORS

(1) lateral incisor

The mandibular lateral incisors are very similar to central incisors, but a few minor distinctions should be emphasized. Which of the two mandibular incisors shown is wider mesiodistally? _____ _____

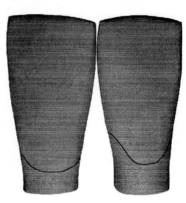

Permanent
Mandibular
Right
1. Lateral Incisor
2. Central Incisor
FACIAL

1   2

no; maxillary central incisor

Does the same relationship hold for the maxillary incisors? _____ (yes/no) Which maxillary incisor is wider mesiodistally? _____ _____

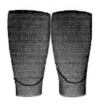

Permanent
1. Maxillary
2. Mandibular
Right Incisors
FACIAL

1

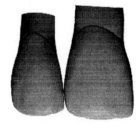

2

The lingual fossa on a mandibular lateral incisor is slightly more evident than that on a mandibular central incisor because of the somewhat more evident mesial and distal _____ ridges.

Permanent
Mandibular
Right
1. Central Incisor
2. Lateral Incisor
LINGUAL

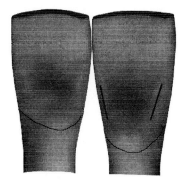

The mandibular lateral incisor also has more curvature on the distal surface than the central incisor. Which of the two figures is a mandibular lateral incisor? _____ (Figure 1/Figure 2)

Permanent
Mandibular
Right Incisors
FACIAL

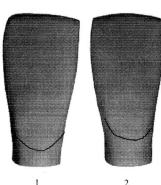

In general, which mandibular incisor has the more evident convexities and concavities? _____

The greater prominence of the lingual fossa on the lateral incisor is _____ (like/unlike) the relationship between the maxillary incisors.

longer

The mesial surface of a mandibular lateral incisor tends to be slightly _____ (shorter/longer) than the distal.

Permanent
Mandibular
Right
Lateral Incisor
1. Lingual
2. Facial

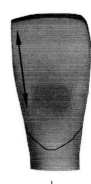
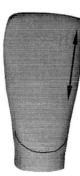

1   2

incisal

Although these general distinctions exist, they are very slight. The best method for distinguishing a mandibular lateral from a central incisor is to examine the functioning surface, that is, the _____ edge.

lingual

The chief identification of a mandibular lateral incisor is made from an incisal view. You will notice a slight rotation of the distal end of the incisal surface toward the _____ surface, due to the location of the tooth in the arch.

Permanent
Mandibular
1. Arch
OCCLUSAL
2. Right
Lateral Incisor
INCISAL

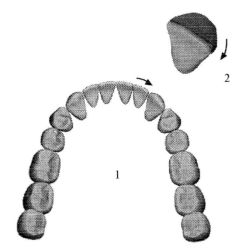

1

2

distal

The cingulum is displaced distally to further add to its appearance of being twisted distally. The cervical line will also follow this _____ displacement.

Which figure is representative of the mandibular right lateral incisor? _____ (Figure 1/ Figure 2)

Permanent
Mandibular
Lateral Incisors
INCISAL

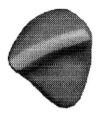   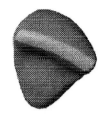

1   2

Figure 2

In the rotation on the incisal edge, which end is rotated lingually? _____

This distal lingual rotation of the lateral is indicative of its placement in the arch, as the arch turns.

distal

For review, identify the lettered areas on the lingual surface of the anterior tooth. Use complete dental terminology.

A. _____
B. _____
C. _____
D. _____
E. _____

A. cingulum; B. mesial
marginal ridge;
C. lingual fossa;
D. lingual pit;
E. distal marginal ridge

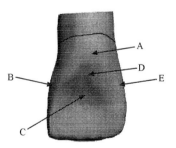

Permanent
Maxillary
Right
Central Incisor
LINGUAL

Which of the following words are spelled correctly?

1. mandibalar   6. incisaly
2. inciser   7. mesiodistal
3. mamilons   8. cingalum
4. cervical   9. mesioincisel
5. mesiel   10. facial

4, 7, 10

TURN TO THE NEXT PAGE AND TAKE REVIEW TEST 2.8.

REVIEW TEST 2.8

1. Choose the *correct* statement.
   a. On the mandibular central incisor, the distofacial line angle is more curved than the mesiofacial line angle.
   b. On the mandibular central incisor, the cervical line is curved more toward the incisal on the distal surface than on the mesial surface.

2. Which of the following anatomical characteristics are found on all incisors? (choose as many as are correct)
   a. lingual fossa
   b. lingual pit
   c. distoincisal angle
   d. mamelons
   e. height of contour in the cervical third on the facial and lingual surfaces of the crown
   f. four lobes

3. The best way to tell the difference between a mandibular lateral incisor and a mandibular central incisor is to inspect which surface?
   a. mesial
   b. lingual
   c. incisal
   d. distal

4. The _____ incisor is wider mesiodistally.
   a. lateral
   b. central

5. The mandibular left lateral incisor is tooth number _____ .
   a. 23
   b. 24
   c. 25
   d. 26

6. The mandibular lateral incisor gives the appearance of being twisted in which direction?
   a. mesiolingual
   b. distolingual
   c. distofacial
   d. mesiofacial

CHECK YOUR ANSWERS IN APPENDIX A.

HEIGHT OF CONTOUR, CONTACTS AND EMBRASURES OF MANDIBULAR LATERAL INCISORS

The mandibular lateral incisors have facial or lingual heights of contour in the _____ third of the crown.

Permanent
Mandibular
Right
Lateral Incisor
MESIAL

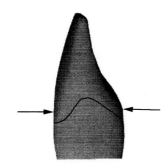

The facial and lingual heights contour of the mandibular lateral incisors are slight. These contours measure

a. more than 1/2 mm
b. 1/2 mm
c. less than 1/2 mm

Permanent
Mandibular
Right
Lateral Incisor
MESIAL

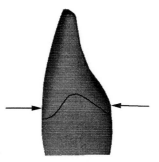

The contacts of the mandibular lateral incisors are located in the _____ third.

Permanent
Mandibular
Right
Lateral Incisor
1. MESIAL
2. DISTAL

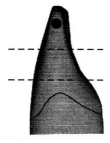
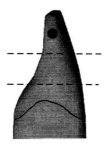

1   2

statement A is correct

Which of the following statements is correct?

A. Incisocervically, each maxillary anterior tooth has a distal contact area that is located more cervically than its mesial contact area.

B. Some of the maxillary anterior teeth have mesial contact areas that are located more cervically than their distal contact areas.

incisal

The mandibular incisors (central and lateral) have both mesial and distal contacts in the _____ third.

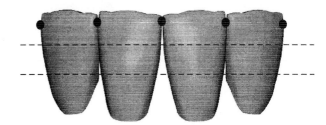

Permanent
Mandibular
Incisors
FACIAL

small

Because of the location of the contacts, the incisal embrasure is very _____ (small/large).

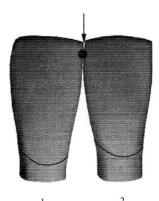

Permanent
Mandibular
Right
1. Lateral Incisor
2. Central Incisor
FACIAL

1   2

smaller

As the incisal edge wears with time, the embrasure will become _____ .

ROOTS OF MANDIBULAR
LATERAL INCISORS

The roots of the mandibular incisors are flattened or pinched from the mesial and distal directions. In which of the two horizontal directions do the roots of the mandibular incisors have the greater measure? _____

Permanent
Mandibular
Right
Lateral Incisor
1. FACIAL
2. MESIAL

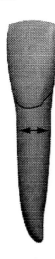
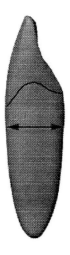

1   2

Viewed from the facial, the root of the mandibular central incisor is symmetrical and straight; that is, the mesial and distal surfaces tend to be relatively straight in the _____ direction.

Permanent
Mandibular
Right
Lateral Incisor
FACIAL

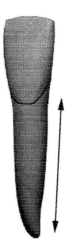

distal

The apical portion of the root on the mandibular lateral incisor may deviate toward the _____ . This distal deviation is the most common, although the deviation shown on these model teeth deviates to the mesial. This would be a very rare deviation.

Permanent
Mandibular
Right
Lateral Incisor
LINGUAL

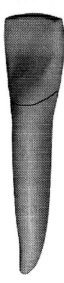

larger

In form, the root of the mandibular lateral incisor resembles that of the mandibular central incisor, the chief distinction being the size of the two roots. In all directions, the root of the mandibular lateral incisor is _____ (larger/smaller) than that of the mandibular central incisor.

Permanent
Mandibular
Right
1. Lateral Incisor
2. Central Incisor
FACIAL

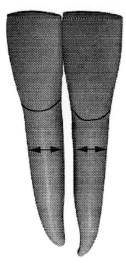

1   2

lateral

The root of which mandibular incisor has the greater circumference? _____

PULP ANATOMY OF MANDIBULAR LATERAL INCISORS

In the mandibular arch, the pulp canals of the two incisors are similar. For most of its incisoapical length, the pulp cavity of the mandibular lateral incisor is wider in the _____ direction.

faciolingual

Permanent
Mandibular
Lateral Incisor
1. FACIOLINGUAL
2. MESIODISTAL

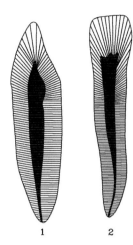

1   2

Examine the series of horizontal sections. Near the roof of the pulp chamber, the elliptical form of the pulp cavity is widest in the _____ direction.

mesiodistal

Permanent
Mandibular
Lateral Incisor
1. MESIODISTAL
2. CROSS SECTIONS

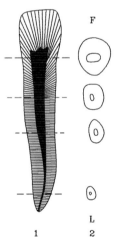

F

L

1   2

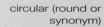

faciolingual

Near mid-root of a mandibular incisor, the elliptical form is widest in the ＿＿＿＿＿ direction.

Permanent
Mandibular
Lateral Incisor
1. MESIODISTAL
2. CROSS SECTIONS

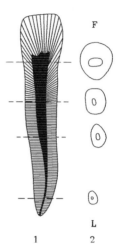

F

L

1 2

circular (round or synonym)

Near the apex of a mandibular incisor, the horizontal form of the pulp cavity is ＿＿＿＿＿ .

Permanent
Mandibular
Lateral Incisor
1. MESIODISTAL
2. CROSS SECTIONS

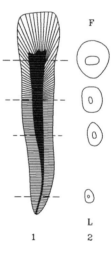

F

L

1 2

facial, lingual

Sometimes a thin wall of dentin divides the flattened root canal of the mandibular incisor. These two root canals are called the ＿＿＿＿＿ and ＿＿＿＿＿ root canals.

Permanent
Mandibular
Incisor
FACIOLINGUAL
Longitudinal Sections

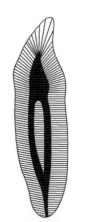

F   L

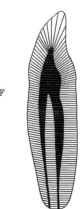

F   L

If two root canals are present, they either have separate apical foramina, as in Figure 2, or they converge apically to form a single canal, as in Figure 1. Mandibular incisors have few accessory canals, relative to maxillary incisors. The incisor with the most variable root and most frequent accessory canals is the _____ .

Permanent
Mandibular
Incisor
FACIOLINGUAL
Longitudinal Sections

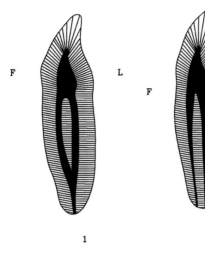

F   L   F   L

1   2

TURN TO THE NEXT AND TAKE REVIEW TEST 2.9.

REVIEW TEST 2.9

1. In which longitudinal section is the pulp chamber widest for most of the mandibular laterals incisoapical length?

   a. faciolingual
   b. mesiodistal

2. When the root canal divides into two root canals instead of one, there will be

   a. only one foramen
   b. one or sometimes two apical foramen present

3. The facial or lingual height of contour on the mandibular lateral incisor is

   a. more than 1/2 mm
   b. less than 1/2 mm
   c. 1/2 mm

4. The contacts of the mandibular lateral incisor are located

   a. in the incisal 1/3
   b. in the cervical 1/3
   c. at the junction of the incisal 1/3 and the middle 1/3

5. In which of the two horizontal directions do the roots of the mandibular incisors have a greater measure?

   a. mesiodistal
   b. faciolingual

6. The apical portion of the root on the mandibular lateral incisor may deviate toward the _____ if it deviates.

   a. mesial
   b. distal
   c. facial
   d. lingual

CHECK YOUR ANSWERS IN APPENDIX A.

MAXILLARY CANINES: FACIAL VIEW

The maxillary canines are the longest, most stable teeth in the mouth (considering crown and root together). The teeth are sometimes referred to as "cuspids"; however, they are more correctly designated the maxillary _____ .

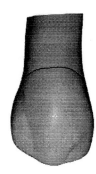

Permanent
Maxillary
Right Canine
FACIAL

The geometric form of the crown is pentagonal. Unlike the other anterior teeth, the crown presents _____ (number) facial borders.

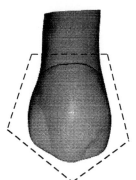

Permanent
Maxillary
Right Canine
FACIAL

The facial surface of the maxillary canine has five borders. Two of these form the incisal edge and are called the mesial and distal cusp ridges; the other three are the _____ , _____ , and _____ borders.

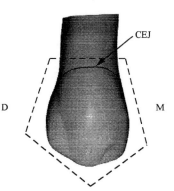

Permanent
Maxillary
Right Canine
FACIAL

CEJ

D   M

three (mesial, facial, distal)

This is the first tooth encountered having a cusp as the prominent crown feature. How many ridges can be seen from a facial view of a maxillary canine? ＿＿＿＿＿＿

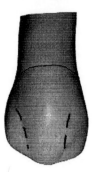

Permanent
Maxillary
Right Canine
FACIAL

ridge, ridge

The cusp tip divides the incisal edge into two parts. These two features are often referred to as the mesial cusp ＿＿＿＿＿＿ and the distal cusp ＿＿＿＿＿＿ .

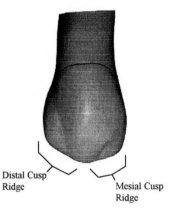

Permanent
Maxillary
Right Canine
FACIAL

Distal Cusp
Ridge

Mesial Cusp
Ridge

incisal

The crowns of all anterior teeth have five surfaces. One surface of a canine is divided into two parts by the cusp tip. Both of these parts combine to make up the one ＿＿＿＿＿＿ surface.

mesial, distal, cervical;
mesial, distal

The facial surface is bounded by five borders, the incisal edge providing two of them. The five are the ＿＿＿＿＿＿ , ＿＿＿＿＿＿ , and ＿＿＿＿＿＿ borders and the ＿＿＿＿＿＿ and ＿＿＿＿＿＿ cusp ridges.

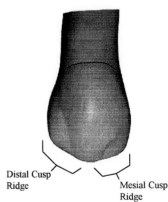

Permanent
Maxillary
Right Canine
FACIAL

Distal Cusp
Ridge

Mesial Cusp
Ridge

The four surfaces and the edge numbered in the illustration are called the

1. _____
2. _____
3. _____
4. _____
5. _____

1. facial, 2. lingual,
3. incisal, 4. mesial,
5. distal

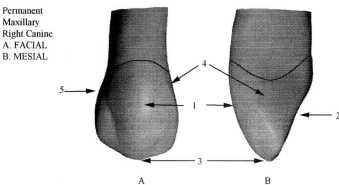

Permanent
Maxillary
Right Canine
A. FACIAL
B. MESIAL

A   B

From the facial view, the cervical line is convex toward the root. Unlike the incisors, the cervical line has its crest of convexity slightly toward the mesial. In the diagram, which is toward the mesial (A/B)? _____

A

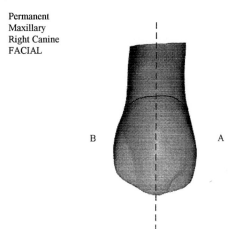

Permanent
Maxillary
Right Canine
FACIAL

B   A

The mesioincisal angle of the maxillary incisors approaches a right angle, especially the central incisors. The mesioincisal angle of the canine, however, is not so well defined. From the facial aspect, the mesioincisal angle is more of a _____ than an angle. (concavity/convexity)

convexity

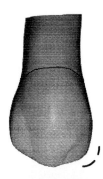

Permanent
Maxillary
Right Canine
FACIAL

mesial

Both the mesial and distal borders are first concave, then convex, from the cervical line to the cusp tip. Which border has the less distinct "S-shape" curvature, the mesial or distal?

_____

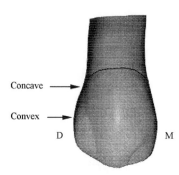

Permanent
Maxillary
Right Canine
FACIAL

Concave ⟶

Convex ⟶

D   M

---

cervical

The distal border has a pronounced convexity at the distoincisal angle that tends to accentuate the degree of concavity found in the _____ (cervical/incisal) third of the distal border.

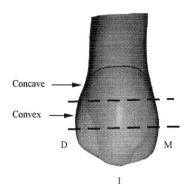

Permanent
Maxillary
Right Canine
FACIAL

Concave ⟶

Convex ⟶

D   M

I

---

straight

The mesial border has less overall convexity than the distal border which makes the cervical concavity on the mesial appear less pronounced, often approaching a _____ (straight/convex) outline in the cervical third.

---

centered

The crest of the cervical line is slightly mesial to the long axis of the tooth (facial view). However, the cusp tip of the incisal edge is _____ (mesial/distal/centered).

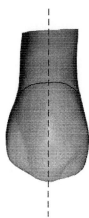

Permanent
Maxillary
Right Canine
FACIAL

The widest portion of the crown, mesiodistally, is located at the proximal contact areas. As is true of all teeth, which proximal contact area is located more cervically? _____

distal

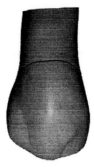

Permanent
Maxillary
Right Canine
FACIAL

The mesial contact area of a maxillary canine is located approximately at the junction of the incisal and middle thirds of the crown. The distal contact area is located in the _____ third of the crown.

middle

Permanent
Maxillary
Right Canine
FACIAL

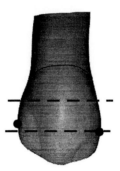

Keeping in mind that the cusp tip is centered mesiodistally, which cusp ridge is longer? _____ _____ _____ (mesial cusp ridge/ distal cusp ridge)

distal cusp ridge

The distal ridge of the canine cusp is _____ (shorter/longer) than the mesial ridge of the cusp.

longer

Permanent
Maxillary
Right Canine
FACIAL

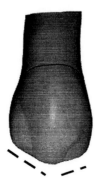

B

Which is the distal cusp ridge? _____ (A/B)

Permanent
Maxillary
Right Canine
FACIAL (Incisal third)

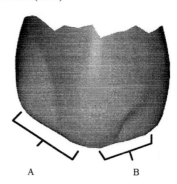

A   B

---

mesial

The facial surface of the maxillary canine is marked by a prominent facial ridge. The facial ridge is not centered on this surface but is located toward the _____ surface.

Permanent
Maxillary
Right Canine
FACIAL

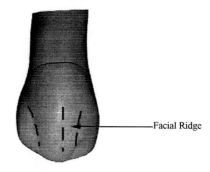

Facial Ridge

---

cusp tip

The shape of the facial surface of the maxillary canine is pentagonal. This is explained by the incisal edge being divided into two ridges by the _____ _____ (cusp tip/facial ridge).

Permanent
Maxillary
Right Canine
FACIAL

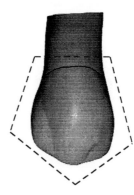

MAXILLARY CANINES: LINGUAL VIEW

Because of the crown form, there are features on the lingual surface of a canine that are generally not present on incisors; i.e., lingual ridge, mesiolingual fossa, and distolingual fossa. Similar to the incisors, however, area A is termed the _____ .

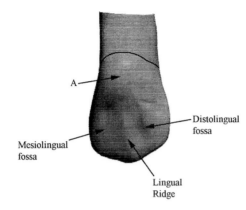

Permanent
Maxillary
Right Canine
LINGUAL

A

Distolingual fossa

Mesiolingual fossa

Lingual Ridge

Typical of most teeth, the lingual surface of a canine is narrower than the facial surface. The lingual surface is marked by a prominent ridge extending from the cusp tip to the cingulum. This ridge is called the _____ _____ .

Cervically, the lingual ridge blends into the well-developed _____ .

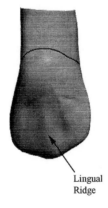

Permanent
Maxillary
Right Canine
LINGUAL

Lingual Ridge

The concavities and convexities (fossae and ridges) on the lingual surface are more prominent than the topographical features of the facial surface. Which of the two surfaces is narrower mesiodistally? _____

Between the lingual ridge and distal marginal ridge is the _____ _____ .

lingual pit. . . . . GO TO FRAME A.

distolingual fossa. . . . . GO TO FRAME B.

lingual pit is incorrect

>Frame A

Unlike the lingual surface of the incisor teeth, the maxillary canine has two distinct fossae, the disto- and mesiolingual fossae.

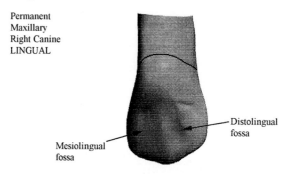

Permanent
Maxillary
Right Canine
LINGUAL

Distolingual fossa

Mesiolingual fossa

RETURN TO THE QUESTION FRAME AND ANSWER AGAIN.

distolingual fossa is correct
E, lingual ridge;
F, distolingual fossa;
A, cervical line;
B, cingulum; C, mesial marginal ridge;
D, mesiolingual fossa

>Frame B

Match each of the terms below with one of the lettered areas on the labeled canine.

_____ lingual ridge

_____ distolingual fossa

_____ cervical line

_____ cingulum

_____ mesial marginal ridge

_____ mesiolingual fossa

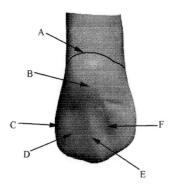

Permanent
Maxillary
Right Canine
LINGUAL

A

B

C

F

D

E

MAXILLARY CANINES: PROXIMAL VIEW

The proximal views of a maxillary canine have several features in common with the incisors. The overall geometric shape is roughly triangular with the cusp tip representing the apex of the triangle. The facial surface appears boldly convex. The lingual surfaces of incisors and canines are "S-shaped" in that they are concave in approximately the middle third and convex in the cervical third. The canine has more bulk however, especially in the faciolingual dimension, than do the incisors.

cervical line, facial

The following refer to proximal views of a maxillary canine.

The lingual surface is both concave and convex from the _____ _____ to the incisal edge. A continuous convexity extends from the cervical line to the incisal edge on the _____ surface.

Permanent
Maxillary
Right
1. Canine
2. Central Incisor
MESIAL

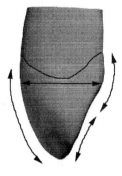
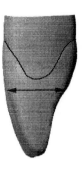

1   2

On which proximal surface does the cervical line show the least amount of curvature?
_____

distal, faciolingual

Compared to the incisors, the canine has a greater measurement from the height of contour on the facial surface to the height of contour on the lingual surface. Thus, the crown of a canine has a greater _____ measurement than the crown of an incisor.

MAXILLARY CANINES: INCISAL VIEW

In the incisal view, the canine tooth shows the marked _____ (convexity/ concavity) of the cingulum.

convexity

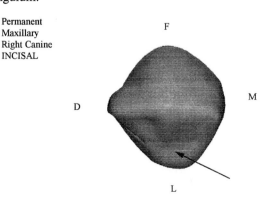

Permanent
Maxillary
Right Canine
INCISAL

F

M

D

L

central facial

Evidence of the four lobes can be seen from the incisal view of a canine. Which of the three lobes of the facial surface is most prominent? _____ _____

Permanent
Maxillary
Right Canine
INCISAL

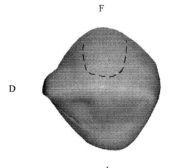

cusp

From the facial view, the cusp tip is formed by the junction of the mesial and distal _____ ridges.

Permanent
Maxillary
Right Canine
FACIAL (Incisal third)

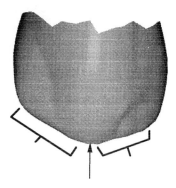

facial and lingual

The cervical line marks the boundary between the anatomical crown and the anatomical root. It consists of a series of arcs that curve either incisally or apically. On which surfaces of the maxillary anterior teeth does the cervical line curve toward the root? _____ _____ _____

Figure 2

Which figure is tooth number 11? _____ (Figure 1/Figure 2)

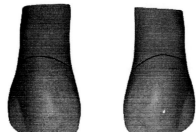

1   2

TURN TO THE NEXT PAGE AND TAKE REVIEW TEST 2.10.

REVIEW TEST 2.10

1. Which cusp ridge of the maxillary canine is shorter?

   a. mesial
   b. distal

2. On which surface is the cervical line more incisally located?

   a. mesial
   b. distal
   c. lingual
   d. facial

3. From the facial view which surface of the maxillary canine is straighter?

   a. distal
   b. mesial

4. The cusp tip of the maxillary canine is placed more

   a. mesial
   b. distal
   c. central

5. The distal contact area is located

   a. at the junction of the incisal and middle thirds
   b. in the middle third
   c. in the incisal third

6. Which surface of tooth number 6 is wider mesiodistally?

   a. facial
   b. lingual

7. The convexity located incisally from the cingulum is the

   a. mesiolingual fossa
   b. lingual ridge
   c. distolingual fossa
   d. mesial marginal ridge

8. The concavity located along the outer mesial border of the lingual surface is the

   a. mesiolingual fossa
   b. distolingual fossa
   c. mesial marginal ridge
   d. distal marginal ridge

9. Which cusp ridge is longer on tooth number 11?

   a. mesial
   b. distal

CHECK YOUR ANSWERS IN APPENDIX A.

HEIGHT OF CONTOUR, CONTACTS AND EMBRASURES OF MAXILLARY CANINES

2.11.0

Maxillary canines have facial and lingual heights of contour on the _____ third of the crown similar to all the anterior teeth.

cervical

Permanent
Maxillary
Right Canine
MESIAL

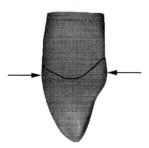

The heights of contour on the facial and lingual of the canines measure _____ , the same as the other anterior teeth.

less than 1/2 mm

Permanent
Maxillary
Right Canine
MESIAL

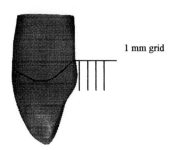

1 mm grid

The contacts of the maxillary canines are located along the height of contour on the mesial and distal surfaces as indicated in the illustration.

Permanent
Maxillary
Right Canine
1. MESIAL
2. DISTAL

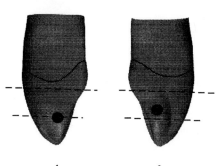

1   2

IJ, JM, JM

The contacts of the maxillary anteriors are reviewed in the illustration.

Permanent
Maxillary
Anteriors
FACIAL

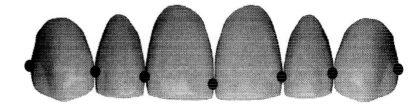

Remember the letter pairs that describe the contacts of the maxillary anterior teeth. Enter the appropriate letter pairs for the central incisor, lateral incisor, and the canine in the maxillary anterior sextant.

	Central Incisor	**Lateral Incisor**	**Canine**
Maxillary	_____	_____	_____

maxillary lateral incisor, canine

The JM pattern of proximal contact locations describe the _____ _____ _____ and _____ .

larger

The incisal embrasure between the maxillary lateral and the maxillary canine is indicated. Is this embrasure area smaller or larger than the one between the mandibular anterior incisors? _____

Permanent
Maxillary
Right
1. Canine
2. Lateral Incisor
FACIAL

1   2

cervically, cervically

The location of the maxillary canine, the rounded distoincisal edge of the lateral incisor, and the contact area are responsible for the larger embrasure area. The contacts are more _____ located in the posterior teeth than in the anterior teeth. Also, the distal contact is located more _____ than the mesial contact.

ROOTS OF MAXILLARY CANINES

The root of the maxillary canine is the _____ (longest/shortest) in the dental arch.

Permanent
Maxillary and
Mandibular
Right Quadrant
FACIAL

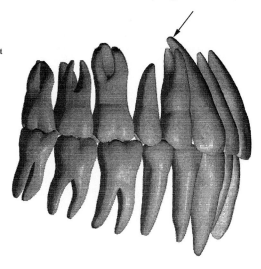

In the faciolingual direction, the mesial and distal surfaces of the maxillary canine are broad and generally flattened in the middle portion. In which view is the root of the maxillary canine wider? _____ (mesiodistal/faciolingual)

faciolingual

Permanent
Maxillary
Right Canine
1. MESIAL
2. FACIAL

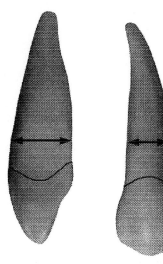

1   2

convex

In the mesiolingual view, the lingual convergence of the root causes the lingual root surface to be _____ .

Permanent
Maxillary
Right Canine
MESIOLINGUAL

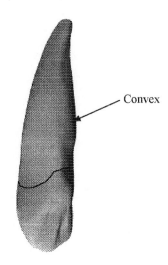

Convex

longitudinal groove

The mesial and distal surfaces may have a concavity in the faciolingual direction. A concavity exists whenever a _____ _____ is present.

Permanent
Maxillary
Right Canine
MESIAL

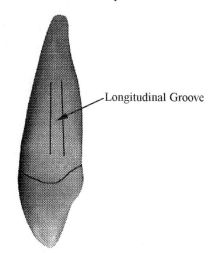

Longitudinal Groove

distal

As is true for the maxillary lateral incisor, the maxillary canine has a longitudinal groove more often on the _____ surface. (mesial or distal)

The apical portion of the root on the maxillary canine tapers to form a blunt apex. This can be seen by comparing the facial and proximal views of the canine. In which view is the canine wider? _____ (Figure 1/Figure 2)

Permanent
Maxillary
Right Canine
1. MESIAL
2. FACIAL

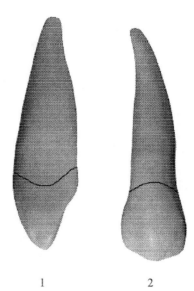

1   2

Figure 1

PULP ANATOMY OF MAXILLARY CANINES   2.11.2

As is true of all teeth, the pulp cavity pattern of the maxillary canine is that of the general form of the tooth. Which longitudinal section(s) shows the roof of the pulp chamber to be pointed? _____ (mesiodistal/faciolingual/both)

Permanent
Maxillary
Right Canine
1. MESIODISTAL
2. FACIOLINGUAL

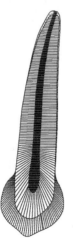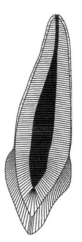

1   2

both

faciolingual

Similar to the horizontal measurements of the root, the cervical portion of the root canal of the maxillary canine is widest in the _____ direction.

Permanent
Maxillary
Right Canine
1. MESIODISTAL
2. FACIOLINGUAL

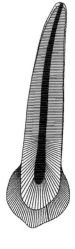
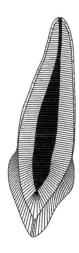

1   2

cervical, faciolingual

A series of horizontal sections through the root of the maxillary canine show the form of the root canal gradually changing from elliptical to nearly circular. The elliptical form is most evident in the _____ (cervical/apical) portion of the root, and is widest in the _____ direction.

Permanent
Maxillary
Right Canine
1. MESIODISTAL
2. CROSS SECTIONS

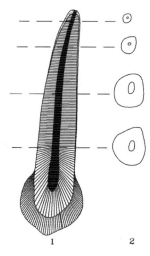

1   2

In the cervical portion of the root of the maxillary canine, a cross section shows the root canal to have an _____ form; but a cross section in the apical portion shows the root canal form to be nearly _____ .

Permanent
Maxillary
Right Canine
1. MESIODISTAL
2. CROSS SECTIONS

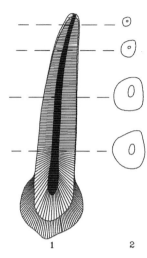

1   2

If the drawings illustrate a representative sample, about _____ % of the maxillary canines will have accessory canals which usually run in a _____ direction.

Permanent
Maxillary
Right Canine
FACIOLINGUAL SECTIONS

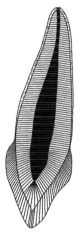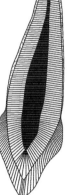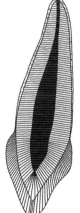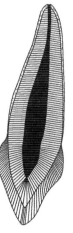

TURN TO THE NEXT PAGE AND TAKE REVIEW TEST 2.11.

REVIEW TEST 2.11

1. In which direction is the pulp chamber of the maxillary canine widest at the roof?

    a. mesiodistal
    b. faciolingual
    c. neither

2. What is the approximate shape of the root canal as seen in a cross section taken at the mid-root?

    a. elliptical
    b. circular
    c. neither

3. The height of contour of the facial and lingual surfaces is located in the _____ third of the crown.

    a. incisal
    b. middle
    c. cervical

4. The contacts of the maxillary canine are identified by which two-letter combinations?

    a. II
    b. JJ
    c. JM
    d. MM

5. The root of the maxillary canine is widest in which longitudinal direction?

    a. mesiodistal
    b. faciolingual

6. If a concavity exists on the root of the maxillary canine, it will be concave in which direction?

    a. longitudinal
    b. horizontal

7. The maxillary canine has the longest _____ in the dental arch.

    a. root
    b. crown

8. The incisal embrasure between the maxillary canine and the lateral is _____ than the embrasures found between the incisors.

    a. larger
    b. smaller

CHECK YOUR ANSWERS IN APPENDIX A.

2.12.0

narrower

The form and outline of the maxillary and mandibular canines are practically alike. Although the crown lengths of the two teeth are nearly the same (the mandibular canine is slightly longer than the maxillary), the mandibular canine is _____ (narrower/wider) mesiodistally than the maxillary canine.

Permanent
Right Canine
1. Mandibular
2. Maxillary
FACIAL

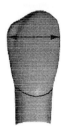
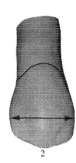

1   2

A

The lingual surface of the mandibular canine is smoother, the cingulum less developed, and the lingual and marginal ridges are less prominent than those of the maxillary canine. The cingulum is area _____ . (A/B/C)

Permanent
Mandibular
Right Canine
LINGUAL

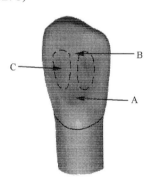

---

straight

From the facial aspect, the line formed by the mesial outline of the crown and root of a maxillary canine is definitely curved. On a mandibular canine this line has less curvature; in fact it is nearly _____ .

Permanent
Right Canine
1. Mandibular
2. Maxillary
FACIAL

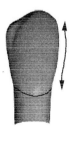
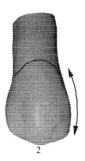

1   2

incisal

When compared with a maxillary canine, a mandibular canine has a distal contact area that is more toward the _____ (cervical/incisal).

Permanent
Right Canine
1. Mandibular
2. Maxillary
FACIAL

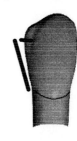
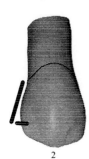

1   2

shorter

Because the distal contact is more cervical than the mesial, the incisocervical length of the distal surface is _____ (longer/shorter) than the mesial.

Permanent
Mandibular
Right Canine
FACIAL

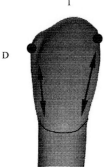

facial

Running cervically from the cusp tip in the center of the facial surface is the _____ ridge.

Permanent
Mandibular
Right Canine
FACIAL

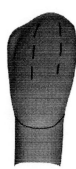

Facially, which cusp tip is shorter? _____

mesial

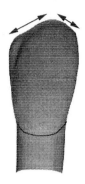

Permanent
Mandibular
Right Canine
FACIAL

MANDIBULAR CANINE: LINGUAL VIEW

2.12.1

The lingual features of a mandibular canine are less prominent than those of a maxillary canine. The cingulum is relatively smooth, and the marginal ridges are less distinct. Are the comparisons between the lingual surfaces of a maxillary and mandibular canine similar to or the opposite of the comparisons between the lingual surfaces of the maxillary and mandibular incisors? _____

similar

Permanent
Mandibular
Right Canine
LINGUAL

M   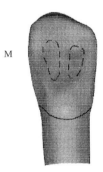   D

Running from the cusp tip to the cervical line and dividing the lingual surface to form two shallow fossae is a prominence called the _____ .

mesial marginal ridge . . . . GO TO FRAME A.

lingual ridge. . . . . GO TO FRAME B.

mesial marginal ridge
is incorrect
lingual ridge is correct

>Frame A

The mesial marginal ridge runs from the mesioincisal angle to the linguocervical ridge, but it does not divide the lingual surface to form the mesial and distal lingual fossa.

Permanent
Mandibular
Right Canine
LINGUAL

Mesial ——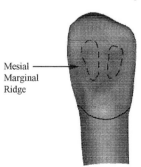
Marginal
Ridge

RETURN TO THE QUESTION FRAME AND ANSWER AGAIN.

mesiolingual fossa,
distolingual fossa

>**Frame B**

Mesial and distal to the lingual ridge are the _____ _____ and
_____ _____ .

Permanent
Mandibular
Right Canine
LINGUAL

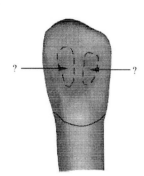

---

lingual ridge,
distolingual fossa

Area A is called the _____ _____ ; area B is the _____
_____ .

Permanent
Mandibular
Right Canine
LINGUAL

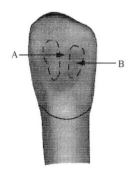

---

mesial cusp ridge,
distal cusp ridge

The areas marked A and B are the _____ _____ _____ and
_____ _____ _____ respectively.

Permanent
Mandibular
Right Canine
LINGUAL

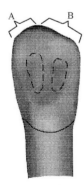

The distal cusp ridge is _____ (longer/shorter) than the mesial cusp ridge.

longer

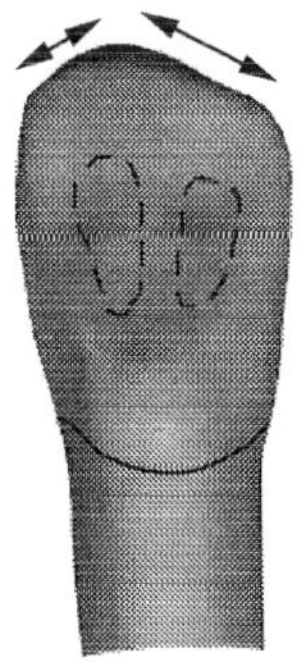

Permanent
Mandibular
Right Canine
LINGUAL

M   D

Compared with the features of the maxillary canine (lingual surface), those of the mandibular canine are _____ (more/less) prominent.

less

MANDIBULAR CANINE: PROXIMAL VIEW

2.12.2

The cingulum on the mandibular canine appears _____ (more/less) prominent than on the maxillary canine.

less

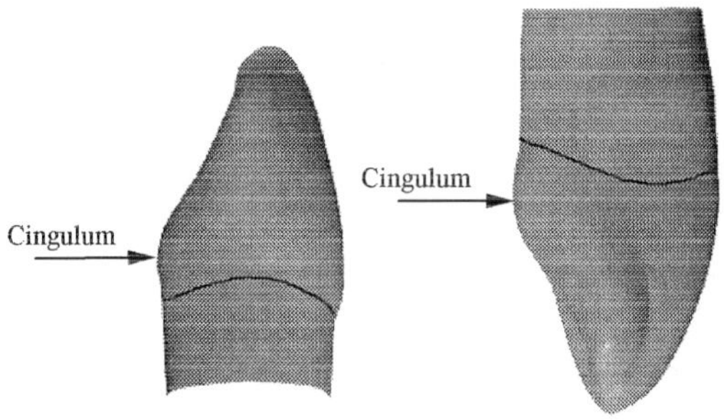

Permanent
Right Canine
1. Mandibular
2. Maxillary
DISTAL

Cingulum

Cingulum

1   2

The incisal portion of the crown of a mandibular canine is _____ (thinner/thicker) faciolingually than that of the maxillary canine.

thinner

lingually

The cusp tip of the mandibular canine is displaced _____ (facially/lingually) from the long axis of the tooth. This displacement is illustrated in the incisal view.

Permanent
Mandibular
Right Canine
INCISAL

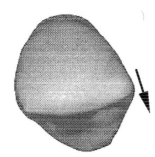

mesial

The cervical lines (mandibular canine, mesial and distal surfaces) are more convex incisally than those on the maxillary canine. On both canines, the cervical line is more convex on the _____ (mesial/distal) surface.

Permanent
Mandibular
Right Canine
1 and 2

Permanent
Maxillary
Right Canine
3 and 4

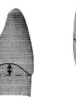 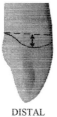

MESIAL	DISTAL	MESIAL	DISTAL
1	2	3	4

distal

The cusp tip divides the mesial and distal cusp ridges. Which is slightly longer?

_____

distal

From an incisal view, the incisal edge of a mandibular canine appears to slant toward the lingual. Which end of the incisal edge is located more lingually? _____

Permanent
Mandibular
Right Canine
INCISAL

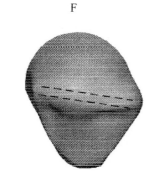

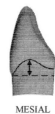

In the illustration, A is the _____ cusp ridge, and B is the _____ cusp ridge.

mesial, distal

Permanent
Mandibular
Right Canine
INCISAL

A

B

From a facial view, the incisal edge on a newly erupted mandibular canine has a cusp tip that is more pointed than that of a maxillary canine. With wear, the cusp tip on a mandibular canine flattens.

facial, lingual

The cervical line curves toward the root on the _____ and _____ surfaces of the canines.

TURN TO THE NEXT PAGE AND TAKE REVIEW TEST 2.12.

REVIEW TEST 2.12

Below are four sets of statements concerning the canine teeth. Choose the *correct* one from each pair.

1.
    a. The mandibular canine has a more prominent cingulum than does the maxillary canine.
    b. The incisal edge (proximal view) of the mandibular canine is thinner than that of the maxillary canine.

2.
    a. The cusp tip of the mandibular canine is displaced slightly to the lingual.
    b. The cusp tip of the maxillary canine is displaced slightly to the lingual.

3.
    a. On its facial surface, the mandibular canine has a more smooth, semicircular cervical line.
    b. The mandibular canine has the more prominent lingual features.

4.
    a. The mandibular canine has a shorter distofacial line angle (distal border) than the maxillary canine.
    b. The mandibular canine has a straighter mesial border then the maxillary canine.

CHECK YOUR ANSWERS IN APPENDIX A.

HEIGHT OF CONTOUR, CONTACTS AND EMBRASURES OF MANDIBULAR CANINES

As with all incisors and canines, the mandibular canines have both the facial and lingual height of contour in the _____ third of the crown.

cervical

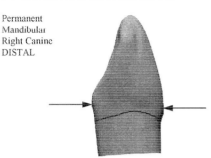

Permanent
Mandibular
Right Canine
DISTAL

The facial and lingual contours of the mandibular anteriors are slight. Mandibular canines have facial and lingual contours that measure _____.

a. more than 1/2 mm
b. 1/2 mm
c. less than 1/2 mm

less than 1/2 mm

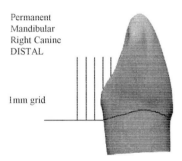

Permanent
Mandibular
Right Canine
DISTAL

1mm grid

As with mandibular incisors, mandibular canines have mesial contacts incisocervically in the _____ third of their crowns.

incisal

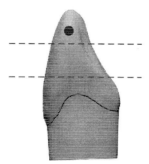

Permanent
Mandibular
Right Canine
MESIAL

middle

Mandibular canines have distal contacts that are located slightly cervical to the junction of the incisal and middle thirds. The contact, therefore, is located in the _____ third of the crown.

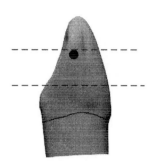

Permanent
Mandibular
Right Canine
DISTAL

larger

The distal ridge of the canine cusp contributes to the size of the occlusal embrasure between the canine and first premolar. The occlusal embrasure between the canine and first premolar is _____ (smaller/larger) than the embrasures between the incisors.

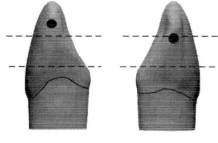

Permanent
Mandibular
Right
1. First Premolar
2. Canine
FACIAL

1   2

cervical

The distal contact of mandibular canines is located _____ (cervical/incisal) to the junction of the incisal and middle thirds.

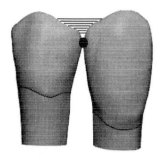

Permanent
Mandibular
Right Canine
1. MESIAL
2. DISTAL

1   2

Review the locations of the proximal contacts of anterior teeth with the aid of the pairs of letters given below. For example, "IJ" means that the mesial contact is located in the incisal third (I) and the distal contact is located at the junction (J) of the incisal and middle thirds.

	Central Incisor	**Lateral Incisor**	**Canine**
Maxillary	IJ	JM	JM
Mandibular	II	II	IM

ROOTS OF MANDIBULAR CANINES

The permanent mandibular canine has the longest root of any tooth in the _____ .

a. permanent dentition
b. mandibular arch

Permanent
Mandibular
Right
Quadrant
FACIAL

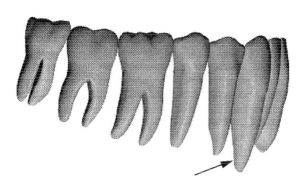

The maxillary canine has the longest root of any tooth in the dental arch. It is true, however, that the mandibular canine has the longest root of any tooth in the _____ arch.

Permanent
Maxillary and
Mandibular
Right Quadrant
FACIAL

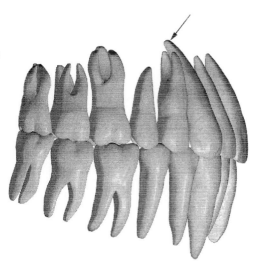

The mesiodistal width of the root of the mandibular canine is less than that of the maxillary canine and greater than that of the mandibular incisor.

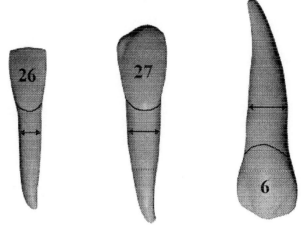

Similar to the root of the maxillary canine, the apical portion of the root of the mandibular canine tapers toward the apex. Which of the two canines has the more pointed apex?

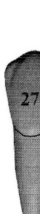
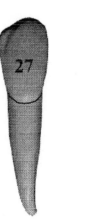
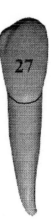

When the apex of the mandibular canine shows a deviation from the tooth axis, it is often toward the incisors or in a _____ direction.

mesial

Permanent
Mandibular
Right
1. Canine
2. Lateral
FACIAL

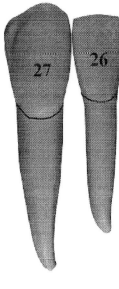

1   2

As concerns the mesial or distal deviations of the apical portions of the roots of anterior teeth, the mesial deviation of the mandibular canine is _____ .

a. unique
b. the same as other anterior teeth

unique

Longitudinal grooves are generally present on the mesial and distal root surfaces of the mandibular canine. Because of these grooves, the mesial and distal root surfaces are concave in the _____ direction.

faciolingual

Permanent
Mandibular
Right Canine
1. DISTAL
2. MESIAL

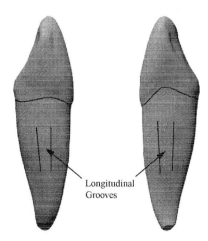

Longitudinal
Grooves

1   2

facial, lingual

Occasionally, the root of the mandibular canine will be bifurcated. As suggested by the longitudinal grooves, whenever a bifurcation exists, the two terminal roots are called the _____ and _____ roots.

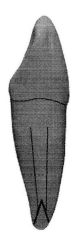

Permanent
Mandibular
Right Canine
DISTAL

mandibular canine,
maxillary central
incisor

Of the anterior teeth, which is most likely to have longitudinal grooves? Which is least likely to have longitudinal grooves?

most likely _____ _____
                    (arch)   (tooth name)

least likely _____ _____
                     (arch)   (tooth name)

2.13.2   PULP ANATOMY OF MANDIBULAR CANINES

faciolingual

The pulp cavity of the mandibular canine follows the same pattern as that of the maxillary canine, in that it follows the same general outline of the tooth. In which longitudinal section will the pulp cavity be widest? _____ (faciolingual/mesiodistal)

Permanent
Mandibular
Right Canine
1. MESIODISTAL
2. FACIOLINGUAL

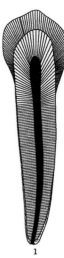 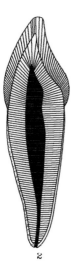

1   2

A series of horizontal sections through the root of the mandibular canine show the form of the root canal gradually changing from elliptical to nearly circular. The elliptical form is most evident in the _____ (cervical/apical) portion of the root, and is widest in the _____ direction.

cervical, faciolingual

Permanent
Mandibular
Right Canine
1. MESIODISTAL
2. CROSS SECTIONS

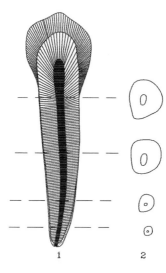

Of all anterior teeth, the mandibular canine is the most likely to have _____ (number) root canals, that may end in a common foramen or separate foramina.

two

Permanent
Mandibular
Right Canine
FACIOLINGUAL

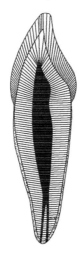

mesial lingual fossa

Review the information presented in the summary illustration. What is the name of the structure indicated with a dashed circle on the lingual of the mandibular canine?

_____   _____   _____

Permanent Mandibular Canine - Summary

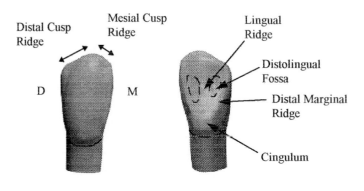

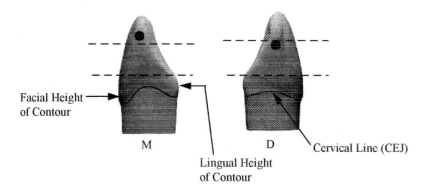

Remember that the mandibular canine has the longest root in the mandibular arch and that it deviates to the mesial.

Permanent Mandibular Right Canine (27)

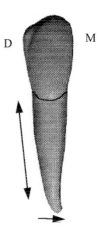

Review the information in this longitudinal section of the mandibular right canine.

Permanent Mandibular Right Canine: FACIOLINGUAL

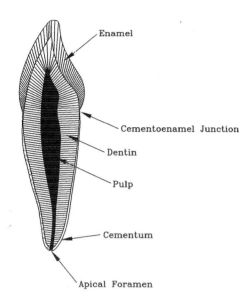

Enamel

Cementoenamel Junction

Dentin

Pulp

Cementum

Apical Foramen

TURN TO THE NEXT PAGE AND TAKE REVIEW TEST 2.13.

REVIEW TEST 2.13

1. In which arch(es) do the anterior teeth have facial and lingual amounts of contour that measure less than 1/2 mm?

   a. mandibular
   b. maxillary
   c. both arches

2. Choose the *correct* statement.

   a. The incisal embrasure between the maxillary lateral incisor and maxillary central incisor is larger than the occlusal embrasure between the mandibular canine and first premolar.
   b. The process of attrition can completely eliminate the incisal embrasures between the mandibular central incisors.

3. In which arch(es) do the facial and lingual heights of contour occur in the cervical third of the crowns of all anterior teeth?

   a. mandibular
   b. maxillary
   c. both arches

4. The canine with the more pointed apex is the

   a. maxillary canine
   b. mandibular canine

5. The roots of all but one anterior tooth are likely to have longitudinal grooves on the mesial and distal surfaces. The tooth that is not likely to have longitudinal grooves is the

   a. mandibular lateral incisor
   b. maxillary canine
   c. maxillary central incisor

6. Which of the following pairs of terms best completes the statements below?
   When the apex of a root shows a deviation, it is generally toward the _____ (mesial/distal).
   Whenever a deviation in the opposite direction occurs, the tooth is generally a _____ (maxillary/mandibular) canine.

7. Of the two mandibular incisors, which has a root that is larger in all dimensions?
   a. mandibular central incisor
   b. mandibular lateral incisor

8. If you were involved in clinical operations on several patients' root canals, you would have to be alert to the possibility of double root canals on which anterior teeth?

   _____   _____
   _____   _____
   _____   _____
   (arch)   (tooth name)

9. Choose the *correct* statement.
   a. When anterior teeth have two root canals they have two apical foramina.
   b. When anterior teeth have two root canals they have either one or two apical foramina.

10. For each of the anterior teeth listed below, write down the number of pulp horns typically found on the roof of their pulp chambers.
    a. maxillary canine   _____
    b. maxillary lateral incisor _____
    c. maxillary central incisor _____

CHECK YOUR ANSWERS IN APPENDIX A.

Permanent Premolars

MAXILLARY PREMOLARS

Although the surfaces of posterior crowns are actually smoothly contoured, we can imagine the crown as a cube sitting on its root. The five visible sides of the cube are the facial, lingual, mesial, distal, and occlusal surfaces. The sides intersect at right angles and form the edges (or lines) of the cube.

In correct dental terminology, these edges are called line _____ .

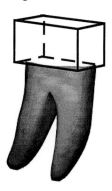

Although line angles do not appear as distinct lines on the tooth crown, these lines provide a useful reference in describing the crown. How many line angles are present on a posterior tooth? _____

eight

distofacial

The eight line angles of a posterior tooth are:

mesiofacial mesiocclusal
distofacial   distocclusal
mesiolingual faciocclusal
distolingual   linguocclusal

Which line angle is indicated by label a? _____

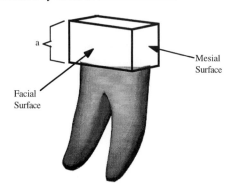

occlusal

Another term in dental anatomy is point angle. A point angle is formed by the intersection of three surfaces, similar to the point that is formed by the intersection of three surfaces on a cube (point B is formed by the intersection of surfaces a, b, c). Although the crown of a tooth does not exhibit distinct points, the concept of a crown as a modified cube with point angles at the "corners" is used for descriptive purposes.

The crown of a posterior tooth has four point angles. One point angle is located at each of the four "corners" of the _____ surface as indicated by the arrows in the illustration.

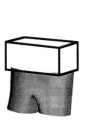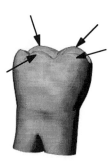

The four point angles of a posterior tooth are named by the three surfaces that intersect to form the "point." The names are

mesiofaciocclusal   mesiolinguoocclusal
distofaciocclusal   distolinguoocclusal

Which point angle is indicated by label a? _____

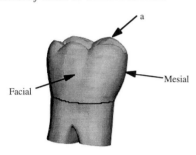

mesiolinguoocclusal

Before describing each posterior tooth, let's clarify the term marginal ridge. The two marginal ridges of an anterior tooth can be viewed from a lingual aspect, but the marginal ridges of a posterior tooth are viewed from an occlusal aspect. Just as the marginal ridges form the mesial and distal borders of the lingual surface for an incisor, the mesial and distal marginal ridges of a posterior tooth form the mesial and distal borders of the _____ surface.

occlusal

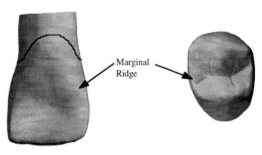

Pemanent
Maxillary
Right
1. Central Incisor
   LINGUAL
2. First Premolar
   OCCLUSAL

Marginal
Ridge

1   2

Similar to the cusp of the canines, each cusp of a posterior tooth has four ridges. Using the cusp tip as the starting point, the ridges are named for the direction they run as seen from the occlusal view. The ridge labeled a is a facial ridge; the ridge labeled b is a _____ ridge.

lingual

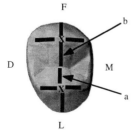

Permanent
Maxillary
Right
First Premolar
OCCLUSAL

mesial

The cusp labeled X is located on the mesial portion of the crown. The cusp labeled Y is on the distal portion of the crown. Ridge a is the distal ridge of cusp X; ridge b is the _____ ridge of cusp Y.

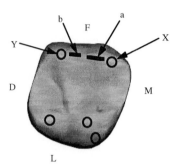

Permanent
Maxillary
Right
First Molar
OCCLUSAL

a

Of the two ridges labeled, which is a mesial ridge? _____ (a/b)

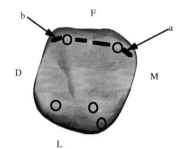

Permanent
Maxillary
Right
First Molar
OCCLUSAL

table

On posterior teeth, the *occlusal surface,* bounded by the mesial and distal ridges of the cusps and the two marginal ridges is often referred to as the *occlusal table.* Although the two terms name the same part of the tooth, they are not used interchangeably. "Occlusal table" is used when discussing the functional aspects of the crown, as in occlusion. "Occlusal surface" is used in more general discussions, such as anatomical descriptions of the tooth.

Because the lingual cusp of the mandibular first premolar is nonfunctional, the lingual portion of the facial cusp contributes more significantly to the occlusal _____ .

six

A maxillary first premolar has two cusps. How many ridges form the boundary of its occlusal table? _____ (four/six).

The boundary of the occlusal table is formed by the two marginal ridges, the two ridges of the facial cusp, and the two ridges of the lingual cusp for a total of six.

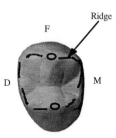

Permanent
Maxillary
Right
First Premolar
OCCLUSAL

There are eight permanent premolar teeth, two in each quadrant. They lie behind the canines and in front of the permanent _____ .

molars

Permanent
Maxillary
Right Quadrant
FACIAL

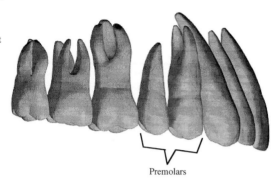

Premolars

The permanent premolars assume the positions formerly occupied by the deciduous molars. The permanent premolars and all permanent anterior teeth are called succedaneous teeth. A succedaneous tooth is a permanent tooth that assumes a position previously occupied by a _____ tooth.

deciduous (primary)

Permanent
Maxillary
Right Quadrant
FACIAL

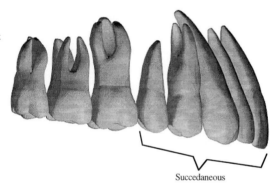

Succedaneous

The permanent molars are not preceded by deciduous teeth; therefore, they are called _____ teeth.

non-succedaneous

Permanent
Maxillary
Right Quadrant
FACIAL

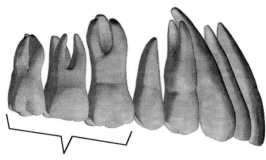

Non-succedaneous

Anterior teeth have incisal edges, but the posterior teeth have occlusal surfaces. On premolar teeth, the view corresponding to the incisal view of the anteriors is called the _____ view.

occlusal

3.1.1 MAXILLARY FIRST PREMOLAR

The permanent maxillary premolars show evidence of four lobes. The lobes are positioned and named in a manner similar to the lobes described on the maxillary anterior teeth. How many lobes are there on the facial surface of a maxillary premolar? _____

Permanent
Maxillary
Right
First Premolar
1. FACIAL
2. LINGUAL

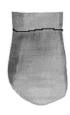 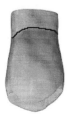

1   2

The three lobes that form the facial portion of a maxillary premolar are called the _____ , _____ , and _____ lobes. The fourth lobe is the _____ lobe.

Permanent Maxillary
Right
First Premolar
FACIAL

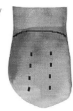

In each quadrant, the two teeth immediately anterior to the first molar generally contain two cusps. However, in the mandibular quadrants one of these teeth frequently contains three cusps. Thus, the preferred term for each of the eight teeth is _____ (bicuspid or premolar).

Since **bi** denotes *two,* the term **bicuspid** means two-cusped. *Premolar* means in front of or anterior to the molars. Since the mandibular second premolar often has three cusps, the term premolar is preferred and will be used in the remainder of this text.

The mesial and distal borders (occlusal view) converge toward the lingual, which is _____ (narrower/wider) than the facial.

Permanent
Maxillary
Right
First Premolar
OCCLUSAL

F

D   M

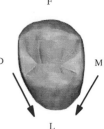

L

On the two-cusped premolars, one of the cusps is located toward the facial, called the facial cusp. The other cusp is located toward the lingual and is called the _____ cusp.

Permanent
Maxillary
First Premolar
1. OCCLUSAL
2. DISTAL

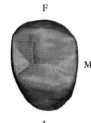
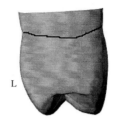

1   2

When two or more cusps are compared, the cusp with the greatest mesiodistal measurement is the widest. As seen from the occlusal view, which of the two cusps on a maxillary first premolar is the widest? _____

Permanent
Maxillary
Right
First Premolar
OCCLUSAL

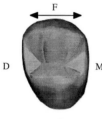

The length of a cusp is determined by its length in the occlusocervical direction. Which view of a maxillary first premolar best shows the comparative length of its two cusps? _____

Permanent
Maxillary
Right
First Premolar
1. OCCLUSAL
2. DISTAL

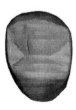
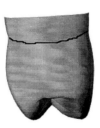

1   2

The occlusocervical measurement of a cusp is the perpendicular distance from the cusp tip to the plane that contains the point of deepest cut by an occlusal groove. If *a* passes through the deepest cut of an occlusal groove, what is the length of the facial cusp? _____

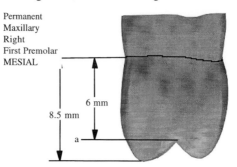

Permanent
Maxillary
Right
First Premolar
MESIAL

6 mm

8.5 mm

a

The facial cusp of a maxillary first premolar is wider than the lingual cusp because it has a greater measurement in the _____ direction.

a. mesiodistal
b. occlusocervical
c. mesiolingual

The facial cusp of the maxillary first premolar has a greater measurement in the occlusocervical direction, but it is the measurement in the mesiodistal direction that determines which cusp is wider. The term "wider" means the "greater mesiodistal measurement" when it is used to compare cusp size. The cusp with the greater measurement in the occlusocervical direction is the "longer" cusp.

When one considers the size of the two cusps of the maxillary first premolar, the facial cusp is both _____ and _____ than the lingual cusp.

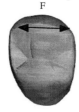
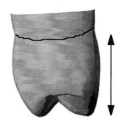

Permanent
Maxillary
Right
First Premolar
1. OCCLUSAL
2. DISTAL

F

F

1   2

The ridges of the facial cusp descend from the cusp tip in a pattern that is common to most cusps. How many ridges are in this pattern? _____

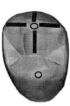

Permanent
Maxillary
Right
First Premolar
OCCLUSAL

Name the ridges of the facial cusp.

1. _____

2. _____

3. _____

4. _____

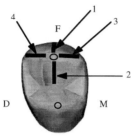

Permanent
Maxillary
Right
First Premolar
OCCLUSAL

Some textbooks use the names listed in the second column in place of the names in the first column.

facial ridge of the facial cusp	Facial (buccal) cusp ridge
lingual ridge of the facial cusp	lingual cusp ridge
mesial ridge of the facial cusp	mesial cusp ridge
distal ridge of the facial cusp	distal cusp ridge

The terms in the first column are much more descriptive, but sometimes more confusing.

Four ridges are located on the larger of the two cusps of the maxillary first premolar, the _____ cusp.

facial

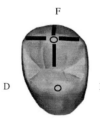

Permanent
Maxillary
Right
First Premolar
OCCLUSAL

The facial ridge of the facial cusp is broad and prominent. It descends in a cervical direction onto the _____ surface.

facial

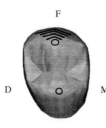

Permanent
Maxillary
Right
First Premolar
OCCLUSAL

no

Does the lingual ridge of the facial cusp descend onto the lingual surface? _____

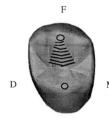

Permanent
Maxillary
Right
First Premolar
OCCLUSAL

occlusal

The lingual ridge of the facial cusp runs from the tip of the cusp to the central area of the _____ surface.

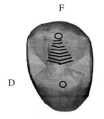

Permanent
Maxillary
Right
First Premolar
OCCLUSAL

no

Any ridge on a posterior tooth that descends from the cusp tip and runs to the central area of the occlusal surface is called a triangular ridge. Does the facial ridge of the facial cusp on a permanent maxillary first premolar qualify as a triangular ridge?
_____ (yes/no)

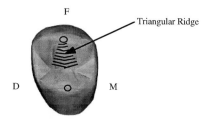

Permanent
Maxillary
Right
First Premolar
OCCLUSAL

Triangular Ridge

occlusal

The facial ridge of the facial cusp on a maxillary first premolar is not a triangular ridge, for it does not run toward the central area of the _____ surface.

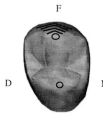

Permanent
Maxillary
Right
First Premolar
OCCLUSAL

On the maxillary first premolar, the mesial ridge of the facial (buccal) cusp descends from the cusp tip and is continuous with the mesial marginal ridge near the _____ point angle.

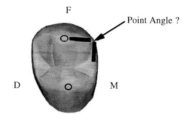

Permanent
Maxillary
Right
First Premolar
OCCLUSAL

F

Point Angle ?

D

M

L

The mesial ridge of the facial cusp joins at an acute angle with the _____ _____ ridge.

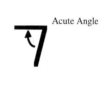

Permanent
Maxillary
Right
First Premolar
OCCLUSAL

F

Acute Angle

D

M

L

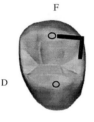

The distal ridge descends from the facial cusp tip and joins at an acute angle with the _____ _____ ridge.

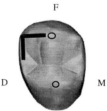

Permanent
Maxillary
Right
First Premolar
OCCLUSAL

F

D

M

L

Like the facial cusp, the smaller lingual cusp also has _____ (number) ridges emerging from its tip.

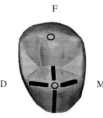

Permanent
Maxillary
Right
First Premolar
OCCLUSAL

F

D

M

L

mesial marginal

The mesial ridge of the lingual cusp joins the ＿＿＿＿＿ ＿＿＿＿＿ ridge to form a rounded, sweeping curve at the mesiolinguocclusal point angle.

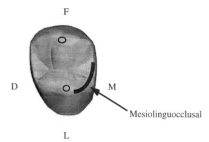

Permanent
Maxillary
Right
First Premolar
OCCLUSAL

F

D   M

Mesiolinguocclusal

L

---

distolinguocclusal

The distal ridge of the lingual cusp joins the distal marginal ridge near the ＿＿＿＿＿ point angle.

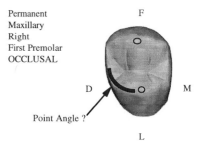

Permanent
Maxillary
Right
First Premolar
OCCLUSAL

F

D   M

Point Angle ?

L

---

lingual ridge

One of the four ridges of the lingual cusp descends to the lingual surface, becoming the prominence of that surface. Extending to the lingual surface from the lingual cusp tip is the ＿＿＿＿＿ ＿＿＿＿＿ .

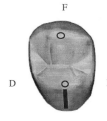

Permanent
Maxillary
Right
First Premolar
OCCLUSAL

F

D   M

L

---

occlusal

The facial ridge of the lingual cusp runs from the tip of the lingual cusp to the central area of the ＿＿＿＿＿ surface.

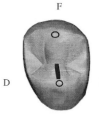

Permanent
Maxillary
Right
First Premolar
OCCLUSAL

F

D   M

L

Which ridge of the lingual cusp is a triangular ridge? _____

Permanent
Maxillary
Right
First Premolar
OCCLUSAL

F

D   M

L

How many triangular ridges are present on a maxillary first premolar? _____

Some texts use a slightly different nomenclature for the triangular ridges of the premolars. The lingual ridge of the facial cusp may be called the facial triangular ridge because it is located on the facial cusp. The facial ridge of the lingual cusp may be called the lingual triangular ridge.

Name the following ridges:

a. _____ ridge of the _____ cusp, _____ _____
_____

b. _____ ridge of the _____ cusp, _____ _____
_____

Permanent
Maxillary
Right
First Premolar
OCCLUSAL

F

a

D   M

b

L

The large depression (or valley) on the occlusal surface is called the occlusal sulcus. The sulcus is included within the limits of the occlusal table. The inclines that meet at an angle form the sulcus. Thus, the occlusal sulcus is surrounded by the cusps and the inclines of the two _____ ridges. (The occlusal table and occlusal sulcus are indicated in the illustration.)

Permanent
Maxillary
Right
First Premolar
OCCLUSAL

F

Occlusal Table

D   M

Occlusal Sulcus

L

triangular

The bottom of the occlusal sulcus is marked by developmental grooves. At the central area of the sulcus, the central groove divides the two _____ ridges.

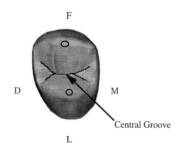

Permanent
Maxillary
Right
First Premolar
OCCLUSAL

Central Groove

b. mesiofacial
triangular groove

Two grooves meet the central groove at its mesial end, the mesial marginal groove and the mesiofacial triangular groove. Which groove is located more toward the facial? _____ _____ _____ (The mesial marginal groove is some-times called the mesial marginal developmental groove.)

a. mesial marginal groove
b. mesiofacial triangular groove

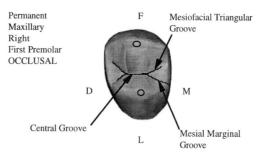

Permanent
Maxillary
Right
First Premolar
OCCLUSAL

Mesiofacial Triangular
Groove

Central Groove

Mesial Marginal
Groove

mesial marginal

The mesial marginal groove extends onto the mesial surface, but first it crosses the _____ _____ ridge.

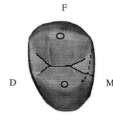

Permanent
Maxillary
Right
First Premolar
OCCLUSAL

The central groove extends distally to the distal marginal ridge, where it branches to form the distofacial triangular groove and the distal marginal groove. Which is the distofacial triangular groove, a or b? _____

a

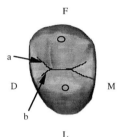

Permanent
Maxillary
Right
First Premolar
OCCLUSAL

F

a

D

M

b

L

The distal marginal groove extends onto the distal marginal ridge but not onto the _____ surface.

distal

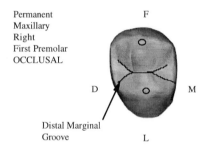

Permanent
Maxillary
Right
First Premolar
OCCLUSAL

F

D

M

Distal Marginal
Groove

L

Label the five grooves (A through E) on the occlusal surface of a maxillary first premolar.

A. _____
B. _____
C. _____
D. _____
E. _____

A. mesiofacial triangular groove;
B. mesial marginal groove; C. central groove; D. distal marginal groove;
E. distofacial triangular groove

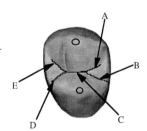

Permanent
Maxillary
Right
First Premolar
OCCLUSAL

A

B

E

C

D

central

At the confluence of these grooves, a small pit is often found. On the maxillary first premolar, there are two pits, one at each end of the _____ groove.

Permanent
Maxillary
Right
First Premolar
OCCLUSAL

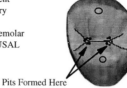

Pits Formed Here

pit

Whenever two or more developmental grooves meet, a _____ is likely to be formed.

mesial

The pits at either end of the central groove are named the distal and the _____ pit.

Permanent
Maxillary
Right
First Premolar
OCCLUSAL

5

The universal code number for the permanent maxillary right first premolar is _____ .

GO TO THE NEXT PAGE AND TAKE REVIEW TEST 3.1.

REVIEW TEST 3.1

1. Name the ridge indicated by the arrow.

   a. distal ridge of the lingual cusp
   b. distal ridge of the facial cusp
   c. mesial ridge of the facial cusp

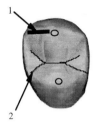

2. Name the groove indicated by the arrow.

   a. distofacial triangular groove
   b. distal marginal groove
   c. mesial marginal groove

3. The wider of two cusps is the cusp with the greater measurement in which direction?

   a. occlusocervical
   b. mesiodistal

4. The triangular ridge of a lingual cusp extends from the cusp tip to the

   a. central groove
   b. mesial marginal ridge
   c. distal marginal groove

5. Which cusp is the longest?

   a. facial
   b. lingual

6. A developmental groove extends onto which proximal surface?

   a. mesial
   b. distal

7. From an occlusal view, the maxillary first premolar converges

   a. lingually
   b. facially

8. The ridge that runs from the cusp tip of the lingual cusp into the central groove is the

   a. lingual ridge of the facial cusp
   b. facial ridge of the lingual cusp

9. Which ridge of the lingual cusp is a triangular ridge?

   a. facial
   b. lingual

10. Which ridge of the lingual cusp joins the distal marginal ridge near the distolinguocclusal point angle?

    a. mesial
    b. distal

CHECK YOUR ANSWERS IN APPENDIX A.

mesial, distal, cervical

3.2.0 MAXILLARY FIRST PREMOLAR: FACIAL VIEW

The facial aspect of the permanent maxillary first premolar is outlined by four borders, one being the occlusal. The other three borders are the _____ , _____ , and _____ .

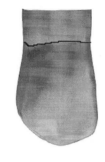

Permanent
Maxillary
Right
First Premolar
FACIAL

D   M

shorter

The facial aspect of the maxillary first premolar is similar to that of the maxillary canine. Occlusocervically, the maxillary first premolar is slightly _____ (longer/shorter) than the canine.

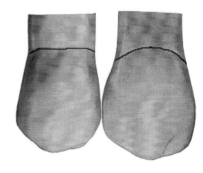

Permanent
Maxillary
Right
1. First Premolar
2. Canine
FACIAL

1   2

mesial, distal

The tip of the facial cusp separates the occlusal border into two parts. These are the _____ and _____ ridges of the facial cusp.

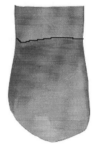

Permanent
Maxillary
Right
First Premolar
FACIAL

D   M

The mesial and distal ridges of the facial cusp can be distinguished by their shape. Which of the two is straighter? _____ Which is convex? _____

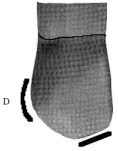

Permanent
Maxillary
Right
First Premolar
FACIAL

D   M

The tip of the facial cusp is not centered with the long axis of the tooth; instead, it is located _____ (mesially/distally) from the long axis. This distal displacement of the cusp tip is unique to this arch.

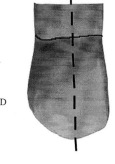

Permanent
Maxillary
Right
First Premolar
FACIAL

D   M

On the maxillary first premolar, the proximal contacts are located in the middle third of the crown, slightly _____ (cervical/occlusal) to the junction of the middle and occlusal thirds.

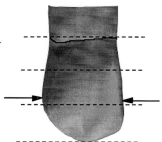

Permanent
Maxillary
Right
First Premolar
FACIAL

In the incisocervical or occlusocervical direction, the location of the proximal contacts varies with the tooth. On some teeth, the contacts are in the incisal third of the crown, on others in the middle third. However, on all teeth, the widest part of the crown (mesiodistally) is at the level of the _____ _____ .

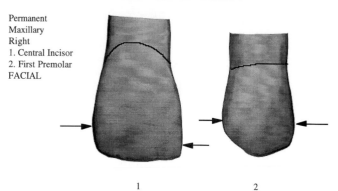

Permanent
Maxillary
Right
1. Central Incisor
2. First Premolar
FACIAL

1   2

From the facial aspect of a maxillary first premolar, which distance is greater? _____

A. The distance between the tip of the facial cusp and the mesiocclusal angle
B. The distance between the tip of the facial cusp and the distocclusal angle

Since the tip of the facial cusp is located toward the distal from the midline of the crown, the distance between the cusp tip and the mesiocclusal angle is greater. In other words, the mesial ridge of the facial cusp is longer than the distal ridge.

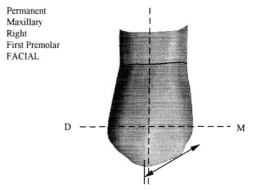

Permanent
Maxillary
Right
First Premolar
FACIAL

D — — — — — — — — — M

From the facial aspect, which of the two contact areas is formed by a sharper angle?

_____

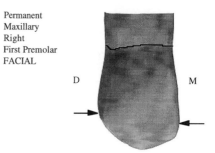

Permanent
Maxillary
Right
First Premolar
FACIAL

D   M

On the maxillary first premolar, the mesial surface joins the facial surface to form the rounded but distinct _____ line angle. The mesial aspect bulges more than the distal.

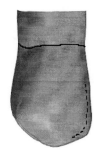
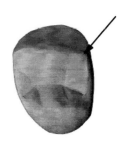

Permanent
Maxillary
Right
First Premolar
1. FACIAL
2. OCCLUSAL

1 2

The distofacial line angle is less distinct than the mesiofacial line angle. The distal and facial surfaces blend together to create a rounded form that contributes to the broad, rounded distal contact area.

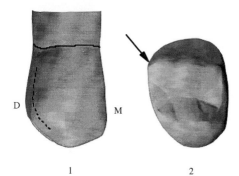

Permanent
Maxillary
Right
First Premolar
1. FACIAL
2. OCCLUSAL

D M

1 2

The discussion of the anatomical features of the teeth describes the average as determined by observing a large sample of individual teeth. A specimen tooth can deviate from the average and remain within the classification of a typical specimen.

Compare the two heavily shaded areas. From the contact area cervically, which border is more nearly straight? _____

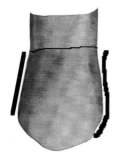

Permanent
Maxillary
Right
First Premolar
FACIAL

mesial

Of the mesial and distal borders of the facial surface, which is concave? _____

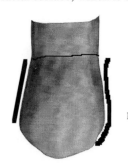

Permanent
Maxillary
Right
First Premolar
FACIAL

M

Use the guidelines to sketch a drawing of the maxillary first premolar, but follow this description: distal straight; rounded distal angle; slightly curved distal cusp ridge; straight mesial cusp ridge; rounded but distinct mesial angle; concave mesial border.

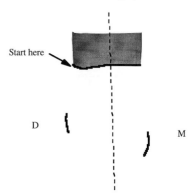

Start here

D

M

Now compare your sketch with the premolar in this frame.

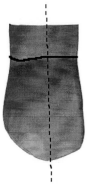

Permanent
Maxillary
Right
First Premolar
FACIAL

The prominent facial ridge of the facial cusp gives the facial surface its great bulk. The facial ridge runs continuously to the cervical line. Cervically, the facial ridge blends with the ____________ ridge.

Permanent
Maxillary
Right
First Premolar
FACIAL

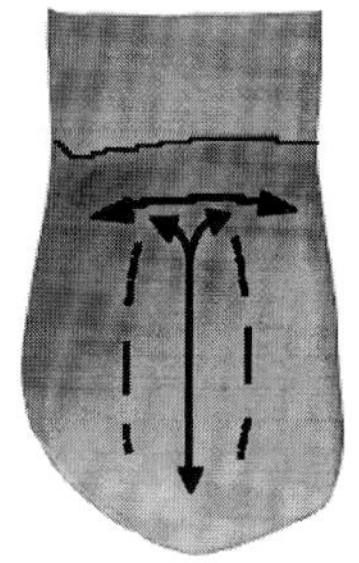

faciocervical

On either side of the facial ridge, facial grooves mark the boundaries of the three facial lobes. On the facial surface of a maxillary first premolar, which lobe is the most prominent? ____________ - ____________

Permanent
Maxillary
Right
First Premolar
FACIAL

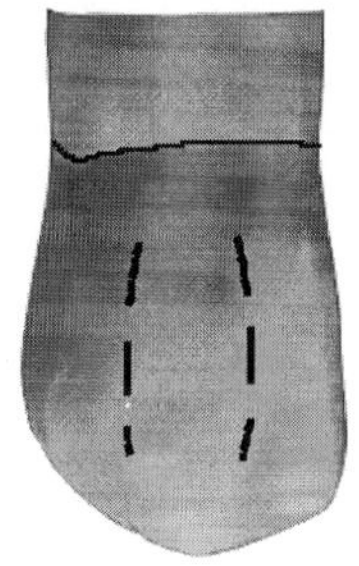

central-facial

On the facial surface, the two faint ____________ ____________ separate the facial lobes.

Permanent
Maxillary
Right
First Premolar
FACIAL

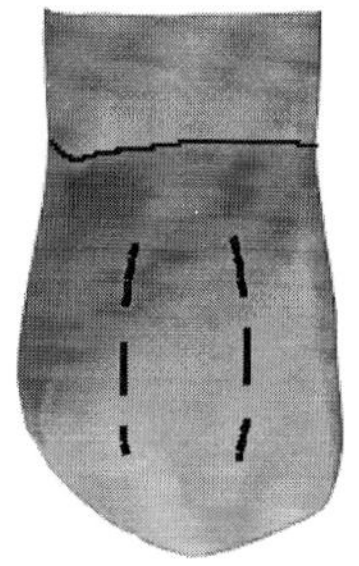

facial grooves

At the cervical border, the facial surface is convex. The cervical line has its crest of convexity toward the ____________ (occlusal/apical).

apical

3.2.1

converges, shorter

MAXILLARY FIRST PREMOLAR: LINGUAL VIEW

The facial view of the maxillary first premolar completely hides the mesial, distal, and lingual portions of the crown. From the lingual view, the lingual surface, parts of the mesial and distal surfaces, and a portion of the facial cusp are visible. This is because the crown _____ toward the lingual, and, in length, the lingual cusp is _____ than the facial cusp.

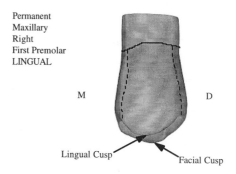

Permanent
Maxillary
Right
First Premolar
LINGUAL

M   D

Lingual Cusp   Facial Cusp

facial, lingual

Mesial and distal ridges are found on both the _____ and _____ cusps.

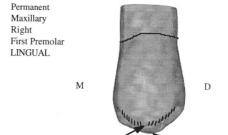

Permanent
Maxillary
Right
First Premolar
LINGUAL

M   D

Lingual Cusp   Facial Cusp

indistinct

Unlike the ridges of the facial cusp, the mesial and distal ridges of the lingual cusp form a rounded curve in joining the mesial and distal marginal ridges. Following this pattern, the lingual surface is rounded mesiodistally, making the mesiolingual and distolingual line angles _____ (sharp/indistinct).

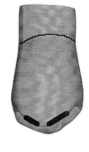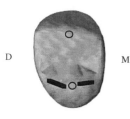

Permanent
Maxillary
Right
First Premolar
1. LINGUAL
2. OCCLUSAL

M   D   M

1   2

The lingual cusp tip is not in the same faciolingual plane as the facial cusp tip. Compared with the facial cusp tip, is the lingual cusp tip located more toward the mesial or distal?

_____

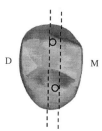

Permanent
Maxillary
Right
First Premolar
OCCLUSAL   D   M

On the maxillary first premolar, which two line angles are more distinct? (mesiofacial and distofacial/mesiolingual and distolingual) _____   _____   _____

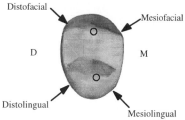

Permanent   Distofacial
Maxillary   Mesiofacial
Right
First Premolar
OCCLUSAL   D   M

Distolingual

Mesiolingual

Compare the cervical lines of the facial and lingual views. The convexity of the cervical line on the facial surface is directed in the (occlusal/apical) _____ direction; also the curvature is greater on the _____ surface.

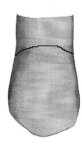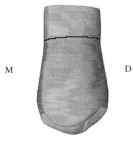

Permanent
Maxillary
Right
First Premolar
1. FACIAL
2. LINGUAL   D   M   D

1   2

3.2.2 MAXILLARY FIRST PREMOLAR: PROXIMAL VIEW

line

A portion of the facial and lingual surfaces of the crown can be seen from a mesial or distal view of a maxillary first premolar. The point angles (A, B, C, D) and line angles (a, b, c, d) mark the limits of the proximal surfaces. The facial and lingual borders of the two proximal surfaces are the four _____ angles.

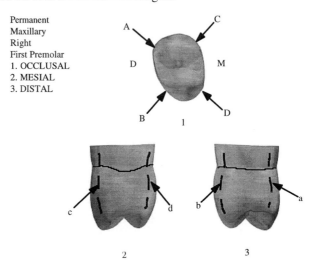

Permanent
Maxillary
Right
First Premolar
1. OCCLUSAL
2. MESIAL
3. DISTAL

mesial

One major difference between the mesial and distal surfaces of the maxillary first premolar is the presence of a mesial marginal groove that extends from the occlusal surface onto the _____ surface.

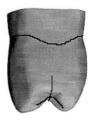
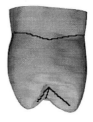

Permanent
Maxillary
Right
First Premolar
1. MESIAL
2. DISTAL

1   2

mesial

As is generally true of all teeth, the cervical line has a crest of curvature that is more occlusally (or incisally) located on the _____ (mesial/distal) surface.

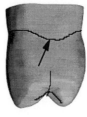
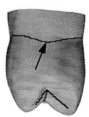

Permanent
Maxillary
Right
First Premolar
1. MESIAL
2. DISTAL

1   2

The mesial marginal groove extends onto the mesial surface of the maxillary first premolar. To do so, this groove passes through the _____ _____ ridge.

Permanent
Maxillary
Right
First Premolar
MESIAL

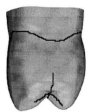

The end of the mesial marginal groove is lingual to the contact area and terminates in the _____ third of the crown.

Permanent
Maxillary
Right
First Premolar
MESIAL

F   L

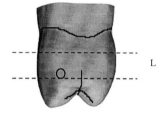

Is the extension of the mesial marginal groove located to the facial or lingual of the contact area? _____

Permanent
Maxillary
Right
First Premolar
MESIAL

F   L

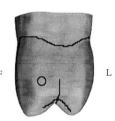

From a mesial view, the facial outline is convex. The height of contour is located in the _____ third of the crown.

Permanent
Maxillary
Right
First Premolar
MESIAL

F   L

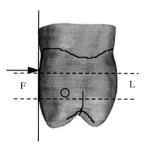

middle

The lingual outline is also convex, the height of contour occurring in the _____ third.

Permanent
Maxillary
Right
First Premolar
MESIAL

F   L

A

The mesial surface of the maxillary first premolar is both convex and concave. The convexity occurs in the area of the marginal ridge and includes the contact area. The concavity occurs between the contact area and cervical line. Identify the mesial surface in the illustration. _____ (A or B)

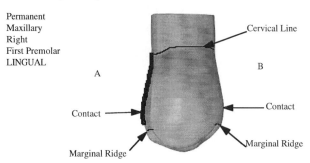

Permanent
Maxillary
Right
First Premolar
LINGUAL

Cervical Line

A   B

Contact   Contact

Marginal Ridge   Marginal Ridge

Figure 2

Three characteristic features of the maxillary first premolar are: (a) the extension of the mesial marginal groove onto the mesial surface, (b) the lingual cusp is shorter (smaller) than the facial cusp, and (c) there is a mesial concavity or depression cervical to the contact area. Which of the two teeth in this frame represents a maxillary first premolar? _____ (Figure 1/Figure 2)

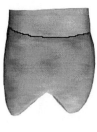
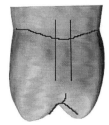

1   2

If the facial and lingual cusps of a specimen tooth appeared approximately equal in height, perhaps due to wear, the tooth could be identified as a maxillary first premolar by the _____ _____ located cervical to the mesial contact area.

Permanent
Maxillary
Right
First Premolar
MESIAL

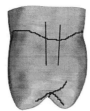

mesial concavity

In contrast to the mesial surface, the distal surface of the crown of a maxillary first premolar does not characteristically have a concavity cervical to the proximal contact area. In the drawing, the distal is toward _____ (A or B).

Permanent
Maxillary
Right
First Premolar
LINGUAL

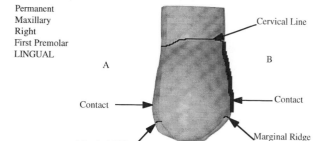

A

Cervical Line

B

Contact

Contact

Marginal Ridge

Marginal Ridge

B

The distal marginal groove does not cut across the distal marginal ridge and onto the distal surface. On a few teeth, an extension of the distal marginal groove may be visible, but it is slight. The illustration shows a maxillary first premolar seen from the _____ view.

Permanent
Maxillary
Right
First Premolar

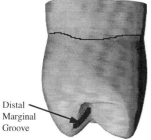

Distal
Marginal
Groove

distal

occlusal, mesial

The curvature of the cervical line on the mesial and distal is consistent with the pattern established by anterior teeth. From both the mesial and distal views, the cementoenamel junction curves toward the _____ with the greater amount of curvature on the _____ .

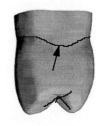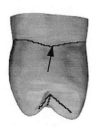

Permanent
Maxillary
Right
First Premolar
1. MESIAL
2. DISTAL

1   2

Figure 1

Of the four illustrations, which one shows the maxillary left first premolar from the distal aspect? _____

Permanent
Maxillary
First Premolars

1   2   3   4

Figure 1: 12; Figure 2: 12; Figure 3: 5; Figure 4: 5

What are the universal (military) code numbers for the teeth shown in Figures 1 through 4?

Figure 1 _____
Figure 2 _____
Figure 3 _____
Figure 4 _____

Permanent
Maxillary
First Premolars

1   2   3   4

GO TO THE NEXT PAGE AND TAKE REVIEW TEST 3.2.

REVIEW TEST 3.2

Write the correct response (one or more words) under the appropriate term on the right.

Maxillary First Premolar   *Mesial*   *Distal*

Which ridge of the facial cusp is shorter and which is longer?   _____ _____

Which surface has a cervical line with more curvature?   _____ _____

Occlusocervical location of this contact area . . .   _____ _____

Does the developmental groove extend onto this surface?   _____ _____

1. The lingual cusp tip is displaced from the facial cusp slightly to the
   a. distal
   b. mesial

2. The cervical line is more convex on which surface?
   a. facial
   b. lingual

3. The more distinct line angle is the
   a. mesiofacial
   b. distofacial

4. The shape of the mesial surface (from contact area to cervical line) is
   a. concave
   b. convex
   c. straight

5. List the three distinguishing characteristics of the maxillary first premolar.
   a. _____
   b. _____
   c. _____

6. In which third (cervical, middle, or occlusal) is the height of contour located on each of these surfaces?
   a. lingual _____
   b. facial _____

CHECK YOUR ANSWERS IN APPENDIX A.

3.3.0 PROXIMAL CONTACTS, EMBRASURES, AND CROWN CONTOURS OF MAXILLARY FIRST PREMOLARS

Recall that the proximal contacts provide stability to the dental arch by providing support to the individual tooth. The proximal contacts between posterior teeth are _____ _____ (centered/facially located) in the faciolingual dimension.

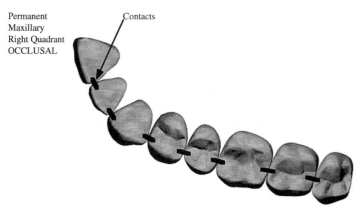

Permanent
Maxillary
Right Quadrant
OCCLUSAL

Contacts

Because the contacts are located more facially, the embrasure with the greater depth is the _____ embrasure.

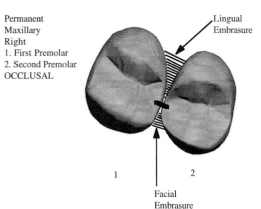

Permanent
Maxillary
Right
1. First Premolar
2. Second Premolar
OCCLUSAL

Lingual
Embrasure

1   2

Facial
Embrasure

The relative depth of facial and lingual embrasures is determined by the location of the contact in the _____ dimension.

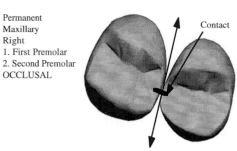

Permanent
Maxillary
Right
1. First Premolar
2. Second Premolar
OCCLUSAL

Contact

1   2

The contacts of the mesial and distal surfaces of the maxillary first premolar have contacts in the _____ third.

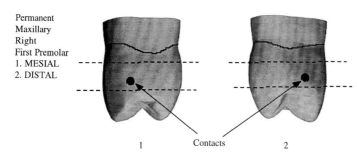

Permanent
Maxillary
Right
First Premolar
1. MESIAL
2. DISTAL

1   Contacts   2

The contacts of the maxillary first premolar are located _____ (facially/centered) in the faciolingual dimension and in the middle third of the tooth in the _____ (occlusocervical/faciolingual) dimension.

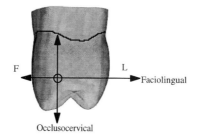

Permanent
Maxillary
Right
First Premolar
MESIAL

F

L

Faciolingual

Occlusocervical

One of the best ways to study the contours of a crown is to focus on the height of contour. The height of contour is an imaginary line encircling the entire crown of the tooth. The proximal contacts of a tooth lie _____ (along/above) the height of contour.

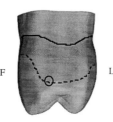

Permanent
Maxillary
Right
First Premolar
MESIAL

F

L

The maxillary first premolar has a height of contour in the middle third on the _____ surface.

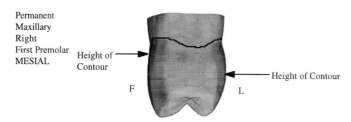

Permanent
Maxillary
Right
First Premolar
MESIAL

Height of
Contour

Height of Contour

F

L

cervical

The height of contour on the facial surface is located in the _____ third. (See illustration in the previous frame.)

1/2

The amount of contour on the maxillary first premolar measures _____ mm.

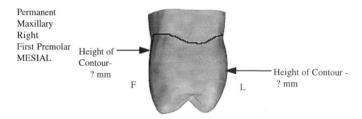

Permanent
Maxillary
Right
First Premolar
MESIAL

Height of Contour-
? mm

F   L

Height of Contour -
? mm

3.3.1 ROOT ANATOMY OF MAXILLARY FIRST PREMOLARS

bifurcated

The maxillary first premolar is the only premolar that commonly occurs in the _____ root type. In some instances the root will be single-rooted.

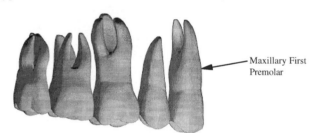

Permanent
Maxillary
Right
Sextant
FACIAL

Maxillary First
Premolar

apical

The bifurcation may occur in either the apical or middle third of the root. The bifurcation shown in the illustration occurs in the _____ third of the root.

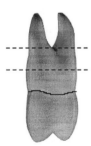

Permanent
Maxillary
Right
First Premolar
MESIAL

The bifurcation is in the mesiodistal direction, therefore the two terminal roots are the

_____ and _____ .

facial, lingual

Permanent
Maxillary
Right
First Premolar
MESIAL

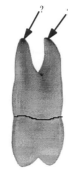

F   L

The mesial surface of the root trunk on a maxillary first premolar has a deep developmental groove that runs from the bifurcation to the cervical line and continues onto the cervical portion of the mesial crown surface as a concavity.

On the distal surface, the longitudinal groove is greatly reduced. In the cervical region of the distal surface of the root trunk, the faciolingual curvature is flat or slightly convex.

Permanent
Maxillary
Right
First Premolar
1. DISTOFACIAL
2. MESIOFACIAL

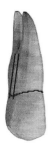   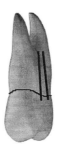

1   2

This mesiofacial and mesiolingual view of the maxillary first premolar shows that the facial and lingual surfaces are convex. Which surface is more narrow—the facial or lingual? _____

lingual

Permanent
Maxillary
Right
First Premolar
1. MESIOFACIAL
2. MESIOLINGUAL

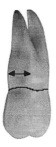   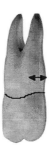

1   2

mesial

The mesial and distal surfaces on the single-rooted form of the maxillary first premolar are marked by longitudinal grooves similar to those on the root trunk of the bifurcated form. The longitudinal groove is more highly developed on the _____ surface.

convex

The cervical portion of the root structure on the two forms of the maxillary first premolar is generally similar. In the longitudinal direction, the cervical portions of the facial and lingual surfaces are _____ (straight/convex).

Permanent
Maxillary
Right
First Premolar
MESIAL

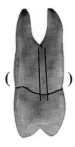

facial, lingual

The mesial and distal surfaces have longitudinal curvatures in the cervical portion that are nearly straight or very slightly convex. Of the two pairs of opposite root surfaces (mesial, distal/facial, lingual), on which pair is the longitudinal curvature more pronounced?

_____ _____

Permanent
Maxillary
Right
First Premolar
1. MESIAL
2. FACIAL

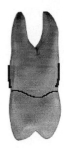   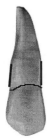

1   2

PULP ANATOMY OF MAXILLARY
FIRST PREMOLARS

A maxillary first premolar may have one or two terminal roots, but in either case two root canals are generally present. Similar to the relative positions of the terminal roots on a bifurcated root structure, the root canals are located toward the _____ and _____ .

facial, lingual

Permanent
Maxillary
Right
First Premolar
FACIOLINGUAL SECTIONS

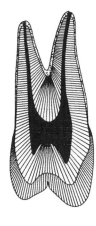
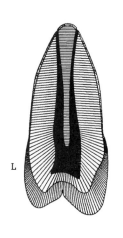

L   F L   F

If the drawings constitute a representative sample of all maxillary first premolars, you may deduce that about _____% have only one canal.

20

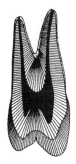
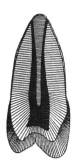
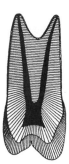
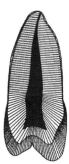
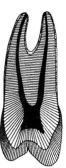

In which direction is the root canal wider? (mesiodistal/faciolingual)

faciolingual

Permanent
Maxillary
Right
First Premolar
1. MESIODISTAL
2. FACIOLINGUAL

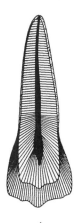
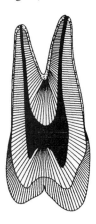

1   2

two

Whether a maxillary premolar has one or two terminal roots, the number of pulp horns corresponds to the number of cusps. How many pulp horns will be present in the pulp chamber of a maxillary premolar? _____

canine

As seen in mesiodistal section, the pulp cavity form of the maxillary first premolar is similar to that of a maxillary _____ (canine/incisor).

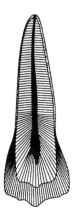

Permanent
Maxillary
Right
First Premolar
MESIODISTAL

apical

A horizontal section taken at the level of the cervical line on a maxillary premolar cuts through the pulp chamber. On maxillary premolars, the floor of the pulp chamber is located _____ (apical/occlusal) to the cervical line.

Permanent
Maxillary
Right
First Premolar
1. FACIOLINGUAL
2. CROSS SECTION

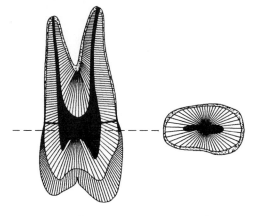

1   2

Review the anatomical features of the maxillary first premolar from the facial, lingual, mesial and distal:

Permanent Maxillary Right First Premolar - Summary

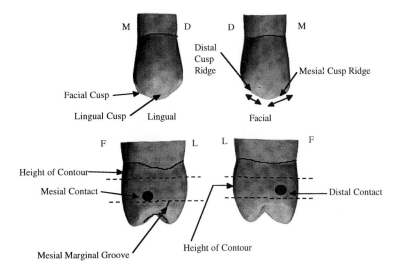

This illustration summarizes the maxillary first premolar from the occlusal view.

Permanent Maxillary Right First Premolar Occlusal - Summary

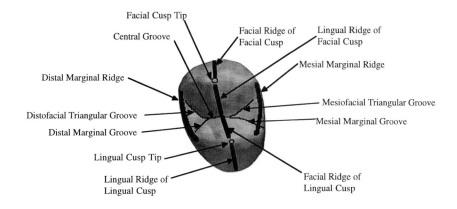

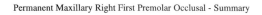

Which ridges are triangular ridges? _____

and _____

Lingual Ridge of Facial Cusp & Facial Ridge of Lingual Cusp

On which surface is the longitudinal groove more highly developed? _____

Mesial

Review root anatomy and pulp anatomy in the illustrations.

Permanent Maxillary Right First Premolar Root Anatomy - Summary

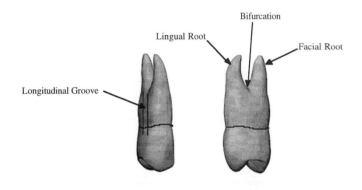

Distofacial View   Distal View

Permanent
Maxillary
Right
First Premolar
1. MESIODISTAL
2. FACIOLINGUAL

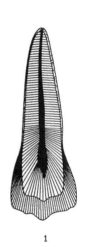

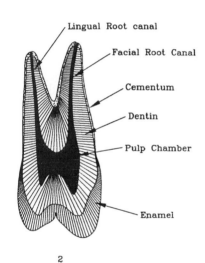

1   2

GO TO THE NEXT PAGE AND TAKE REVIEW TEST 3.3.

REVIEW TEST 3.3

1. The maxillary first premolar most commonly has _____ roots.

    a. one
    b. two
    c. three
    d. four

2. If a maxillary premolar is bifurcated, what is the location of the bifurcation?

    a. middle or apical
    b. apical only

3. Which longitudinal groove on a maxillary first premolar is most prominent?

    a. mesial
    b. distal

4. What percentage of maxillary first premolars have only one root canal?

    a. 80
    b. 20
    c. 50
    d. 10

5. In which longitudinal view will the root canals of a maxillary first premolar with two canals be seen?

    a. mesiodistal
    b. faciolingual

6. Which surface of the maxillary premolar (cervical portion), is narrower?

    a. facial
    b. lingual

7. Which surface of the crown of the maxillary premolar has a groove extending onto the surface?

    a. mesial
    b. distal

8. Which cusp of the maxillary premolar is longer?

    a. lingual
    b. facial

9. On which surface is the height of contour located in the middle third?

    a. facial
    b. lingual

10. Which primary tooth does the maxillary first premolar replace?

    a. canine
    b. first molar
    c. second molar

CHECK YOUR ANSWERS IN APPENDIX A.

3.4.0 MAXILLARY SECOND PREMOLARS

first premolar

The size and shape of the maxillary second premolar is generally similar to the maxillary first premolar.

Variation in the relative sizes of the two maxillary premolars will occur because the second premolar deviates from the average form more often than the first premolar. Although the crown size of a maxillary second premolar is variable, it generally has approximately the same dimensions as the maxillary _____ _____ .

5, 13

The universal code number for the maxillary right first premolar is _____ . The universal code number for the maxillary left second premolar is _____ .

equal (or synonym)

On the maxillary first premolar, the lingual cusp is shorter than the facial cusp. However, in relative length, the two cusps of the second premolar are approximately _____ .

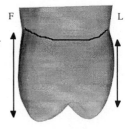
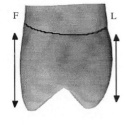

Permanent
Maxillary Right
1. First Premolar
2. Second Premolar
MESIAL

1   2

lingual

On the maxillary second premolar, if one cusp is slightly shorter, the shorter of the two is the _____ cusp.

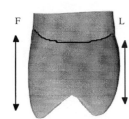

Permanent
Maxillary
Right
Second Premolar
MESIAL

The facial cusp of the second premolar lacks the pointed cusp tip seen on the first premolar. Thus, in length (depth of occlusal groove to cusp tip), the facial cusp of the second premolar is _____ than that of the first premolar.

shorter

Permanent
Maxillary
Right
1. First Premolar
2. Second Premolar
MESIAL

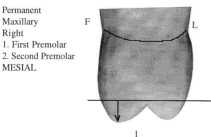
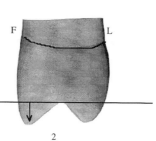

1   2

On the occlusal, the groove pattern of the second premolar is less distinct than that of the first premolar. On the maxillary second premolar, the central groove is short and _____ (straight/irregular).

irregular

Permanent
Maxillary
Right
1. First Premolar
2. Second Premolar
OCCLUSAL

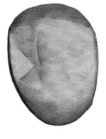
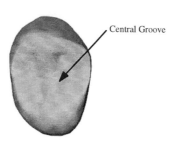

Central Groove

1   2

On the occlusal surface of the second premolar, shallow linear supplemental grooves radiate from the central groove. With the presence of these supplemental grooves, the mesiofacial and distofacial triangular grooves are less positive and may be more difficult to identify. Which of the two illustrations represents the occlusal view of the maxillary second premolar? _____ (Figure 1 or Figure 2)

Figure 2

Permanent
Maxillary
Right
Premolars

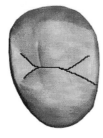
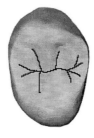

1   2

first premolar

On the second premolar, a developmental groove does not cross the mesial marginal ridge and descend onto the mesial surface. The extension of a developmental groove onto the mesial surface is a characteristic only of the maxillary _____ _____ .

Permanent
Maxillary
Right
1. First Premolar
2. Second Premolar
OCCLUSAL

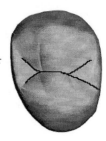
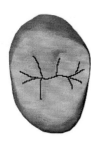

1   2

The facial and lingual cusps on the maxillary second premolar are nearly equal in length.

What is the difference between the relative length of the facial and lingual cusps on the maxillary first premolar when compared to the relative length of the facial and lingual cusps on the maxillary second premolar? _____

Permanent
Maxillary
Right
1. First Premolar
2. Second Premolar
DISTAL

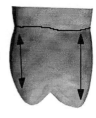
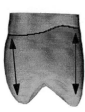

1   2

---

first

Of the two maxillary premolars, which has the longer facial cusp? _____

Permanent
Maxillary
Right
1. First Premolar
2. Second Premolar
DISTAL

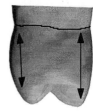
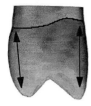

1   2

The mesial surface of the maxillary second premolar differs from the mesial surface of the first premolar. As mentioned, the mesial marginal groove does not extend onto the mesial surface on the maxillary _____ premolar.

Permanent
Maxillary Right
1. First Premolar
2. Second Premolar
MESIAL

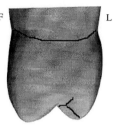

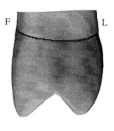

1   2

The mesial surface on the crown of the maxillary second premolar shows less overall curvature when viewed from the facial or lingual as shown by the mesiolingual line angle. In this respect, the mesial surfaces of the two maxillary premolars are _____ (similar/dissimilar).

Permanent
Maxillary
Right
1. First Premolar
2. Second Premolar
LINGUAL

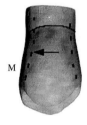

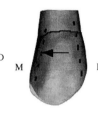

M   D   M   D

1   2

On the facial and lingual surfaces, the cervical line is curved toward the _____ ; on the mesial and distal surfaces, it is slightly curved toward the _____ .

second premolar

Which maxillary premolar has cervical lines that are slightly less curved? _____
_____

Permanent
Maxillary
1. First Premolar
2. Second Premolar
a. FACIAL
b. LINGUAL
c. MESIAL
d. DISTAL

1   2

GO TO THE NEXT PAGE AND TAKE REVIEW TEST 3.4.

REVIEW TEST 3.4

Place an X in the square that matches the left hand column with the top row.

	First Premolar	*Second Premolar*	*Neither/ Both*
Longer buccal cusp	☐	☐	☐
Mesial marginal groove extends onto mesial surface	☐	☐	☐
More supplemental grooves	☐	☐	☐
Cervical line less contoured	☐	☐	☐
Mesial surface has less curvature	☐	☐	☐

1. The tooth shown is the maxillary _____ premolar (mesial view).
   a. first
   b. second

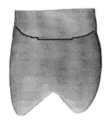

2. This cusp is the
   a. buccal
   b. lingual

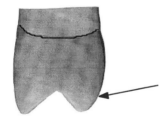

3. This maxillary premolar is the
   a. first
   b. second

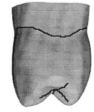

4. The tooth shown is the maxillary
   a. second premolar
   b. first premolar

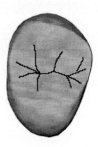

CHECK YOUR ANSWERS IN APPENDIX A.

PROXIMAL CONTACTS, EMBRASURES, AND CROWN CONTOURS OF MAXILLARY SECOND PREMOLARS

3.5.0

As is true for all posterior teeth, the proximal contact areas on the maxillary premolars are not centered in the faciolingual direction. In the faciolingual direction, the proximal contacts of posterior teeth are located slightly toward the _____ .

facial

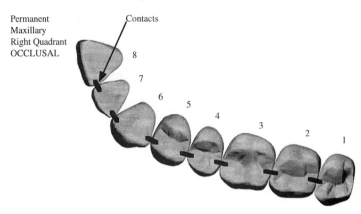

Permanent
Maxillary
Right Quadrant
OCCLUSAL

Contacts

8 7 6 5 4 3 2 1

Similar to the maxillary first premolars, the occlusocervical location of the mesial and distal contact areas on the second premolar is slightly _____ to the junction of the _____ and _____ thirds.

cervical, occlusal, middle

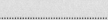

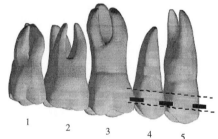

Permanent
Maxillary
Right Sextant
1. Third Molar
2. Second Molar
3. First Molar
4. Second Premolar
5. First Premolar
FACIAL

1 2 3 4 5

Universal Code Numbers

The relative depth of facial and lingual embrasures is determined by the location of the contact in the _____ dimension. Which embrasures are deeper? _____

faciolingual, lingual

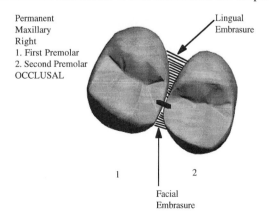

Permanent
Maxillary
Right
1. First Premolar
2. Second Premolar
OCCLUSAL

Lingual
Embrasure

1 2

Facial
Embrasure

middle

The contacts on the maxillary premolars are located in the _____ third, along the height of contour.

lingual, cervical

The maxillary second premolars have the height of contour in the middle third on the _____ surface, and in the _____ third on the facial surface.

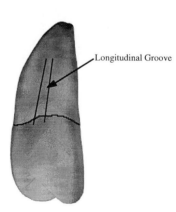

Permanent
Maxillary
Right
Second Premolar
MESIAL

F   L

1/2

Similar to the other maxillary teeth, the height of contour measures _____ mm.

3.5.1 ROOT ANATOMY OF MAXILLARY SECOND PREMOLARS

concave

The longitudinal groove of the maxillary second premolar is not as highly developed as the first premolar. Both proximal root surfaces on the maxillary second premolar have longitudinal grooves and, therefore, a curvature in the faciolingual direction that is nearly flat to

_____ .

Permanent
Maxillary
Right
Second Premolar
DISTOFACIAL

Longitudinal Groove

The apex of the maxillary second premolar (proximal view) is _____ (rounded/pointed).

Permanent
Maxillary
Right
Second Premolar
DISTAL

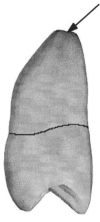

Compare the facial view and the proximal view in the illustration. Which root surface is narrower? _____ (facial/lingual) In which direction is the root wider? _____ (faciolingual/mesiodistal)

Permanent
Maxillary
Right
Second Premolar
1. DISTAL
2. FACIAL

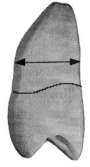
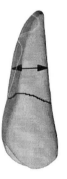

3.5.2

PULP ANATOMY OF MAXILLARY SECOND PREMOLARS

mesiodistal

The illustration is representative of the _____ (mesiodistal/faciolingual) section of the maxillary second premolar.

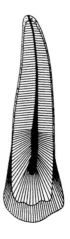

```
Permanent
Maxillary
Right
Second Premolar
MESIODISTAL SECTION
```

apical

A horizontal section taken at the level of the cervical line on a maxillary second premolar cuts through the pulp chamber. On maxillary premolars, the floor of the pulp chamber is located _____ (apical/oclusal) to the cervical line.

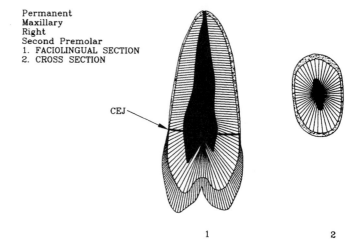

```
Permanent
Maxillary
Right
Second Premolar
1. FACIOLINGUAL SECTION
2. CROSS SECTION
```

CEJ

1   2

With the exception of the relative frequency of teeth with a single root canal, the form of the pulp chamber on the maxillary second premolar is similar to that of the maxillary first premolar. As suggested by the relative frequency of the bifurcated roots, which maxillary premolar is most likely to have a single root canal? _____ _____

These illustrations summarize the permanent maxillary second premolar:

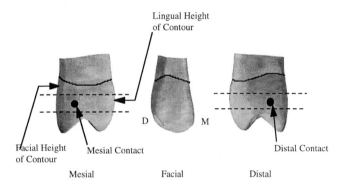

Permanent Maxillary Right Second Premolar - Summary

Notice the root width is wider and the apex is blunt in the mesial view. Also note the narrow root width and the distal displacement of the root in the facial view in this summary illustration.

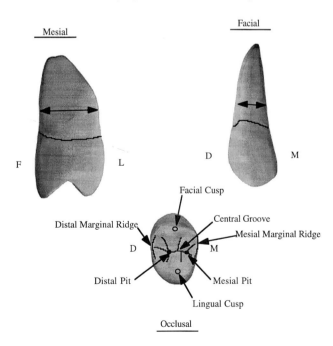

Permanent Maxillary Right Second Premolar - Summary

TURN TO THE NEXT PAGE AND TAKE REVIEW TEST 3.5.

REVIEW TEST 3.5

1. The proximal contacts on the maxillary premolars are
   a. centered faciolingually
   b. facially located

2. In the occlusocervical direction the contacts are located
   a. in the cervical third
   b. in the occlusal third
   c. cervical to the junction of the occlusal and middle thirds

3. The height of contour on the maxillary second premolar is located in the _____ third on the lingual.
   a. occlusal
   b. middle
   c. cervical

4. The amount of contour mentioned in 3 above, is approximately _____ mm.
   a. 1/2
   b. 1
   c. 3/4
   d. 2

5. There are _____ grooves on the proximal root surfaces of the maxillary second premolar.
   a. horizontal
   b. longitudinal
   c. oblique

6. From the proximal view of the maxillary second premolar, the apex is
   a. pointed
   b. blunted
   c. bifurcated

7. The maxillary second premolar is most likely to have _____ root canal(s).
   a. one
   b. two
   c. three

8. Which cusp of the maxillary first premolar is shorter?
   a. facial
   b. lingual
   c. mesial
   d. distal

9. Which premolar is most likely to have a bifurcated root?
   a. first
   b. second

10. Which groove of the maxillary first premolar passes onto the mesial surface?
    a. mesial marginal
    b. mesiofacial triangular groove

CHECK YOUR ANSWERS IN APPENDIX A.

MANDIBULAR FIRST PREMOLAR

The mandibular premolars are located immediately posterior to the permanent mandibular canines. Since the permanent mandibular central incisors are teeth numbers 24 and 25 (universal code), what numbers are assigned to the permanent mandibular first premolars? _____

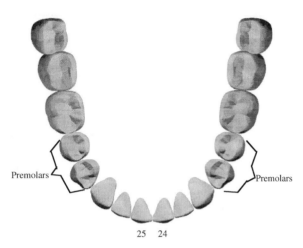

Permanent
Mandibular
Arch
OCCLUSAL

Premolars

Premolars

25   24

Similar to the maxillary premolars, the mandibular first premolar has a four-lobe pattern. Three of the lobes are seen on the _____ portion of the crown; the fourth lobe represents the _____ portion.

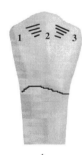
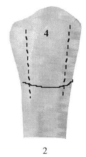

Permanent
Mandibular
Right
First Premolar
1. FACIAL
2. LINGUAL

1   2

Like the maxillary premolars, the mandibular first premolar has two cusps, called the _____ and _____ cusps.

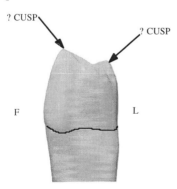

Permanent
Mandibular
Right
First Premolar
MESIAL

? CUSP

? CUSP

F   L

facial

Only one of the two cusps of the mandibular first premolar is functional. The shorter, non-functional cusp does not usually occlude with maxillary teeth. Which is the functional cusp? _____

Permanent
Mandibular
Right
First Premolar
MESIAL

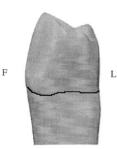

F   L

lingual cusp

In some respects, the mandibular first premolar resembles a canine. The lingual feature of a mandibular first premolar that resembles a large cingulum on a canine is the _____ _____ .

Permanent
Mandibular
Right
First Premolar
MESIAL

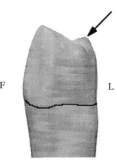

F   L

non-centric

The facial cusp of the mandibular first premolar is large and considered a centric cusp; however, the lingual cusp is small and considered a _____ cusp.

Permanent
Mandibular
Right
First Premolar
MESIAL

Centric
Cusp

Lingual
Cusp

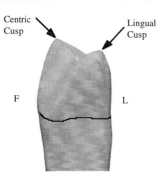

F   L

Centric cusps of mandibular premolars are those that contact their antagonists and determine the position of the mandible in maximum opposing tooth contact (centric occlusion).

Choose the letter (a or b) corresponding to the centric cusp as shown in the illustration.

_____

Permanent
Mandibular
Right
First Premolar
MESIAL

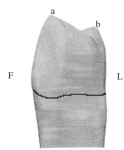

a

Viewed from the distal, the premolars normally occlude so that the mandibular facial cusps strike the _____ portion.

a. central portion of the occlusal surface of their antagonists.
b. facial portion of the facial cusps of their antagonists.

Permanent
Maxillary and
Mandibular
Premolars
DISTAL

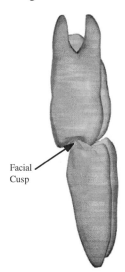

Facial
Cusp

a

a

From the occlusal view, the geometric outline of the crown is nearly a rounded diamond shape with a mesiodistal width that is narrower in the _____ (facial/lingual) portion.

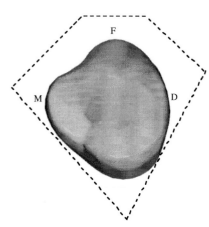

Permanent
Mandibular
Right
First Premolar
OCCLUSAL

Which crown surface (occlusal view) combines with the occlusal surface to form the major part of the tooth? _____

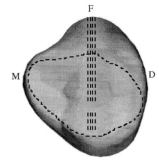

Permanent
Mandibular
Right
First Premolar
OCCLUSAL

Compared to the maxillary premolars, the large facial surface coupled with the large triangular ridge of the facial cusp on the mandibular first premolar results in an occlusal surface that is relatively _____ (small/large).

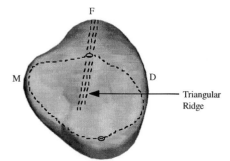

Permanent
Mandibular
Right
First Premolar
OCCLUSAL

Triangular
Ridge

The facial ridge of the facial cusp descends in the cervical direction as part of the facial surface. It adds to the prominence of the _____ - _____ lobe.

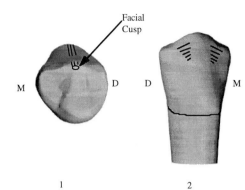

Permanent
Mandibular
Right
First Premolar
1. OCCLUSAL
2. FACIAL

Facial
Cusp

M   D   D   M

1   2

The mesial and distal ridges of the facial cusp descend toward the proximal surface where they become continuous with the mesial and distal _____ _____ .

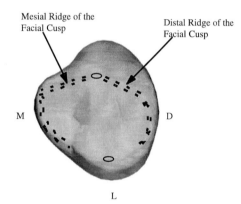

Permanent
Mandibular
Right
First Premolar
OCCLUSAL

Mesial Ridge of the
Facial Cusp

Distal Ridge of the
Facial Cusp

M   D

L

smaller (less rounded)

From the occlusal view, the large arc of the distal outline creates a broad contact area. The mesial outline turns more acutely than the distal and forms a _____ (relative size) contact area. (The teeth are identified by universal code number.)

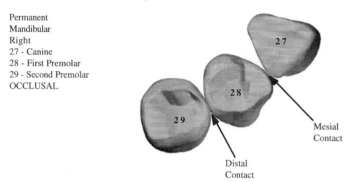

Permanent
Mandibular
Right
27 - Canine
28 - First Premolar
29 - Second Premolar
OCCLUSAL

27

28

29

Mesial
Contact

Distal
Contact

The maxillary premolars have central grooves that separate the triangular ridges. Notice, however, that the mandibular first premolar does not usually have a division of the two triangular ridges. Instead, the triangular ridges characteristically cross the occlusal surface uninterrupted. Any union of two triangular ridges produces a single ridge called the transverse ridge.

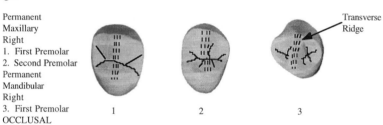

Permanent
Maxillary
Right
1. First Premolar
2. Second Premolar
Permanent
Mandibular
Right
3. First Premolar
OCCLUSAL

Transverse
Ridge

1

2

3

transverse

In the most common form of the mandibular first premolar the occlusal table (bounded by the cusp ridges and marginal ridges) is triangular-shaped and bisected by a prominent _____ ridge. The first premolar model tooth used in this illustration has a transverse ridge that is displaced slightly to the mesial.

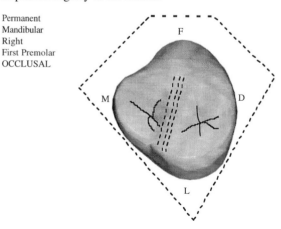

Permanent
Mandibular
Right
First Premolar
OCCLUSAL

F

M

D

L

Because of the reduced form of the lingual cusp, the major portion of the lingual half of the occlusal table is bounded by the mesial and distal _____   _____ .

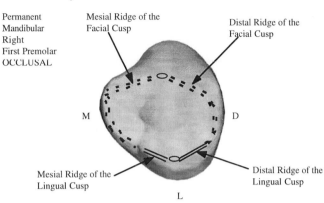

Permanent
Mandibular
Right
First Premolar
OCCLUSAL

Mesial Ridge of the
Facial Cusp

Distal Ridge of the
Facial Cusp

M

D

Mesial Ridge of the
Lingual Cusp

Distal Ridge of the
Lingual Cusp

L

The prominent triangular ridge of the facial cusp and the small facial ridge of the lingual cusp unite to form a _____ ridge.

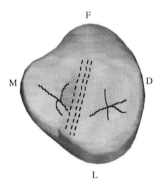

Permanent
Mandibular
Right
First Premolar
OCCLUSAL

F

M

D

L

You may occasionally find specimens of mandibular first premolars that do not have an uninterrupted transverse ridge, because they have a more prominent central _____ .

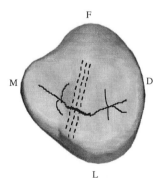

Permanent
Mandibular
Right
First Premolar
OCCLUSAL

F

M

D

L

Of the maxillary premolars and the mandibular first premolar, which usually has an uninterrupted transverse ridge? _____ _____ _____

Permanent
Maxillary
Right
1. First Premolar
2. Second Premolar
Permanent
Mandibular
Right
3. First Premolar
OCCLUSAL

1   2   3

The _____ ridge of the _____ cusp contributes the largest part to the transverse ridge of the mandibular first premolar.

Permanent
Mandibular
Right
First Premolar
OCCLUSAL

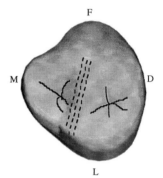

The occlusal surface of the mandibular first premolar has two fossae (the mesial and distal fossae). The mesial and distal ridges of the cusps and the marginal ridges surround the two occlusal fossae which are separated by the _____ _____ .

Permanent
Mandibular
Right
First Premolar
OCCLUSAL

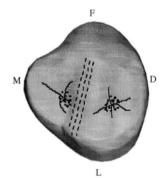

Since the two occlusal fossae of the mandibular first premolar are separated by the transverse ridge, the groove patterns of the maxillary premolars and mandibular first premolar are _____ (similar/different).

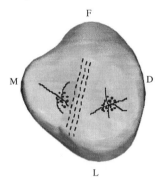

Permanent
Mandibular
Right
First Premolar
OCCLUSAL

F

M   D

L

Although the groove pattern is variable, most mandibular first premolars have a mesial groove contained within the mesial fossae. The mesial groove runs in a faciolingual direction and is continuous with its lingual extension, the mesiolingual groove.

Which groove separates the mesial marginal ridge from the mesial ridge of the lingual cusp? _____

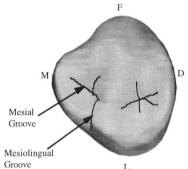

Permanent
Mandibular
Right
First Premolar
OCCLUSAL

F

M   D

Mesial
Groove

Mesiolingual
Groove   L

Which of the following grooves is not usually present on a mandibular first premolar? _____

a. mesial
b. central
c. mesiolingual

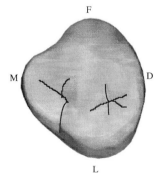

Permanent
Mandibular
Right
First Premolar
OCCLUSAL

F

M   D

L

3.6.1 MANDIBULAR FIRST PREMOLAR: FACIAL VIEW

first premolar

The facial aspect of the mandibular first premolar has a general resemblance to the facial aspect of the mandibular canine. On which of the two teeth is the cusp tip slightly more rounded? _____

Permanent
Mandibular
Right
1. First Premolar
2. Canine
FACIAL

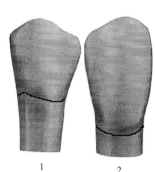

1   2

distal

Of the mesial and distal ridges on the facial cusp of the mandibular first premolar, which is longer? _____

Permanent
Mandibular
Right
First Premolar
FACIAL

D   M

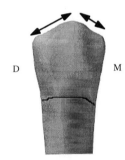

maxillary

In which arch is the tip of the facial cusp on the first premolar located toward the distal (from the longitudinal axis of the crown)? _____

Permanent
Maxillary
Right
4. Second Premolar
5. First Premolar
6. Canine
Mandibular
Right
27. Canine
28. First Premolar
29. Second Premolar
FACIAL

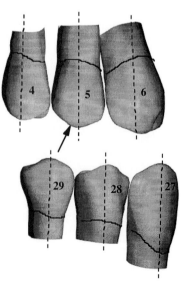

Question Frame

Examine teeth 5, 6, 27, and 28 from the facial (see preceding illustration). How many have cusps with a distal ridge longer than the mesial ridge? _____

two.. GO TO FRAME A.
three.. GO TO FRAME B.

>Frame A

From the facial, both the mandibular canine and the mandibular first premolar have cusps with a distal ridge longer than the mesial ridge. In the maxillary arch, a similar relationship exists between the mesial and distal ridges of the canine. Of the four teeth, 5, 6, 27, and 28, only tooth number 5, the maxillary first premolar, has a facial cusp with the mesial ridge longer than the distal ridge.

Permanent
Maxillary
Right
4. Second Premolar
5. First Premolar
6. Canine
Mandibular
Right
27. Canine
28. First Premolar
29. Second Premolar
FACIAL

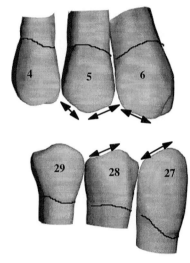

two is incorrect

>Frame B

The facial surface of the mandibular first premolar exhibits two concave areas called facial grooves. The two facial grooves are evidence of the three anatomical divisions called _____ .

Permanent
Mandibular
Right
First Premolar
FACIAL   D   M

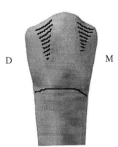

three is correct

lobes

central-facial

On the mandibular first premolar, the facial grooves are particularly evident because of the prominence of the _____ - _____ lobe.

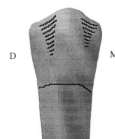

Permanent
Mandibular
Right
First Premolar
FACIAL   D   M

cervical, occlusal

The mesial and distal contact areas are broad, rounded areas located approximately at the same level in the occlusocervical direction. Occlusocervically, the proximal contacts of the mandibular first premolar are located in the middle third of the crown, usually slightly _____ to the junction of the middle and _____ thirds.

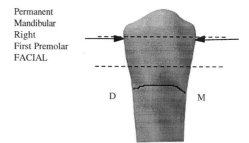

Permanent
Mandibular
Right
First Premolar
FACIAL

D   M

3.6.2   MANDIBULAR FIRST PREMOLAR: LINGUAL VIEW

occlusal

Because of the distinct lingual convergence of the crown and the reduced development of the lingual cusp, more than the lingual surface is visible from the lingual aspect of the mandibular first premolar. The surfaces visible are the lingual surface, most of the mesial and distal surfaces, and a large portion of the _____ surface.

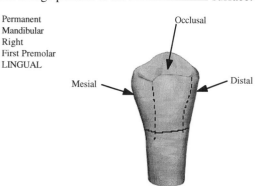

Permanent
Mandibular
Right
First Premolar
LINGUAL

Occlusal

Mesial   Distal

From the lingual view, the most visible occlusal feature of the mandibular first premolar is the well-developed _____ ridge of the facial cusp.

Permanent
Mandibular
Right
First Premolar
LINGUAL

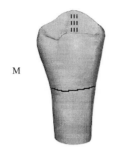

M   D

From the lingual aspect, the lingual surface of the crown includes only that part of the crown lying between the _____ and _____ _____ .

Permanent
Mandibular
Right
First Premolar
LINGUAL

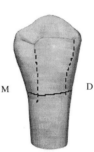

M   D

In the mesiodistal direction, the lingual surface of the mandibular first premolar is best described by which two of the following adjectives: wide, narrow, convex, flat, long?

_____ , _____

Permanent
Mandibular
Right
First Premolar
1. LINGUAL
2. OCCLUSAL

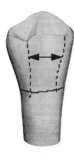
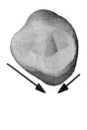

1   2

mesiolingual

Originating in the mesial fossa of the occlusal surface, a developmental groove extends lingually to separate the mesial marginal ridge from the lingual cusp. This groove, a unique feature of the mandibular first premolar, is called the _____ groove.

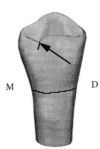

Permanent
Mandibular
Right
First Premolar
LINGUAL

M   D

lingual

From the proximal views, sometimes the tip of the facial cusp is slightly inclined toward the _____ , making it nearly centered over the root.

Permanent
Mandibular
Right
First Premolar
1. MESIAL
2. DISTAL

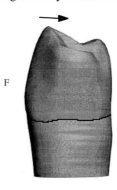
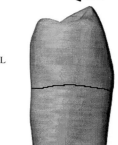

F   L   F

1   2

facial

In position in the arch (Figure 1), the first premolar has a slight facial tilt. The shape of the facial surface as seen from a proximal view appears to allow the contour of the crown to be continuous with the surrounding gingival tissue. When viewed out of the mouth, in an upright position (Figure 2), however, the facial height of contour appears accentuated by the sharp inclination of the _____ cusp.

Permanent
Mandibular
Right
1. First Premolar
2. First Premolar
MESIAL

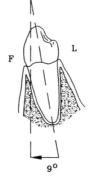
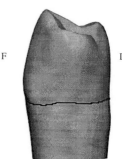

F   L   F   L

9°

1

From a proximal view in relation to the long axis of the tooth, the tip of the lingual cusp is located in a very _____ (central/lingual) position.

lingual

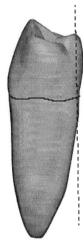

Permanent
Mandibular
Right
First Premolar
MESIAL

In the faciolingual direction, perpendicular to the long axis of the tooth, the lingual height of contour _____ (extends beyond/is in line with) the root of the mandibular first premolar.

extends beyond

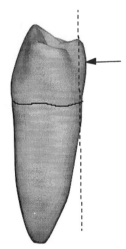

Permanent
Mandibular
Right
First Premolar
MESIAL

A key distinction between the mesial and distal surfaces of the mandibular first premolar is the degree of linguocervical inclination of the marginal ridges. Which marginal ridge more nearly parallels the slope of the lingual ridge of the facial cusp? _____

Permanent
Mandibular
Right
First Premolar
1. MESIAL
2. DISTAL

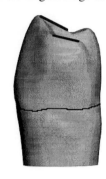   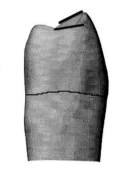

F   L   F

1   2

The cervical line is slightly curved toward the occlusal on both the mesial and distal surfaces. From which proximal aspect does the cervical line exhibit less curvature? _____

Permanent
Mandibular
Right
First Premolar
1. MESIAL
2. DISTAL

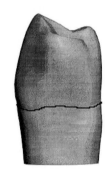   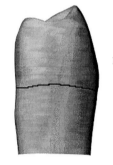

F   L   F

1   2

The features of the mandibular first premolar show a great deal of variation between different people. The prominence of the transverse ridge and the size of the lingual cusp are features which vary. For example, the model tooth representing the mandibular first premolar has a large lingual cusp, an off-center transverse ridge, and a large mesial marginal ridge. You will see other variations between people. Which drawing in this illustration shows a more prominent transverse ridge from a mesial view, Figure 1 or Figure 2? _____

Permanent
Mandibular
Right
1. First Premolar
2. First Premolar
MESIAL

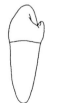   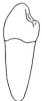

1   2

Identify the mesial marginal ridge and the transverse ridge on tooth number 28 in the illustration. The illustration shows the relationship of the mandibular first premolar to the canine and second premolar. Notice, the curve of the arch causes the mandibular first premolar to have a large mesial marginal ridge. _____ , _____

Permanent
Mandibular
Right
Canine
First Premolar
Second Premolar
OCCLUSAL

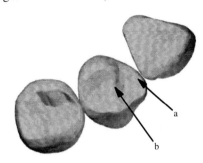

TURN TO THE NEXT PAGE AND TAKE REVIEW TEST 3.6.

a. mesial marginal ridge, b. transverse ridge

REVIEW TEST 3.6

Choose the correct statement from each pair.

1. a. Mandibular first premolars usually have no central groove.
   b. All permanent first premolars usually have no central groove.

2. a. In the facial view of the mandibular first premolar, the tip of the facial cusp is displaced slightly toward the distal from the midline of the crown.
   b. Of all the premolars you have studied so far, the mandibular first premolar has the smallest lingual cusp.

3. a. On the mandibular first premolar, the transverse ridge is made up of the lingual ridge of the facial cusp and the facial ridge of the lingual cusp.
   b. The transverse ridge of the mandibular first premolar is made up of the mesial and distal ridges of the facial cusp.

4. a. From a proximal view, in relation to the long axis of the tooth, the tip of the facial cusp is lingually located.
   b. On the mandibular first premolar, the tip of the lingual cusp is in line with the height of contour on the lingual surface.

5. The longer facial cusp ridge of the mandibular first premolar is
   a. mesial
   b. distal

6. The broader contact area on the mandibular first premolar is the
   a. mesial
   b. distal

7. The occlusal fossa of the mandibular first premolar that contains a developmental groove with a lingual extension is the
   a. mesial
   b. distal

8. The marginal ridge of the mandibular first premolar with a slope most nearly parallel to the slope of the lingual ridge of the facial cusp is the
   a. mesial
   b. distal

9. The proximal aspect showing least curvature of the cervical line is the
   a. mesial
   b. distal

CHECK YOUR ANSWERS IN APPENDIX A.

PROXIMAL CONTACTS, EMBRASURES, AND CROWN CONTOURS OF MANDIBULAR FIRST PREMOLARS

3.7.0

The proximal contacts of the mandibular first premolars are located cervical to the junction of the occlusal and middle thirds. Indicate the location of the proximal contacts in the illustration.

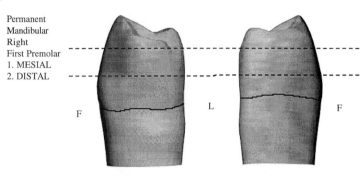

Permanent
Mandibular
Right
First Premolar
1. MESIAL
2. DISTAL

The contacts are facially located.

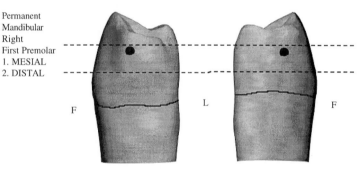

Permanent
Mandibular
Right
First Premolar
1. MESIAL
2. DISTAL

Your contacts should
be placed similar to
the ones in this
illustration.

The embrasures are named according to their location in relation to the contact. The embrasure located incisally or occlusally of the contact are called the incisal or occlusal embrasure. The embrasures located facially are called _____ embrasures, and those located lingually are called _____ _____ .

facial, lingual
embrasures

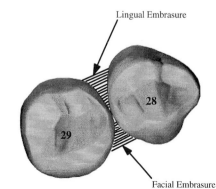

Permanent
Mandibular
Right
28 - First Premolar
29 - Second Premolar
OCCLUSAL

Lingual Embrasure

28

29

Facial Embrasure

lingual

The relative depth of the facial and lingual embrasures is determined by the location of the contact faciolingually. Because the contact is located more facially, the embrasure with the greater depth is the _____ embrasure.

Permanent
Mandibular
Right
28 - First Premolar
29 - Second Premolar
OCCLUSAL

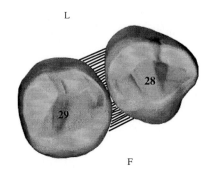

along

One of the best ways to study the contour of crowns is to focus on the height of contour. The height of contour is an imaginary line encircling the entire crown of the tooth. The proximal contacts of a tooth lie _____ (along/above) the height of contour.

Permanent
Mandibular
Right
First Premolar
MESIAL

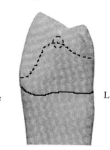

lingual, cervical

Mandibular first premolars have the height of contour in the middle third on the _____ surface, and in the _____ third on the facial surface.

Permanent
Mandibular
Right
First Premolar
MESIAL

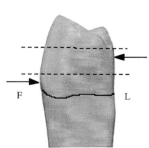

ROOT ANATOMY OF MANDIBULAR FIRST PREMOLARS

The mandibular first premolar is normally _____ -rooted.

Permanent
Mandibular
Right
First Premolar
1. FACIAL
2. MESIAL

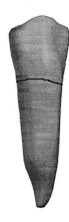
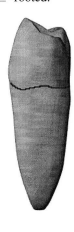

1   2

Most frequently the mesial and distal surfaces on a mandibular premolar tend to be convex in the faciolingual direction. A shallow longitudinal groove may be present on the proximal root surfaces. When present, the grooves cause the central part of these surfaces to be slightly concave or nearly flat in the faciolingual direction. Which surface (mesial or distal) generally has a more prominent root depression? _____

Permanent
Mandibular
Right
First Premolar
1. DISTAL
2. MESIAL

L   F   L

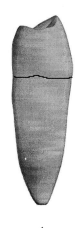
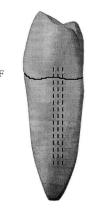

1   2

The mandibular first premolar root tends to be narrow and pointed. The illustration indicates a slight root deviation toward the _____ .

Permanent
Mandibular
Right
First Premolar
FACIAL

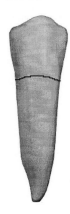

3.7.2 PULP ANATOMY OF MANDIBULAR FIRST PREMOLARS

Because of the cusp development on the mandibular first premolar, which pulp horn is usually absent or very small? _____

Permanent
Mandibular
Right
First Premolar
FACIOLINGUAL

F   L

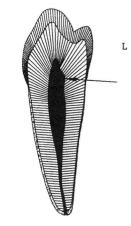

A faciolingual longitudinal section of the mandibular first premolar shows a spindle-shaped pulp canal with one horn, the _____ pulp horn.

```
Permanent
Mandibular
Right
First Premolar
FACIOLINGUAL        F                    L
```

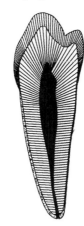

Because the mandibular premolar has a single root canal, the division between the pulp chamber and root canal is indistinct. Premolars with a single root canal have a pulp chamber with no _____ (roof/floor/walls).

```
Permanent
Mandibular
Right
First Premolar
FACIOLINGUAL        F                    L
```

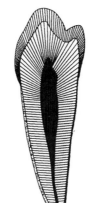

faciolingual

Similar to the root canals of the mandibular canine, the root canal of a mandibular premolar is widest in the _____ horizontal direction?

Permanent
Mandibular
Right
First Premolar
1. FACIOLINGUAL
2. MESIODISTAL

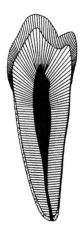
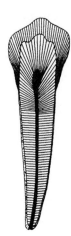

1   2

apical

A bifurcated root canal is rare in the mandibular premolars. When found, the bifurcation generally occurs in the _____ portion of the root.

Permanent
Mandibular
Right
First Premolar
FACIOLINGUAL

F   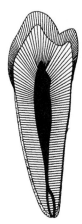   L

Occasionally, lateral branches of the root canal will be present in the apical portion of the root. These branches are called _____ _____ .

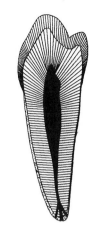

```
Permanent
Mandibular
Right
First Premolar
FACIOLINGUAL
```
F   L

Figure 1

Which figure represents the form of the pulp cavity of a mandibular first premolar as seen in faciolingual section? _____

```
Permanent
Mandibular
Right
First Premolar
PULP ANATOMY
```

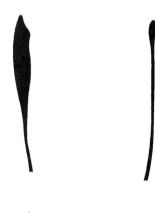

1   2

The following illustrations summarize the information about the permanent mandibular first premolar.

Permanent Mandibular Right First Premolar - Summary

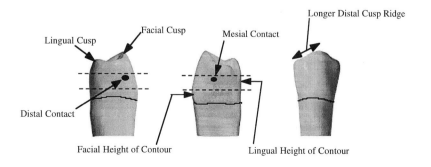

Permanent Mandibular Right First Premolar OCCLUSAL - Summary

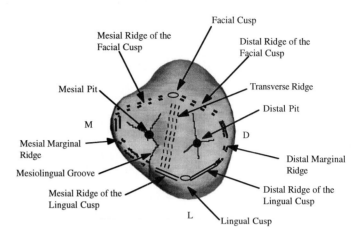

Facial Cusp

Mesial Ridge of the Facial Cusp

Distal Ridge of the Facial Cusp

Mesial Pit

Transverse Ridge

Distal Pit

M

Mesial Marginal Ridge

D

Distal Marginal Ridge

Mesiolingual Groove

Mesial Ridge of the Lingual Cusp

Distal Ridge of the Lingual Cusp

L

Lingual Cusp

Permanent
Mandibular
Right
First Premolar
1. FACIAL
2. MESIAL

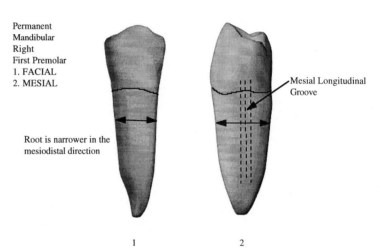

Mesial Longitudinal Groove

Root is narrower in the mesiodistal direction

1   2

Permanent
Mandibular
Right
First Premolar
1. FACIOLINGUAL
2. MESIODISTAL

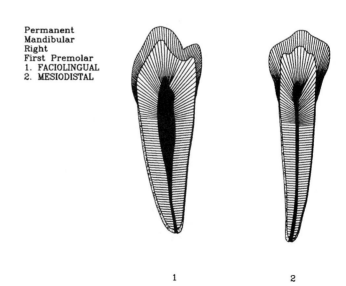

1   2

GO TO THE NEXT PAGE AND TAKE REVIEW TEST 3.7.

REVIEW TEST 3.7

1. The proximal contacts of the mandibular first premolar are located at the

    a. incisal third
    b. cervical third
    c. junction of the occlusal and middle thirds
    d. middle third

2. In the faciolingual direction the contacts are more _____ located.

    a. facially
    b. lingually

3. The mandibular first premolars have the height of contour in the middle third on the _____ surface.

    a. lingual
    b. facial

4. The mandibular first premolar has _____ roots.

    a. one
    b. two

5. Which root surface normally has the more prominent root depression?

    a. mesial
    b. distal

6. The root canal of the mandibular first premolar is widest in which direction?

    a. mesiodistal
    b. faciolingual

7. If accessory canals are present, they are usually in the _____ portion of the root.

    a. cervical
    b. middle
    c. apical

CHECK YOUR ANSWERS IN APPENDIX A.

3.8.0   MANDIBULAR SECOND PREMOLAR

five

The mandibular second premolar often shows one more lobe than the other premolars. Therefore, how many lobes would you expect to find on the mandibular second premolar? _____

Permanent
Mandibular
Right
Second Premolar
1. FACIAL
2. LINGUAL

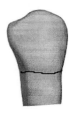
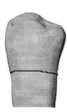

1   2

two

The facial portion of the mandibular second premolar has three lobes, and the lingual portion often has _____ lobes.

Permanent
Mandibular
Right
Second Premolar
1. FACIAL
2. LINGUAL

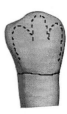
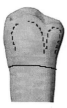

1   2

A

In the occlusal view, the mandibular second premolar is nearly square in shape with little of the lingual convergence seen on the mandibular first premolar. Which illustration is of a second premolar, A or B? _____

Permanent
Mandibular
Premolars
OCCLUSAL

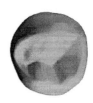
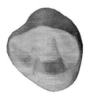

A   B

When you examine all of the permanent premolars, you see that two of the four show less amounts of lingual convergence in an occlusal view, the maxillary second premolar and the _____ second premolar. (The latter premolar also has three rather than two cusps, typically.)

Permanent
Maxillary
Right
5 - First Premolar
4 - Second Premolar
Mandibular
Right
28 - First Premolar
29 - Second Premolar

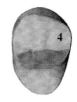

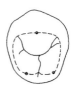

Actually, the occlusal surface of the mandibular second premolar occurs as one of three types. Each "Y," "H," and "U type," is named for its occlusal groove pattern. Figure 1 shows the _____ type, Figure 2 the _____ type, and Figure 3 the _____ type.

Permanent
Mandibular
Right
Second Premolar
OCCLUSAL

1   2   3

Of the three types of mandibular second premolars, the most common is the three-cusp or _____ type.

Permanent
Mandibular
Right
Second Premolar
OCCLUSAL

"U"   "H"   "Y"

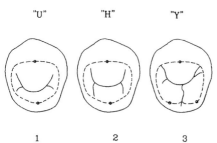

1   2   3

two

In contrast to the "Y" type, the "H" and "U" types have _____ (number) cusps.

Permanent
Mandibular
Right
Second Premolar
OCCLUSAL

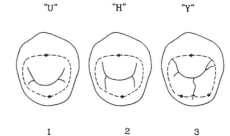

"U"   "H"   "Y"

1   2   3

"Y", "U"

On two-cusped mandibular premolars, the "H"-type groove pattern is the more common. Therefore, the most common type on mandibular second premolars is the _____ type; the least common is the _____ type.

Permanent
Mandibular
Right
Second Premolar
OCCLUSAL

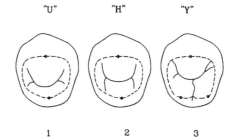

"U"   "H"   "Y"

1   2   3

lingual

When three cusps are present, which portion of the crown has two cusps? _____ (facial/lingual)

Permanent
Mandibular
Right
Second Premolar
OCCLUSAL

F

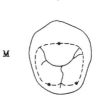

M   D

L

square

The two lingual cusps on the "Y" type result in a greater lingual development. Which one of the following terms best describes the outline of the occlusal table on the "Y" type? (circular, square, ovoid)

Permanent
Mandibular
Right
Second Premolar
OCCLUSAL

F

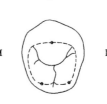

M   D

L

Because the "Y" type of groove pattern is the most common of the three types, it will be described in detail. Although the "H" and "U" types are less common, they are considered as typical specimens of the mandibular second premolar.

Of the two lingual cusps (the mesiolingual and distolingual), which is the largest? _____

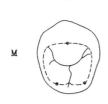

Permanent
Mandibular
Right
Second Premolar
OCCLUSAL

F

M   D

L

Arrange the three cusps of the mandibular second premolar in order according to size, largest to smallest.

Largest   _____
Next largest   _____
Smallest   _____

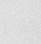

On the "Y"-type mandibular second premolar, how many triangular ridges run toward the center of the occlusal surface? _____ (The model tooth used in the illustration is representative of the "Y" type.)

Permanent
Mandibular
Right
Second Premolar
OCCLUSAL

M   D

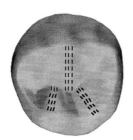

The three triangular ridges partition the occlusal table. A mesial fossa is bound mesially by the mesial marginal ridge and distally by the triangular ridges of the _____ and _____ cusps.

Permanent
Mandibular
Right
Second Premolar
OCCLUSAL

M   D

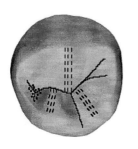

The mesial border of the distal fossa is formed by the triangular ridges of the _____ and _____ cusps.

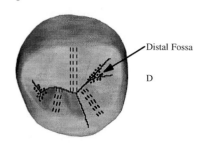

Permanent
Mandibular
Right
Second Premolar
OCCLUSAL

M

Distal Fossa

D

One of three developmental grooves, the lingual groove passes between the two lingual cusps, ending on the _____ surface.

Permanent
Mandibular
Right
Second Premolar
OCCLUSAL

M

D

Lingual Groove

The mesial groove originates at the central pit and runs in a mesiofacial direction through the mesial _____ .

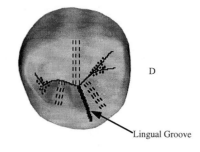

Permanent
Mandibular
Right
Second Premolar
OCCLUSAL

M

D

Mesial Groove

The distal groove originates at the central pit and runs in a distofacial direction through the _____ _____ .

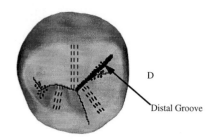

Permanent
Mandibular
Right
Second Premolar
OCCLUSAL

M

D

Distal Groove

Similar to that of the mandibular first premolar, the facial surface of the mandibular second premolar is inclined toward the lingual. Because of the increased faciolingual diameter of the second premolar, the tip of the facial cusp is located slightly toward the _____ from the faciolingual midline of the crown.

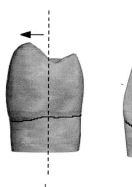
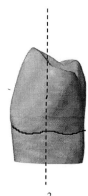

Permanent
Mandibular
Right
1. Second Premolar
2. First Premolar
MESIAL

1   2

From which proximal view of the mandibular second premolar is a greater portion of the occlusal surface visible? _____

Permanent
Mandibular
Right
Second Premolar
1. DISTAL
2. MESIAL

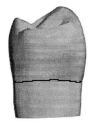
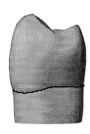

1   2

Which is the smallest cusp? _____

Permanent
Mandibular
Right
Second Premolar
LINGUAL

M

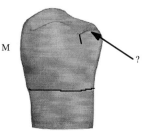

?

The three developmental grooves on the three-cusped mandibular second premolar originate at the point of common intersection called the _____ _____ .

mesial, distal, lingual

Name the three developmental grooves of the three-cusped mandibular second premolar.

1. _____
2. _____
3. _____

most common: Y, 3
less common: H, 2
least common: U, 2

Complete the following matrix by supplying the appropriate letter or numeral for each space.

PERMANENT MANDIBULAR SECOND PREMOLAR GROOVE PATTERN TYPES

	name of type	*number of cusps*
most common		
less common		
least common		

triangular

The occlusal table of the two-cusped mandibular second premolars is partitioned by two _____ ridges.

Permanent Mandibular Right Second Premolar OCCLUSAL   "U"   "H"

On the two-cusped mandibular second premolar, 43% have a transverse ridge. On the 3-cusped type, 54% do not have a transverse ridge.

central

On the "H" and "U" occlusal types, a groove separates the triangular ridges and terminates in the mesial and distal fossae. As on the maxillary premolars, this groove is called the _____ groove.

Permanent Mandibular Right Second Premolar OCCLUSAL   "U"   "H"

MANDIBULAR SECOND PREMOLAR: FACIAL VIEW

From the facial aspect most features of the mandibular second premolar are similar to the first premolar. However, there is a small difference in the length of their facial cusps. Recall that cusp length is defined as the measurement from the cusp tip to the depth of the occlusal grooves. On which of these teeth is the facial cusp slightly shorter?

Permanent
Mandibular
Right
1. Second Premolar
2. First Premolar
FACIAL

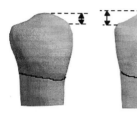

1   2

On the mandibular second premolar, the angle formed by the mesial and distal ridges of the facial cusp is less pointed. This blunter angulation is a result of the cusp tip of the second premolar being _____ (shorter/longer).

Permanent
Mandibular
Right
1. Second Premolar
2. First Premolar
FACIAL

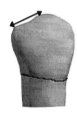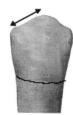

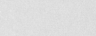

1   2

Compared to the mandibular first premolar, the position of the facial cusp of the mandibular second premolar is more toward the _____ (lingual/facial).

Permanent
Mandibular
Right
1. , 3. Second Premolar
2. , 4. First Premolar
1. , 2. OCCLUSAL
3. , 4. MESIAL

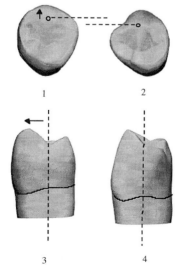

1   2

3   4

3.8.2

MANDIBULAR SECOND PREMOLAR: LINGUAL VIEW

The lingual aspects of the mandibular first and second premolars are distinctly different. On the illustration of the lingual aspect, indicate which portion of the second premolar is the lingual surface by sketching in the mesiolingual and distolingual line angles.

Permanent
Mandibular
Right
Second Premolar
1. LINGUAL
2. OCCLUSAL

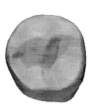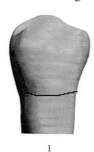

1   2

Compare your drawing with this illustration

Permanent
Mandibular
Right
1. Second Premolar
2. First Premolar
LINGUAL

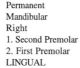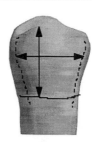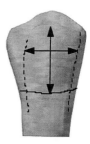

1   2

Your description should indicate that the lingual surface of the second premolar is wider in the mesiodistal direction and longer in the occlusocervical direction.

In your own words, describe the size of the lingual surface of the mandibular second premolar as compared to the lingual surface of the mandibular first premolar.

lingual

The lingual surface of the mandibular second premolar is marked by a groove running between the cusps. This groove is called the _____ groove.

Permanent
Mandibular
Right
Second Premolar
LINGUAL

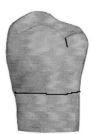

mesiolingual, distolingual

The lingual groove separates the two lingual cusps, the larger _____ cusp and the smaller _____ cusp.

MANDIBULAR SECOND PREMOLAR:
PROXIMAL VIEW

Of the three cusps on the mandibular second premolar, is the widest also the longest? _____ (yes/no)

yes

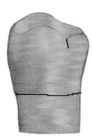

Permanent
Mandibular
Right
Second Premolar
LINGUAL

The greater lingual development on the mandibular second premolar causes the mesial and distal marginal ridges to be nearly

a

a. perpendicular to the long axis of the tooth
b. parallel to the lingual ridge of the facial cusp

Permanent
Mandibular
Right
Second Premolar
1. MESIAL
2. DISTAL

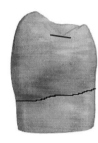 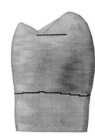

1   2

In place in the mouth, the mandibular first premolar is tipped slightly to the facial (as is the mandibular canine). However, the second premolar, and the mandibular teeth posterior to it, are tipped toward the lingual.

in line

The contours of the premolar crowns become continuous with the surrounding gingival tissue in this way. Also, this makes the occlusal planes of the premolars more _____ (in line/out of line).

Permanent
Mandibular
Right
1. Second Premolar
2. First Premolar
MESIAL

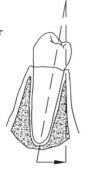 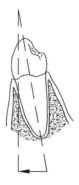

1   2

toward the lingual

From an occlusal view, the location of the central pit in a faciolingual direction, is _____ (central/toward the lingual).

Permanent
Mandibular
Right
Second Premolar
OCCLUSAL

M   D

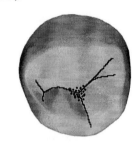

distal

In the mesiodistal direction, the central pit is displaced slightly toward the _____ (mesial/distal).

Permanent
Mandibular
Right
Second Premolar
OCCLUSAL

M   D

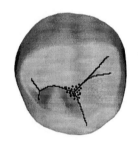

distal

On the mandibular second premolar, which marginal ridge is at a lower level in the occlusocervical direction? _____

Permanent
Mandibular
Right
Second Premolar
1. MESIAL
2. DISTAL

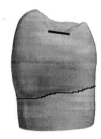 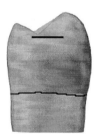

1   2

molar

In the mandibular arch, the premolars somewhat resemble either a canine or a molar. Of these two classes of teeth, the mandibular second premolar more closely resembles a _____ .

Permanent
Mandibular
Right
27 - Canine
28 - First Premolar
29 - Second Premolar
30 - Molar
OCCLUSAL

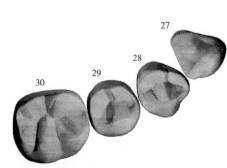

Indicate whether each of the diagrams represents a maxillary or mandibular, first or second premolar. (All are drawn with crowns toward the top of the page even if they are maxillary.)

Figure 1 _____ _____ premolar
Figure 2 _____ _____ premolar
Figure 3 _____ _____ premolar
Figure 4 _____ _____ premolar

Permanent
Premolars

F   1   2   L

3   4

The answers to the previous frame are given in universal code numbers. Translate each code number to proper tooth name.

In position in the mandibular arch, the mandibular second premolar has its crown tipped slightly toward the _____ (facial/lingual).

The second premolar is tipped to the lingual, whereas the crown of the mandibular first premolar is tipped toward the facial.

TURN TO THE NEXT PAGE AND TAKE REVIEW TEST 3.8.

Figure 1 - 29; Figure 2 - 12; Figure 3 - 13; Figure 4 - 28

29 - Permanent mandibular right second premolar
12 - Permanent maxillary left first premolar
13 - Permanent maxillary left second premolar
28 - permanent mandibular right first premolar

lingual

REVIEW TEST 3.8

Place an X in the square that matches the left hand column with the top row.

Mandibular Second Premolar	*Mesial*	*Distal*
Occlusal fossae located at the	☐	☐
Larger of the two lingual cusps	☐	☐
Marginal ridge at lower level	☐	☐
Central pit displaced toward the	☐	☐

Use this diagram for questions 1 through 4.

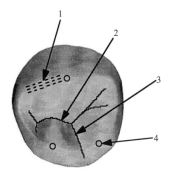

Identify each of the four features.

1. a. mesial ridge of the buccal cusp
   b. distal ridge of the buccal cusp

2. a. central groove
   b. mesial groove

3. a. distolingual groove
   b. lingual groove

4. a. distolingual cusp
   b. distal cusp

5. Which of the following describe the mandibular second premolar as compared to the mandibular first premolar?

   a. composed of five lobes most frequently
   b. most frequently has two lingual cusps
   c. has a less well-developed lingual cusp
   d. has a slightly shorter facial cusp
   e. most frequently has a single highly developed transverse ridge
   f. tipped toward the facial
   g. tipped toward the lingual

CHECK YOUR ANSWERS IN APPENDIX A.

PROXIMAL CONTACTS, EMBRASURES, AND CROWN CONTOURS OF MANDIBULAR SECOND PREMOLARS

Both the mesial and distal contacts on each of the eight premolars are located occlusocervically, just cervical to the junction of the occlusal and middle thirds. Therefore, the contact areas on the second premolars are in the _____ third of the crown.

Permanent
Maxillary
Left
11 - Canine
12 - First Premolar
13 - Second Premolar
14 - First Molar
Mandibular
Left
22 - Canine
21 - First Premolar
20 - Second Premolar
19 - First Molar
FACIAL

It is important to study the curved contours of crowns because there are many occasions for the dentist to operate on these contours in restoring or replacing crown surfaces. There is clinical evidence that smooth and properly contoured (not too convex) crown surfaces promote tooth cleaning and gingival health.

The curved contours of the crown are normally continuous with the gingiva, as shown in the drawing. This form seems to help make the _____ (cervical/occlusal) areas of the teeth cleanable.

Permanent
Mandibular
Right
Second Premolar
MESIAL

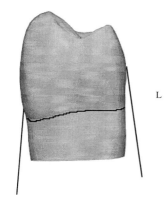

F   L

1/2

The amount of contour on the facial surfaces of mandibular posteriors is similar to that on the facial surfaces of the maxillary posterior teeth. Therefore, the facial contour of the mandibular second premolar measures approximately _____ mm.

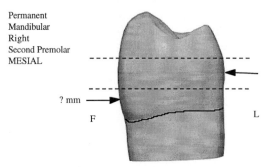

Permanent
Mandibular
Right
Second Premolar
MESIAL

? mm

F   L

1

The mandibular posterior teeth have lingual contours that measure nearly double those of the maxillaries. The amount of contour on the lingual surface of mandibular second premolars approaches _____ mm in measurement.

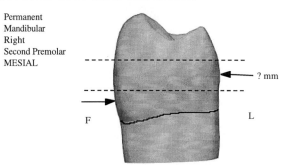

Permanent
Mandibular
Right
Second Premolar
MESIAL

? mm

F   L

lingual

When examining the mandibular second premolar in position in the oral cavity, the observed lingual height of contour may appear closer to the occlusal surface than the anatomical contour would suggest. This is because the mandibular second premolar (and the mandibular molars) are inclined, so that their crowns are tilted toward the _____ (facial/lingual/distal).

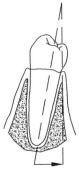

Permanent
Mandibular
Right
Second Premolar
MESIAL

The height of contour is located in the middle third on the lingual surface of all maxillary and mandibular _____ (anterior/posterior) teeth.

posterior

In the region of the posterior teeth, the lingual embrasures are deeper than facial embrasures. This is because the proximal contacts between posterior teeth are toward the _____ (facial/lingual) surface in the faciolingual dimension.

facial

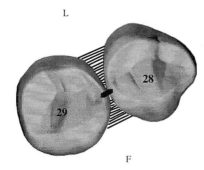

Permanent
Mandibular
Right
28 - First Premolar
29 - Second Premolar
OCCLUSAL

L

F

The embrasures are named according to their location in relation to the contact. The embrasures located incisally or occlusally of the contact are called the incisal or occlusal embrasures. The embrasure located facially are called _____ embrasures and those located lingually are called _____ embrasures.

facial, lingual

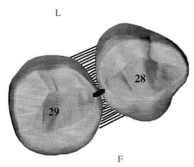

Permanent
Mandibular
Right
28 - First Premolar
29 - Second Premolar
OCCLUSAL

L

F

ROOT ANATOMY OF THE MANDIBULAR
SECOND PREMOLARS

3.9.1

The mandibular second premolar is normally _____ -rooted.

single

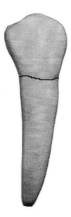

Permanent
Mandibular
Right
Second Premolar
FACIAL

faciolingual

Most frequently the mesial and distal surfaces on a mandibular second premolar tend to be convex in the faciolingual direction. A shallow longitudinal groove may be present on the proximal root surfaces. When present, the grooves cause the central part of these surfaces to be slightly concave or nearly flat in the _____ direction.

Permanent
Mandibular
Right
Second Premolar
MESIAL

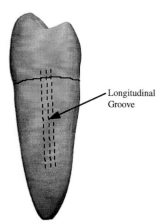

Longitudinal Groove

larger

The root of the mandibular second premolar is similar in form to the mandibular first premolar, but is _____ (larger/smaller) in all directions.

Permanent
Mandibular
Right
Second Premolar
FACIAL

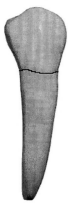

distal

The apex on the permanent mandibular second premolar may have a slight deviation toward the molars. The deviation of the apex is, therefore, in the _____ direction.

Permanent
Mandibular
Right
Second Premolar
FACIAL

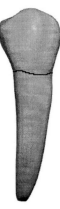

Review of Premolar Roots: Question Frame

The mandibular premolar root tends to have a more oval shape as seen from a cross section (Figure 3), when longitudinal grooves are not present. The longitudinal curvature of the facial surface is irregular, having both convexities and concavities. The lingual, mesial, and distal surfaces are more evenly contoured in the longitudinal direction and tend to be flat or very slightly convex. The longitudinal curvatures result in a root with a distinct taper on all four surfaces and an apex more pointed than the apexes on the single-rooted premolars in the maxillary arch. Considering the root forms on the premolars, in which arch could a premolar be more easily rotated in its alveolus? _____

Mandibular arch. . . . . GO TO FRAME B.
Maxillary arch . . . . GO TO FRAME A.

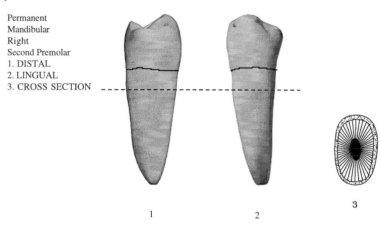

Permanent
Mandibular
Right
Second Premolar
1. DISTAL
2. LINGUAL
3. CROSS SECTION

1   2   3

>Frame A

Recall that the maxillary arch includes the bifurcated first premolar which would be tricky to rotate.

RETURN TO THE QUESTION FRAME AND ANSWER AGAIN.

maxillary arch is
incorrect

>Frame B

Here is a comparison of the root structures of the premolars in each arch.

Maxillary arch

Frequently bifurcated (especially first premolars)
Broad in the faciolingual direction
Distinct longitudinal grooves

Mandibular arch

Single-rooted
Tends to be oval in horizontal section
More slender than those of the maxillary arch
Tapered in longitudinal direction
Shallow or no longitudinal grooves

The root forms of the premolars in the maxillary arch would be generally resistant to rotation in their alveoli. In the mandibular arch, the root forms of the premolars would tend to allow rotation.

mandibular arch is
correct

longitudinal groove

On the mandibular premolars, the facial and lingual surfaces are smoothly convex. The mesial and distal surfaces may show a horizontal curvature with a slight central concavity created by the _____ .

Permanent
Mandibular
Right
Second Premolar
1. FACIAL
2. CROSS SECTION

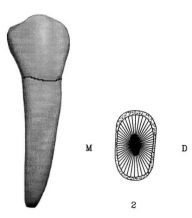

M   D

2

3.9.2 PULP ANATOMY OF MANDIBULAR SECOND PREMOLARS

This is an illustration of the faciolingual, mesiodistal, and cross section of the mandibular second premolar. Notice the outline form of the root canal of the two longitudinal sections. Being able to recognize the two forms will help you identify the teeth in radiographs. It will also assist with radiographic identification of rotated premolars.

Permanent
Mandibular
Right
Second Premolar
1. FACIOLINGUAL
2. MESIODISTAL
3. CROSS SECTION

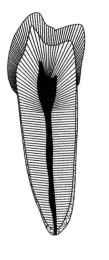
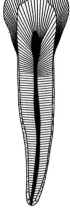
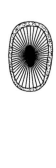

1   2   3

Identify the outline of the mesiodistal view of the root canal.

This would be the view normally seen in radiographs.

Permanent
Mandibular
Second Premolar
Pulp Outlines

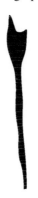

Fig. 1   Fig. 2

How many pulp horns are present on the mandibular second premolar?

Permanent
Mandibular
Right
Second Premolar
FACIOLINGUAL

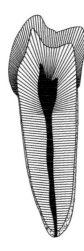

Permanent
Mandibular
Right
Second Premolar
CROSS SECTION

The cross section indicates a generally _____ (oval/round) pulp configuration.

TURN TO THE NEXT PAGE AND TAKE REVIEW TEST 3.9.

REVIEW TEST 3.9

Write in the correct word(s) on the line that matches the left-hand column with the top row.

Pulp of Premolars	*Maxillary First Premolar*	*Mandibular First Premolar*	*Maxillary Second Premolar*	*Mandibular Second Premolar*
Most common number of root canals.	_____	_____	_____	_____
If the tooth has a less common number of root canals, what number of canals would that be?	_____	_____	_____	_____
Number of pulp horns in pulp chamber.	_____	_____	_____	_____
Names of usual root canals (if more than one).	_____	_____	_____	_____
Universal code numbers	_____	_____	_____	_____

The following illustrations summarize the permanent mandibular second premolars.

Permanent Mandibular Right Second Premolar - Summary

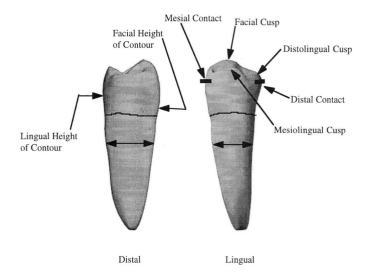

Mesial Contact Facial Cusp
Facial Height of Contour
Distolingual Cusp
Distal Contact
Lingual Height of Contour
Mesiolingual Cusp

Distal   Lingual

Permanent Mandibular Right Second Premolar OCCLUSAL - Summary

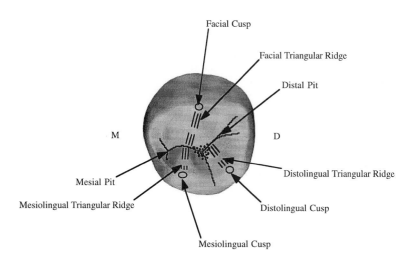

Facial Cusp

Facial Triangular Ridge

Distal Pit

M   D

Mesial Pit

Distolingual Triangular Ridge

Mesiolingual Triangular Ridge

Distolingual Cusp

Mesiolingual Cusp

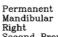

Permanent Mandibular Right Second Premolar
1. FACIOLINGUAL
2. MESIODISTAL
3. CROSS SECTION

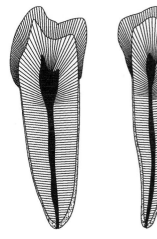

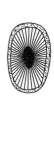

1   2   3

1. When the premolars have a single root canal, that root canal is narrower in which direction?

   a. mesiodistal   c. occlusocervical
   b. faciolingual   d. sideways

2. The mesial and distal contacts of the mandibular second premolars is located

   a. in the occlusal third
   b. at the junction of the occlusal and middle thirds
   c. in the middle third
   d. in the cervical third

3. The height of contour on the facial surface of the mandibular second premolar measures approximately

   a. 1/2 mm   c. 1 1/2 mm
   b. 1 mm   d. 2 mm

4. The height of contour on the lingual surface of the mandibular second premolar is located in the

   a. cervical third
   b. middle third
   c. occlusal third

5. The lingual height of contour on tooth #20 measures approximately

   a. 1/2 mm   c. 1 1/2 mm
   b. 1 mm   d. 2 mm

6. The mandibular second premolars are inclined

   a. facially   c. distally
   b. lingually   d. mesially

7. Which embrasures are the deeper embrasures?

   a. facial
   b. lingual
   c. occlusal

8. The mandibular second premolar is usually

   a. single-rooted
   b. bifurcated
   c. trifurcated

9. A shallow _____ groove may be present on the proximal root surfaces of the mandibular second premolar.

   a. horizontal
   b. longitudinal

10. The universal code numbers for the mandibular second premolars are

   a. 21 and 28
   b. 20 and 29
   c. 19 and 30
   d. 22 and 27

CHECK YOUR ANSWERS IN APPENDIX A.

4

Permanent Molars

ERUPTION OF THE MOLARS

The eruption of the permanent molars is related to the growth and development of the maxilla and mandible. Since the permanent incisors, canines, and premolars succeed the primary dentition, the permanent molars erupt in positions _____ (anterior/posterior) to the original positions of the primary dentition.

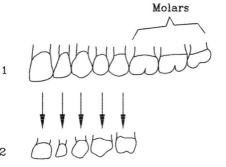

1. Permanent
2. Primary
Maxillary
Left Quadrant
FACIAL

The permanent teeth replacing the primary dentition are called succedaneous teeth. Permanent molars are called _____ teeth.

primary maxillary
second molar

The permanent first molars are the first permanent teeth to erupt. At the time of eruption, the permanent maxillary first molar is in contact mesially with the

_____ _____ _____ _____ .

(dentition)   (arch)   (tooth)

1. Permanent
2. Primary
Maxillary
Left Quadrant
FACIAL

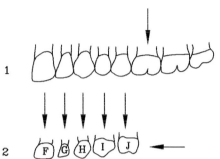

permanent maxillary
second premolar

After the eruption of the permanent dentition, the permanent maxillary first molar is in contact mesially with the _____ _____ _____ _____ .

(dentition)   (arch)   (tooth)

Permanent
Maxillary
Left Quadrant
FACIAL

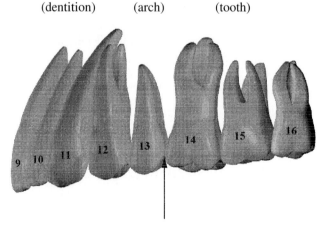

a. six;
b. mandibular

The eruption sequence of the permanent dentition was discussed in Chapter 1. Check your recall by answering these questions.

a. At what age, approximately, do the permanent first molars erupt? _____

b. In which arch does the permanent first molar usually erupt first? _____

1. 3;
2. 14

1. What is the universal code number for the permanent maxillary right first molar?
   _____

2. What is the universal code number for the permanent maxillary left first molar?
   _____

On molar teeth, each lobe is represented by a cusp. Both the permanent maxillary first molar and the permanent mandibular first molar have _____ (number) lobes. (The cusps are indicated with circles in the illustration.)

five

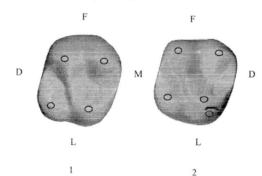

Permanent
1. Maxillary
2. Mandibular
Right
First Molar
OCCLUSAL

MAXILLARY FIRST MOLAR: OCCLUSAL VIEW

4.1.1

There is a great deal of variation in the development of the cusp of Carabelli on the mesiolingual surface of the mesiolingual cusp of the maxillary first molar. It may be completely absent, appear as a groove, or as a cusp. For this reason, the maxillary first molar may be thought of as having only _____ major cusps.

four

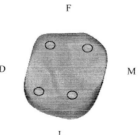

Permanent
Maxillary
Right
First Molar
1. Four Cusps
2. Five Cusps
OCCLUSAL

The two facial cusps of the maxillary first molar are named the _____ cusp and the _____ cusp.

mesiofacial
(mesiobuccal),
distofacial
(distobuccal)

Permanent
Maxillary
Right
First Molar
OCCLUSAL

mesiolingual,
distolingual

The two lingual cusps are called the _____ cusp and the _____ cusp.

Permanent
Maxillary
Right
First Molar
OCCLUSAL

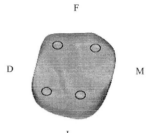

mesiolingual

When highly developed, the fifth cusp of the permanent maxillary first molar (the cusp of Carabelli) is seen lingual to the _____ cusp.

Permanent
Maxillary
Right
First Molar
OCCLUSAL

facial

The occlusal surface of the maxillary first molar varies a good deal from person to person. The occlusal outline may appear square (Figure 1), rhomboidal (Figure 2), or quadrilateral (Figure 3). This means that, unlike any other tooth in the permanent dentition, the mesiodistal width at the lingual is equal to (and at times slightly greater than) the width of the _____ .

Permanent
Maxillary
Right
First Molar
OCCLUSAL
1. Square
2. Rhomboidal
3. Quadrilateral

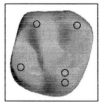
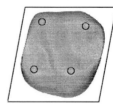
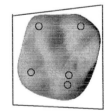

When the occlusal outline is rhomboidal, the junctions of which sides (facial, lingual, mesial, distal) of the rhomboid form acute angles? _____ and _____ , _____ and _____ .

Permanent
Maxillary
Right
First Molar
OCCLUSAL

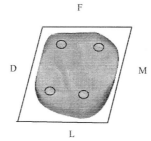

There are several major features that characterize the occlusal view of the maxillary first molar:

1. Lines connecting the cusp tips of the three largest cusps form a triangle.
2. The faciolingual diameter is equal to or greater than the mesiodistal width.
3. There is usually a pronounced oblique ridge from the distofacial cusp to the mesiolingual cusp.
4. The distolingual cusp is less developed than the three larger cusps.
5. A small fifth cusp, the cusp of Carabelli, is frequently present.

Each of these will be discussed in turn.

Permanent
Maxillary
Right
First Molar
OCCLUSAL

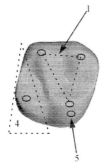
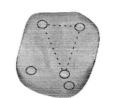
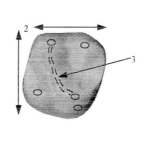

What are the names of the three major cusps that form a triangle if lines are drawn to connect their cusp tips? _____ , _____ , and _____ .

Permanent
Maxillary
Right
First Molar
OCCLUSAL

b. mesiolingual

Of the three major cusps on the maxillary first molar, which is the widest mesiodistally?

_____

a. mesiofacial
b. mesiolingual

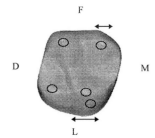

Permanent
Maxillary
Right
First Molar
OCCLUSAL

---

mesiodistal

Maxillary molars have crowns with a faciolingual size that is equal to or greater than the _____ width of the crown.

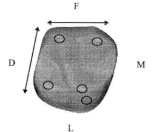

Permanent
Maxillary
Right
First Molar
OCCLUSAL

---

triangular

Maxillary molars have a characteristic oblique ridge. An oblique ridge is the union of two ridges running obliquely across the occlusal surface. On the maxillary first molar, the oblique ridge is made up of the distal ridge of the mesiolingual cusp and the _____ ridge of the distofacial cusp.

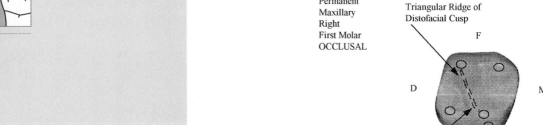

Permanent
Maxillary
Right
First Molar
OCCLUSAL

Triangular Ridge of
Distofacial Cusp

Distal Ridge of
Mesiolingual Cusp

maxillary, distofacial,
mesiolingual

Oblique ridges are found only on the molar teeth in one arch and running in the same direction. Therefore, oblique ridges are found only on the molars of the _____ arch and always run between the _____ cusp and the _____ cusp.

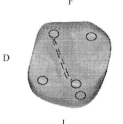

Permanent
Maxillary
Right
First Molar
OCCLUSAL

F · D · M · L

Complete the following list of the five cusps of the maxillary first molar in the order of their size, largest to smallest (mesiodistal measurement).

a. mesiolingual
b. _____
c. _____
d. _____
e. cusp of Carabelli

b. mesiofacial
c. distofacial
d. distolingual

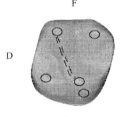

Permanent
Maxillary
Right
First Molar
OCCLUSAL

F · D · M · L

On the illustration of the maxillary right first molar, sketch the path of the oblique ridge.

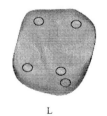

Permanent
Maxillary
Right
First Molar
OCCLUSAL

F · D · M · L

Compare your work with the drawing in this frame.

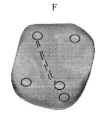

Permanent
Maxillary
Right
First Molar
OCCLUSAL

F · D · M · L

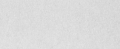

The smaller distolingual cusp of the maxillary first molar forms somewhat of a shelf that is lower in elevation than the rest of the occlusal surface. This triangular shelf has one side that is distolingual to and parallel with the _____ (oblique/marginal) ridge.

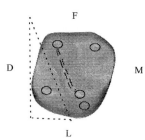

Permanent
Maxillary
Right
First Molar
OCCLUSAL

To review, complete the following list of the three major characteristics of the occlusal view of the maxillary first molar.

1. _____ .
2. _____ .
3. _____ .
4. The distolingual cusp is less developed than the three larger cusps and forms a triangular area distolingual to the oblique ridge.
5. The small fifth cusp is frequently present.

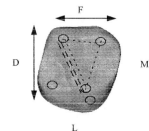

Permanent
Maxillary
Right
First Molar
OCCLUSAL

Name the small fifth cusp which is often present on the permanent maxillary first molar.

_____ _____ _____ .

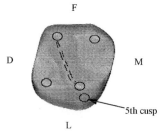

Permanent
Maxillary
Right
First Molar
OCCLUSAL

5th cusp

The facial ridges of the two facial cusps descend in the cervical direction to become part of the _____ _____ .

facial surface

Permanent
Maxillary
Right
First Molar
OCCLUSAL

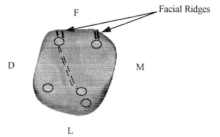

The lingual ridges of the two facial cusps are triangular ridges; therefore, they descend to the central area of the _____ _____ .

occlusal surface

Permanent
Maxillary
Right
First Molar
OCCLUSAL

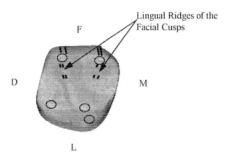

Keeping in mind the rules for naming ridges and the cusps involved, name the four ridges that form the faciocclusal line angle of the maxillary first molar _____ _____ _____ _____ .

mesial and distal ridges of the mesiofacial cusp; mesial and distal ridges of the distofacial cusp

Permanent
Maxillary
Right
First Molar
OCCLUSAL

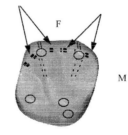

a. distal marginal
ridge; b. distal ridge of
the distolingual cusp;
c. mesial ridge of the
distolingual cusp;
d. mesial ridge of the
mesiolingual cusp;
e. mesial marginal
ridge

Name the ridges labeled in the drawing.

a. _____

b. _____

c. _____

d. _____

e. _____

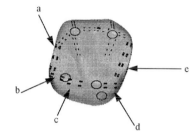

Permanent
Maxillary
Right
First Molar
OCCLUSAL

---

occlusal surface (table)

On the maxillary first molar mesial and distal ridges of the cusps, the mesial marginal ridge and the distal marginal ridge form the boundary of the _____ _____ .

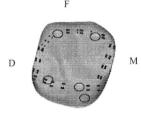

Permanent
Maxillary
Right
First Molar
OCCLUSAL

---

three

The ridges crossing the occlusal surface of the maxillary first molar divide that surface into _____ (number) fossae.

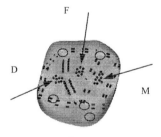

Permanent
Maxillary
Right
First Molar
OCCLUSAL

The fossae on either side of the central fossa are called the mesial and distal fossa. Therefore, the oblique ridge separates the _____ fossa from the _____ fossa.

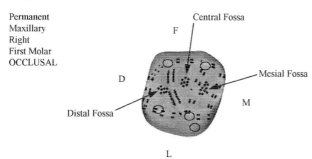

Permanent
Maxillary
Right
First Molar
OCCLUSAL

Central Fossa
F
Mesial Fossa
D
M
Distal Fossa
L

The lingual ridge of the mesiofacial cusp and the facial ridge of the mesiolingual cusp separate the central fossa from the _____ fossa.

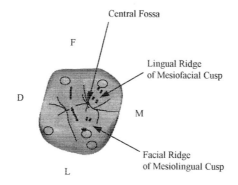

Permanent
Maxillary
Right
First Molar
OCCLUSAL

Central Fossa
F
Lingual Ridge
of Mesiofacial Cusp
D
M
Facial Ridge
of Mesiolingual Cusp
L

Within each of the three fossae, a pointed depression (called a pit) is found at the intersection of two or more developmental _____ .

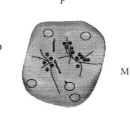

Permanent
Maxillary
Right
First Molar
OCCLUSAL

F
D
M
L

A. central; B. mesial;
C. distal

The occlusal pits of the maxillary first molar are named for the fossa in which they are found. The pits labeled A, B, and C are the _____ pit, _____ pit, and _____ pit.

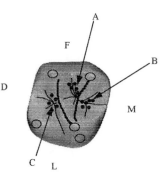

Permanent
Maxillary
Right
First Molar
OCCLUSAL

facial

The coalescence of the mesiofacial and distofacial lobes is marked by the facial groove which originates at the central pit and runs in the _____ direction.

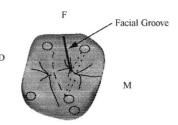

Permanent
Maxillary
Right
First Molar
OCCLUSAL

distal

The oblique ridge, if highly developed, is not crossed by a groove (Figure 1). However, if the oblique ridge is not as prominent (Figure 2), both the mesial and distal grooves originate at the central pit and terminate at the mesial and distal pits. The mesial and distal grooves together form the central groove. Which part of the central groove may cross the oblique ridge? _____

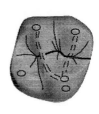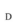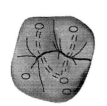

Permanent
Maxillary
Right
First Molar
OCCLUSAL

1 2

The union of the two ridges forming the oblique ridge is relatively complete. Because the distal groove may or may not cross the oblique ridge, the distal groove is often separated into two parts.

Of the mesial and distal developmental grooves which is more distinct? _____

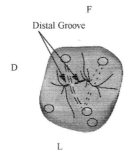

Permanent
Maxillary
Right
First Molar
OCCLUSAL

F

Distal Groove

D

M

L

The mesial and distal grooves form the two parts of the central groove. For the maxillary first molar, the term "central groove" refers to the one running in the mesiodistal direction between the _____ _____ and the _____ _____ .

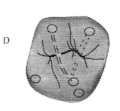

Permanent
Maxillary
Right
First Molar
OCCLUSAL

F

D

M

L

In addition to the mesial groove, the mesial fossa contains three grooves that are confluent at the mesial pit: the mesiofacial triangular groove, the mesiolingual triangular groove, and the mesial marginal groove.

The grooves marked A, B, and C are

A. _____ _____ .
B. _____ _____ .
C. _____ _____ .

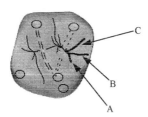

Permanent
Maxillary
Right
First Molar
OCCLUSAL

C

B

A

distolingual

Five grooves run through the distal fossa. One of these is the distal groove. The longest, most distinct is the distolingual groove. It extends onto the lingual surface and separates the mesiolingual cusp from the _____ cusp.

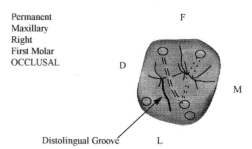

Permanent
Maxillary
Right
First Molar
OCCLUSAL

Distolingual Groove

A. distofacial triangular; B. distal marginal; C. distolingual triangular

The grooves (labeled A, B, and C) originate at the distal pit and are named similar to the corresponding grooves in the mesial fossa; these are the

A. _____ _____ groove,
B. _____ _____ groove, and the
C. _____ _____ groove.

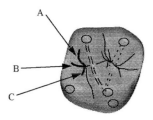

Permanent
Maxillary
Right
First Molar
OCCLUSAL

---

is

The accessory fifth cusp of the maxillary first molar is separated from the mesiolingual cusp by the mesiolingual developmental groove. The mesiolingual developmental groove _____ (is/is not) within the occlusal surface.

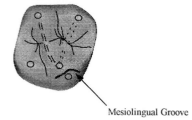

Permanent
Maxillary
Right
First Molar
OCCLUSAL

Mesiolingual Groove

The mesiolingual cusp of the maxillary first molar is separated from the distolingual cusp by the _____ groove and from the fifth cusp by the _____ groove.

Permanent
Maxillary
Right
First Molar
OCCLUSAL

F

D   M

L

TURN TO THE NEXT PAGE AND TAKE REVIEW TEST 4.1.

distolingual,
mesiolingual (in that
order)

REVIEW TEST 4.1

Place an X on the lines that match the left-hand column with the top row.

	Mesiofacial	*Mesiolingual*	*Distolingual*	*Distofacial*
Cusp with widest mesiodistal measurement	_____	_____	_____	_____
Two cusps joined by oblique ridge	_____	_____	_____	_____
The cusp which is least developed of the four major cusps	_____	_____	_____	_____
Cusp nearest the cusp of Carabelli	_____	_____	_____	_____
Cusps with ridges that surround the central fossa	_____	_____	_____	_____

1. Select the *true* statement.

   a. At the time of eruption, the permanent maxillary first molar is in contact mesially with the permanent maxillary second premolar.
   b. From the occlusal aspect of a rhomboid-shaped maxillary first molar, the mesiofacial angle of the rhomboid shape is often acute.

2. Which of the following statements is *more correct*?

   a. The permanent maxillary first molar has three lobes.
   b. An oblique ridge is found only on maxillary molars and always runs between the mesiolingual and distofacial cusps.

3. Select the *true* statement.

   a. On the permanent maxillary first molar, the mesial groove is usually more distinct than the distal groove.
   b. The occlusal fossae of the permanent maxillary first molar are called the mesial, distal, central, and lingual fossae.

4. The faciocclusal line angle of the maxillary first molar is formed by the

   a. mesial and distal ridges of the mesiofacial and distofacial cusps.
   b. Mesial and distal ridges of the mesiofacial cusp and the mesial ridge of the distofacial cusp.

5. Here is an exercise to help you name the grooves on the occlusal portion of the maxillary first molar.

   Write in the names of the lettered grooves as shown in the illustration.

   a. ⎯⎯⎯⎯
   b. ⎯⎯⎯⎯
   c. ⎯⎯⎯⎯
   d. ⎯⎯⎯⎯
   e. ⎯⎯⎯⎯
   f. ⎯⎯⎯⎯
   g. ⎯⎯⎯⎯
   b & g. ⎯⎯⎯⎯

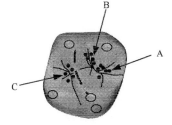

6. Write in the names of the lettered fossae as shown in the illustration.

   A. ⎯⎯⎯⎯
   B. ⎯⎯⎯⎯
   C. ⎯⎯⎯⎯

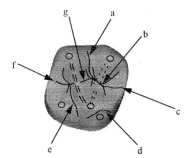

7. Write in the names of the lettered ridges as shown in the illustration.

   A. ⎯⎯⎯⎯
   B. ⎯⎯⎯⎯
   C. ⎯⎯⎯⎯
   D. ⎯⎯⎯⎯
   E. ⎯⎯⎯⎯
   F. ⎯⎯⎯⎯

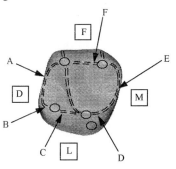

CHECK YOUR ANSWERS IN APPENDIX A.

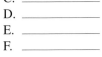

4.2.0

trapezoid

MAXILLARY FIRST MOLAR: FACIAL VIEW

In general, the outline of the facial view of the maxillary first molar is closest to the _____ shape. (circle/trapezoid/square)

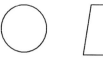

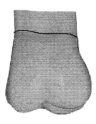

---

facial

Originating at the central pit and emerging from between the two facial cusps is the _____ groove.

Permanent
Maxillary
Right First Molar
1. OCCLUSAL
2. FACIAL

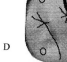

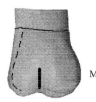

1   2

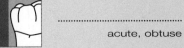

acute, obtuse

The intersection of the mesial and facial surfaces tends to form an _____ angle, while the intersection of the facial and distal surfaces forms an _____ angle.

Permanent
Maxillary
Right First Molar
1. OCCLUSAL
2. FACIAL

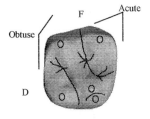

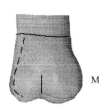

1   2

From a facial view, a portion of the distal surface can be seen, particularly on those maxillary first molars with a rhomboidal occlusal surface.

Permanent
Maxillary
Right
First Molar
FACIAL

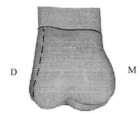

D   M

The facial groove terminates in a dip in the facial contour occlusocervically in the _____ third of the crown.

Permanent
Maxillary
Right
First Molar
FACIAL

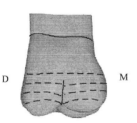

D   M

Facial Groove

As the facial groove progresses in the cervical direction from the occlusal, it gradually becomes _____ (more/less) distinct.

Permanent
Maxillary
Right
First Molar
FACIAL

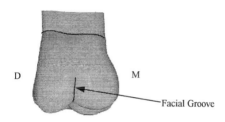

D   M

The terminal end of the facial groove is sometimes marked by a small pointed pit. What is the logical name for that pit? _____ _____

Permanent
Maxillary
Right
First Molar
FACIAL

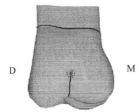

D   M

facial groove

Compare the mesiodistal contour of the facial surface at (a) with (b) in the middle third. The difference in shape is the concavity caused by the _____ _____ .

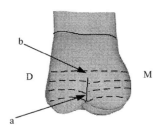

Permanent
Maxillary
Right
First Molar
FACIAL

---

facial ridge

The convexity on either side of the facial groove is formed by the _____ _____ of each facial cusp.

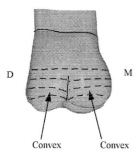

Permanent
Maxillary
Right
First Molar
FACIAL

---

convex

At the height of contour (mesiodistal direction), the form of the facial surface is _____ .

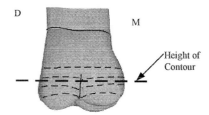

Permanent
Maxillary
Right
First Molar
FACIAL

---

mesiofacial

Of the two facial cusps on the maxillary first molar, which cusp is wider mesiodistally? _____

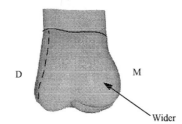

Permanent
Maxillary
Right
First Molar
FACIAL

In the "V"-shaped concavity between the distal ridge of the mesiofacial cusp and the mesial ridge of the distofacial cusp, one sees a portion of one of the lingual cusps. Which cusp is it? _____

Permanent
Maxillary
Right First Molar
1. OCCLUSAL
2. FACIAL

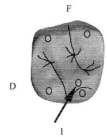
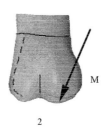

MAXILLARY FIRST MOLAR: LINGUAL VIEW

4.2.1

The lingual outline of the maxillary first molar is the same as the facial outline. A portion of the _____ surface can be seen from the lingual.

Permanent Maxillary
Right
First Molar
LINGUAL

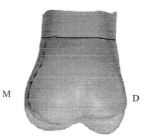

From the lingual view, the crown is trapezoid in outline. The trapezoid is narrower at the _____ (occlusal/cervical).

Permanent Maxillary
Right
First Molar
LINGUAL

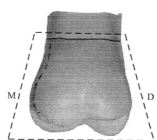

A. distolingual groove;
B. mesiolingual groove

Earlier, you learned the names of the two developmental grooves that appear on the lingual surface of the maxillary first molar: the (A) _____ _____ and the (B) _____ _____ .

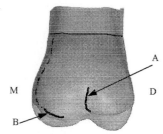

Permanent Maxillary
Right
First Molar
LINGUAL

distal, lingual

The distolingual groove originates at an occlusal pit and terminates in a pit on the lingual surface. Therefore, the distolingual groove of the maxillary first molar runs from the _____ pit to the _____ pit.

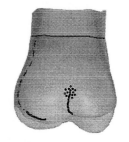

Permanent Maxillary
Right
First Molar
LINGUAL

a. mesiolingual;
d. distolingual

Of the two lingual cusps, one is the longest and the other the shortest of the four major cusps on the maxillary first molar. Complete the list of the four major cusps in order, longest to shortest.

a. _____ (longest)
b. distofacial
c. mesiofacial
d. _____ (shortest)

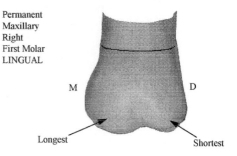

Permanent
Maxillary
Right
First Molar
LINGUAL

MAXILLARY FIRST MOLAR: PROXIMAL VIEW

From the proximal views, the mesiofacial, mesiolingual, distofacial, and distolingual line angles bound the proximal surfaces of the maxillary first molar. To the right and left of these line angles, portions of the _____ and _____ surfaces are visible.

facial, lingual

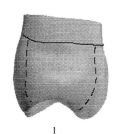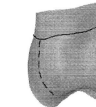

Permanent
Maxillary
Right
First Molar
1. MESIAL
2. DISTAL

F   L   F

1   2

From the proximal views, which surface is more uniformly convex in the occlusocervical direction? _____ (facial/lingual)

lingual

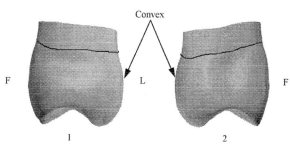

Permanent
Maxillary
Right
First Molar
1. MESIAL
2. DISTAL

Convex

F   L   F

1   2

On the maxillary first molar, the lingual height of contour is in the _____ third of the crown.

middle

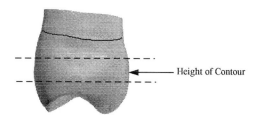

Permanent
Maxillary
Right
First Molar
MESIAL

Height of Contour

mesial marginal ridge

The rounded fold of enamel that forms the occlusal border of the mesial surface is the

_____ _____ _____ .

Permanent
Maxillary
Right
First Molar
1. MESIAL
2. OCCLUSAL

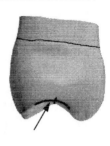 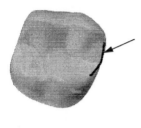

1   2

---

b

Which of the following describes the form of the mesial marginal ridge as seen from the mesial view? _____

a. The mesial marginal ridge nearly parallels the curvature of the cervical line.
b. The mesial marginal ridge has a slight central concavity between the mesiofacial and mesiolingual cusps.

Permanent
Maxillary
Right
First Molar
MESIAL

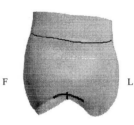

F   L

---

less

Compared to the cervical line on anterior teeth and premolars, the cervical line on the maxillary first molar has _____ (more/less) curvature. (The cervical line is marked on each tooth in the maxillary right quadrant in both the facial view and the mesial view. You can identify the teeth according to the universal code number printed on the tooth. If you are having difficulty identifying which universal code number is associated with a tooth, review would be indicated.)

Permanent
Maxillary
Right Quadrant
FACIAL
MESIAL

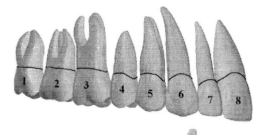

Facial

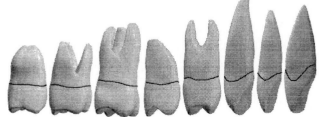

Mesial

The mesial and distal contact areas are located, occlusocervically, in the _____ third of the crown and, faciolingually, slightly _____ to the faciolingual midline of the crown.

middle, facial

Permanent
Maxillary
Right
First Molar
1. MESIAL
2. DISTAL

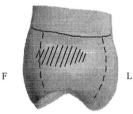

Cervical to the mesial contact area is a shallow, irregular-shaped concave region extending nearly to the cervical line and often crossing the mesiofacial line angle onto the _____ surface.

facial

Permanent
Maxillary
Right
First Molar
MESIAL

F   L

Compare the mesial and distal views of the maxillary first molar. Which exposes more of the occlusal surface? _____

distal

Permanent
Maxillary
Right
First Molar
1. MESIAL
2. DISTAL

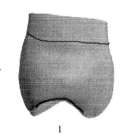
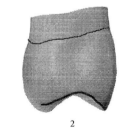

The increased exposure of the occlusal surface from the distal view is due to the short distolingual cusp and the lower level of the _____ _____ _____ .

distal marginal ridge

Permanent
Maxillary
Right
First Molar
1. MESIAL
2. DISTAL

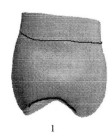
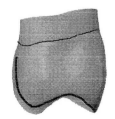

less

Because of the distal taper of the facial surface, the faciolingual measurement of the distal surface is slightly _____ (more/less) than that of the mesial surface.

Permanent
Maxillary
Right
First Molar
OCCLUSAL

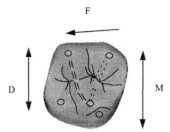

cervical

From a proximal view, the crown of the maxillary first molar is wider, faciolingually at the _____ (occlusal/cervical).

Permanent
Maxillary
Right
First Molar
1. MESIAL
2. DISTAL

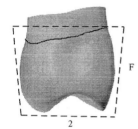
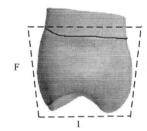

facial, cervical

The distal surface of the maxillary first molar has a small concave area located in the _____ (facial/lingual) portion of its _____ (middle/cervical) third.

Permanent
Maxillary
Right
First Molar
DISTAL

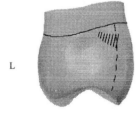

GO TO THE NEXT PAGE AND TAKE REVIEW TEST 4.2.

REVIEW TEST 4.2

Place an X on the lines that match the left-hand column with the top row. Mark your answers in the book, and check them in Appendix A.

Maxillary First Molar	*Facial*	*Lingual*	*Mesial*	*Distal*
What surfaces are visible from the facial aspect? (complete or part)	_____	_____	_____	_____
What surfaces are visible from the lingual aspect? (complete or part)	_____	_____	_____	_____
Which proximal view exposes more of the occlusal?	_____	_____	_____	_____
What surfaces have their widest measurement at the occlusal?	_____	_____	_____	_____
Which surfaces are marked by a developmental groove that terminates in a pit?	_____	_____	_____	_____

1. The order of the four major cusps of the maxillary first molar, longest to shortest is

    a. mesiofacial, mesiolingual, distofacial, distolingual
    b. mesiolingual, distofacial, distolingual, mesiofacial
    c. mesiolingual, distofacial, mesiofacial, distolingual

2. What cusps are visible from the facial view of the maxillary first molar?

    a. mesiofacial, distofacial, distolingual
    b. mesiofacial, distofacial, mesiolingual
    c. mesiofacial, distofacial

3. Which facial cusp of the maxillary first molar is narrower mesiodistally?

    a. mesiofacial
    b. distofacial

4. Which of the following proximal surfaces have contact areas which are displaced somewhat to the lingual from the midline of the crown?

    a. mesial   c. both
    b. distal   d. neither

CHECK YOUR ANSWERS IN APPENDIX A.

4.3.0 PROXIMAL CONTACTS, EMBRASURES, AND CROWN CONTOURS: MAXILLARY FIRST MOLAR

facially, larger

The proximal contacts between the molars (as with all posterior teeth) are located _____ (facially/lingually) in the faciolingual direction. This location creates a _____ (larger/smaller) lingual embrasure. (The teeth are identified with universal code numbers.)

Permanent
Maxillary
Right
4. Second Premolar
3. First Molar
2. Second Molar
1. Third Molar
OCCLUSAL

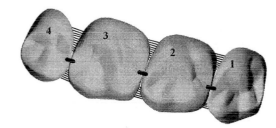

middle

The location of the contacts in the occlusocervical direction is in the _____ third on both the mesial and the distal surfaces of the maxillary molars.

Permanent
Maxillary
Right
1. Third Molar
2. Second Molar
3. First Molar
4. Second Premolar
FACIAL

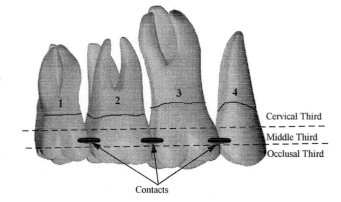

Cervical Third

Middle Third

Occlusal Third

Contacts

lingual, facial

Maxillary posterior teeth have the height of contour in the middle third on the lingual surface and in the cervical third on the facial surface. So the height of contour of the maxillary first molar is located in the middle third on the _____ surface and in the cervical third on the _____ surface.

Permanent
Maxillary
Right
First Molar
DISTAL

L   F

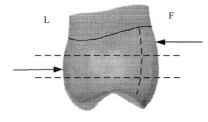

The lingual height of contour measures 1/2 mm. Similarly, the facial height of contour also measures _____ mm.

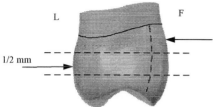

Permanent
Maxillary
Right
First Molar
DISTAL

L   F

1/2 mm

ROOT ANATOMY: MAXILLARY FIRST MOLAR

The maxillary molars generally have three roots. Of the three teeth assigned the universal code numbers 3, 6, and 12, the tooth with the trifurcated root is number _____ , the _____ _____ _____ _____ .

   (universal   (arch)   (quadrant)   (tooth name)
code number)

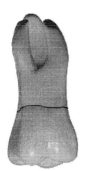

When a tooth has three roots, the root portion of that tooth has one root trunk and three _____ _____ .

Permanent
Maxillary
Right
First Molar
FACIAL

Terminal Roots

Root Trunk

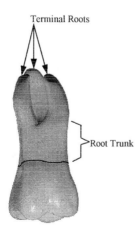

Although the curved contours of the roots do not present distinct surface boundaries, the terms facial, lingual, mesial, and distal are used to indicate root surfaces and directions. Of the three terminal roots on maxillary molars, one is located toward the lingual and two toward the _____ .

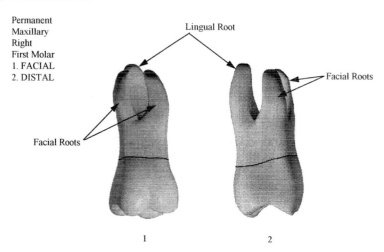

Permanent
Maxillary
Right
First Molar
1. FACIAL
2. DISTAL

Lingual Root

Facial Roots

Facial Roots

1   2

Terminal roots are named for the position they occupy in relation to the surfaces of the crown. Root (A) is the distofacial root, (B) the _____ root, and (C) the _____ root.

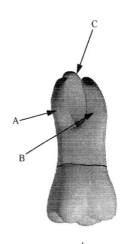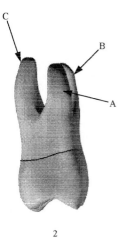

Permanent
Maxillary
Right
First Molar
1. FACIAL
2. DISTAL

C   C

A   B

B   A

1   2

On the roots of the maxillary molars, the level of trifurcation is variable, but the root trunk is almost always short. In the cervico-apical direction, the root trunk will consist of _____ _____ _____ (more than half/less than half) of the total root length.

Permanent
Maxillary
Right
First Molar
FACIAL

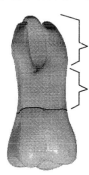

Corresponding to the division of the terminal roots, the three surfaces of the trunk are grooved from the trifurcation nearly to the cervical line. Because of the relative position of the roots, on which three surfaces of the root trunk are these grooves found?

_____

a. facial, lingual, mesial
b. mesial, distal, lingual
c. mesial, distal, facial

Permanent
Maxillary
Right
First Molar
1. FACIAL
2. DISTAL
3. LINGUAL
4. MESIAL

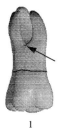

1

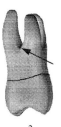

2

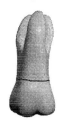

3

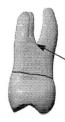

4

On multi-rooted molars, regardless of the number of terminal roots, a general term is often used to designate the division of the common root trunk into terminal root ends. This general term is **furcation.**

lingual

On a maxillary molar, the longest, largest, and strongest of the three roots is the _____ root. (This distolingual view illustrates the size comparison.)

Permanent
Maxillary
Right
First Molar
DISTOLINGUAL

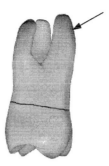

mesiofacial

The two facial roots are nearly the same length, but the more highly developed and some-times longer of the two facial roots is the _____ root.

Permanent
Maxillary
Right
First Molar
FACIAL

D   M

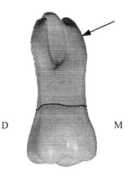

lingual, mesiofacial, distofacial (in that order)

In overall size (all directions), how do the three terminal roots order themselves, largest to smallest?

_____ largest
_____ next largest
_____ smallest

Permanent
Maxillary
Right
First Molar
1. FACIAL
2. DISTAL

Largest

Next Largest

Smallest

Smallest

Next Largest

D   M   L   F

1   2

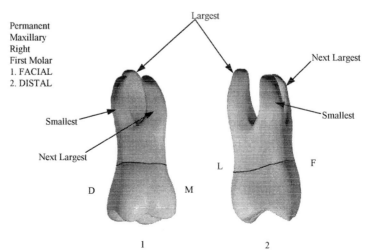

In which of the two horizontal directions are the two facial roots wider? _____

Permanent
Maxillary
Right
First Molar
1. FACIAL
2. MESIAL
3. DISTAL

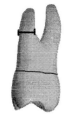

D   M

1

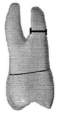

F   L   F

2   3

On the lingual root, the relative width in the faciolingual and mesiodistal directions is reversed from that on the two facial roots. In which horizontal direction is the lingual root the widest? _____

mesiodistal

The wide lingual surface of the lingual root is sometimes marked by a longitudinal groove that is more pronounced in the cervical than at the apical portion.

Permanent
Maxillary
Right
First Molar
LINGUAL

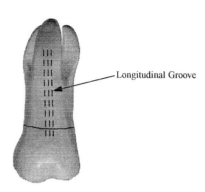

—Longitudinal Groove

The lingual root is somewhat banana-shaped viewed from the mesial or distal, but it is straight when viewed from the lingual.

facial

At the apical third, the lingual root changes directions, inclining slightly toward the _____ .

Permanent
Maxillary
Right
First Molar
1. LINGUAL
2. MESIAL

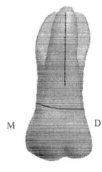
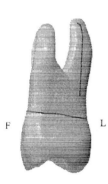

M   D   F   L

1   2

lingual

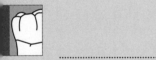

Occasionally, the single lingual root does not change directions at its apical third. When this is the case, it diverges for its entire length in a _____ direction. (An outline drawing illustrates this concept.)

Permanent
Maxillary
Right
First Molar
MESIAL
1. More Common
2. Less Common

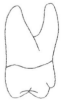
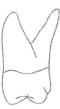

1   2

The terminal roots of the maxillary first molars generally diverge initially but return toward the midline near the _____ third.

Permanent
Maxillary
Right
First Molar
1. FACIAL
2. DISTAL

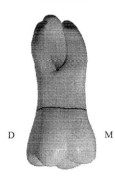
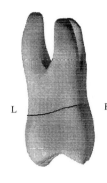

D   M   L   F

1   2

PULP ANATOMY: MAXILLARY FIRST MOLAR

The maxillary first molar has a pulp chamber with four major pulp horns corresponding to its four major cusps. These are called the _____ , _____ , _____ , and _____ pulp horns.

Permanent
Maxillary
Right
First Molar
CROSS SECTION
OCCLUSAL

D   M

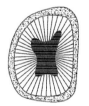

Surprisingly, given the number of roots in a maxillary molar, there are more often _____ (number) root canals.

Permanent
Maxillary
Right
First Molar
MESIODISTAL SECTION

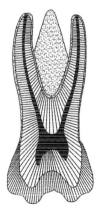

M   D

cervical

The two root canals present (with either one or two foramina) in the mesiofacial root, generally unite near the apical third of the root. A cross section showing two root canals in the mesiofacial root probably was taken in the _____ (cervical/ apical) portion of the root.

Permanent
Maxillary
Right
First Molar
1. FACIOLINGUAL SECTION
2. CROSS SECTION

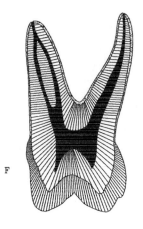

three

About 40% of the time the mesiofacial root is undivided and the total number of root canals is _____ .

Permanent
Maxillary
Right
First Molar
MESIODISTAL SECTION

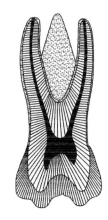

Whether there are three root canals (mesiofacial undivided) or four root canals (mesiofacial divided), the orifice of each major canal serves as a corner of the maxillary first molar pulp chamber. Therefore, the shape of the floor of the pulp chamber is roughly _____ .

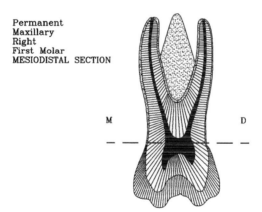

Permanent
Maxillary
Right
First Molar
1. MESIODISTAL SECTION
2. CROSS SECTION

M   D   M   D

triangular

A cross section taken at the level of the cervical line usually cuts through the pulp chamber. Therefore, the floor of the pulp chamber of the maxillary molars is generally located somewhere between the cervical line and the _____ of the root structure.

Permanent
Maxillary
Right
First Molar
MESIODISTAL SECTION

M   D

trifurcation

mesiodistal

A series of cross sections through the lingual root show that the lingual root canal is nearly round at the orifice and near the apex. In the middle portion of the lingual root, the lingual root canal is more elliptical, with the major axis running in the _____ direction.

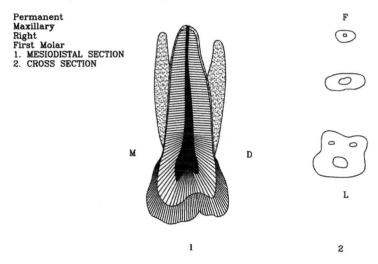

Permanent
Maxillary
Right
First Molar
1. MESIODISTAL SECTION
2. CROSS SECTION

circular (round or synonym)

Similar to the pattern of the distofacial root, the distofacial root canal of a maxillary molar is small and tapered. A cross section through this root shows it to be almost _____ .

Permanent
Maxillary
Right
First Molar
1. MESIODISTAL SECTION
2. CROSS SECTION

When the mesiofacial root has a single root canal (called the mesiofacial root canal) it is usually flattened. It is widest in the _____ direction.

faciolingual

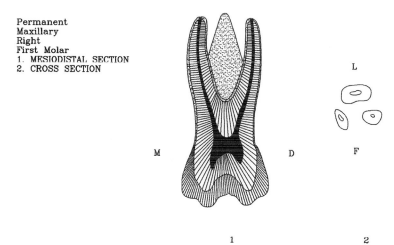

Permanent
Maxillary
Right
First Molar
1. MESIODISTAL SECTION
2. CROSS SECTION

SUMMARY

Permanent Maxillary Right First Molar OCCLUSAL - Summary

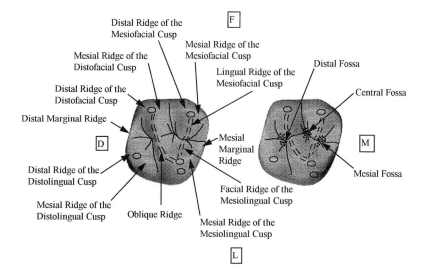

The two missing labels are the mesiolingual groove and the central groove.

Which two grooves are not labeled on this illustration? Find them and mark for future reference.

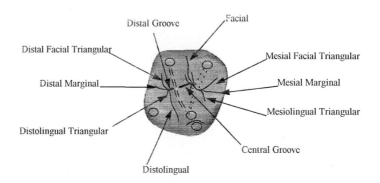

Permanent Maxillary Right First Molar Summary - - Grooves

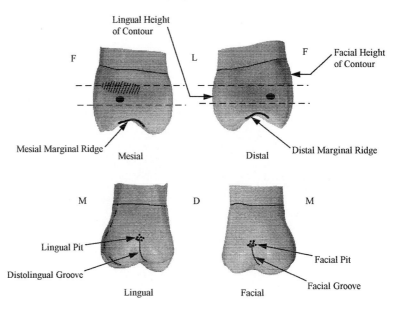

Permanent Maxillary Right First Molar - Summary

Permanent Maxillary Right First Molar - Summary

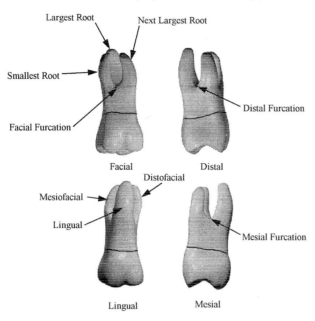

Facial   Distal

Lingual   Mesial

Permanent Maxillary First Molar Pulp Anatomy — Summary

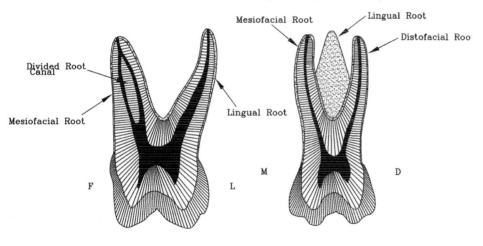

Faciolingual   Mesiodistal

TURN TO THE NEXT PAGE AND TAKE REVIEW TEST 4.3.

REVIEW TEST 4.3

1. The mesial and distal contacts on the maxillary first molar are located
   a. in the occlusal third
   b. in the middle third
   c. in the cervical third

2. In the faciolingual direction, the contacts are located
   a. facially
   b. centered
   c. lingually

3. The lingual height of contour on the maxillary first molar is located
   a. in the cervical third
   b. in the middle third
   c. in the occlusal third

4. The facial and lingual height of contour measures about
   a. 1/2 mm
   b. 1 mm
   c. 1 1/2 mm

5. Which embrasure is larger?
   a. lingual
   b. facial
   c. occlusal

6. The maxillary first molar is
   a. single rooted
   b. bifurcated
   c. trifurcated

7. The largest root of the maxillary first molar is
   a. mesiofacial
   b. distofacial
   c. lingual
   d. none of the above (it is single rooted)

8. Which root commonly has two root canals?
   a. mesiofacial
   b. distofacial
   c. lingual

9. Where are the furcations located on a maxillary first molar?
   a. _____
   b. _____
   c. _____
   d. _____

10. The largest facial root is the
    a. mesiofacial
    b. distofacial

CHECK YOUR ANSWERS IN APPENDIX A.

MAXILLARY SECOND MOLAR

4.4.0

Because the maxillary second molar resembles the maxillary first molar, only the essential differences will be covered.

Permanent
Maxillary
Right
1. Second Molar
2. First Molar
OCCLUSAL

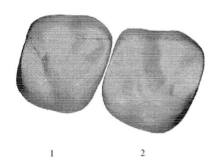

1   2

In the occlusocervical direction, the crown of the second molar is _____ (longer/shorter) than the first molar.

Permanent
Maxillary
Right
1. Second Molar
2. First Molar
FACIAL

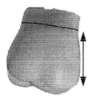 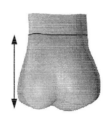

1   2

What is the relationship between the faciolingual measurement of the maxillary first and second molars? _____ (a or b)

a. The first molar has a greater faciolingual measurement.
b. The two molars have nearly equal faciolingual measurement.

Permanent
Maxillary
Right
1. Second Molar
2. First Molar
MESIAL

1   2

In the mesiodistal direction, the maxillary second molar is _____ (wider/narrower) than the first molar.

Permanent
Maxillary
Right
1. Second Molar
2. First Molar
FACIAL

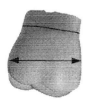 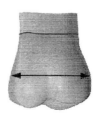

1   2

second molar

In occlusal view, which tooth is more narrow mesiodistally? _____

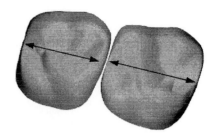

Permanent
Maxillary
Right
1. Second Molar
2. First Molar
OCCLUSAL

1   2

four

How many cusps are visible in occlusal view of the second molar? _____

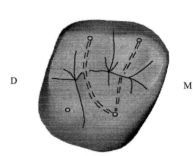

Permanent
Maxillary
Right
Second Molar
OCCLUSAL

F

D   M

L

five, four

Each lobe is represented by a cusp on molar teeth; thus, the maxillary first molar has _____ (number) lobes, and the maxillary second molar has _____ (number) lobes.

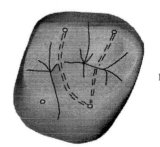

Permanent
Maxillary
Right
Second Molar
OCCLUSAL

F

D   M

L

On the maxillary second molar, the small accessory cusp of Carabelli _____ (is/is not) present.

is not

Permanent
Maxillary
Right
Second Molar
1. OCCLUSAL
2. LINGUAL

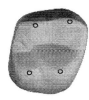

1   2

The cusps of the maxillary second molar are as follows:

A. _____
B. _____
C. _____
D. _____

A. mesiofacial;
B. distofacial;
C. distolingual;
D. mesiolingual

Permanent
Maxillary
Right
Second Molar
OCCLUSAL

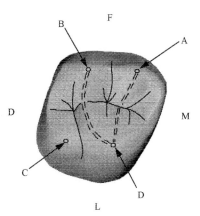

The maxillary second molar has two types of occlusal patterns: (1) the more common rhomboidal type and (2) the "heart-shaped" type. Which occlusal type has more nearly parallel sides which run in the faciolingual direction? _____ (The outline drawings are representative of the different types of occlusal patterns.)

rhomboidal

Permanent
Maxillary
Right
Second Molar
1. Rhomboidal
2. Heart—shaped
OCCLUSAL

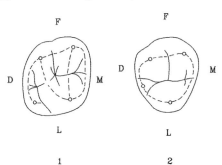

1   2

On the rhomboidal type, the outline formed by joining the four cusp tips is a rhomboid. The longer and more nearly parallel sides run in the _____ direction.

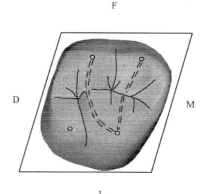

Permanent
Maxillary
Right
Second Molar
OCCLUSAL

F

D

M

L

The two largest cusps on the maxillary second molar are the _____ and _____ cusps.

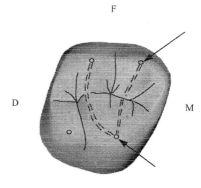

Permanent
Maxillary
Right
Second Molar
OCCLUSAL

F

D

M

L

In the study of the premolars, the difference was drawn between developmental and supplemental grooves. Which of these two types of grooves does not mark the major anatomical division of tooth crowns? _____

The maxillary second molar may have more shallow linear grooves than the first molar. These grooves neither mark the junction of the primary parts of the tooth nor are shown in the standard drawings of the occlusal aspect of the crown. As on the maxillary second premolar, these shallow grooves are called _____ grooves.

Permanent
Maxillary
Right
Second Molar
OCCLUSAL

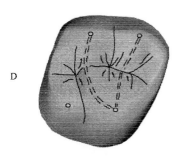

F

D   M

L

The less common "heart-shaped" occlusal type results from the poor development of the _____ cusp.

Permanent
Maxillary
Right
Second Molar   D   M
OCCLUSAL

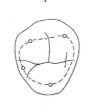

F

L

The rhomboidal occlusal pattern of the maxillary second molar resembles the maxillary first molar, but the "heart-shaped" occlusal pattern resembles the maxillary _____ _____ (compare Figures 3 and 4). (The outline drawings are representative of the different shapes.)

Permanent
Maxillary
Right
1. First Molar
2. Second Molar (Rhomboid)
3. Second Molar (Heart–shaped)
4. Third Molar
OCCLUSAL

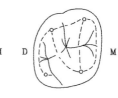

D   M   D   M

1   2

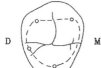
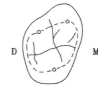

D   M   D   M

3   4

a. equal; b. smaller; c. smaller

How do the measurements of the maxillary second molar compare to those of the maxillary first molar in the following directions?

a. faciolingual   ————————— (larger/smaller/equal)
b. mesiodistal   ————————— (larger/smaller/equal)
c. occlusocervical —————————— (larger/smaller/equal)

distolingual

The mesiolingual and distolingual cusps show a progressive shift in position from the maxillary first to third molar. Which cusp has the greater amount of variability in position? ———————— (The teeth are labeled 1, 2, and 3, which also coincides with their universal code numbers.)

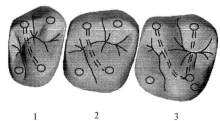

Permanent
Maxillary
Right
1. Third Molar
2. Second Molar
3. First Molar
OCCLUSAL

1   2   3

facial

The mesiolingual cusp shifts slightly toward the distal. The distolingual cusp shifts toward the mesial and ———————— directions.

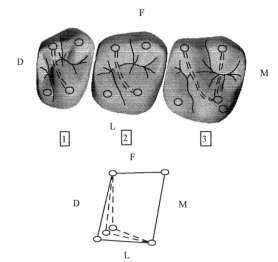

Permanent
Maxillary
Right
1. Third Molar
2. Second Molar
3. First Molar
OCCLUSAL

Compared to the first molar, the facial groove of the maxillary second molar is slightly
_____ _____ (more distinct/less distinct).

Permanent
Maxillary
Right
1. Second Molar
2. First Molar
FACIAL

1   2

A part of the oblique ridge is seen in the concavity between the two facial cusps, the
_____ ridge of the _____ cusp.

Permanent
Maxillary
Right
Second Molar
FACIAL

D   M

The two distal cusps of the maxillary second molar are not only smaller than those of the
first molar, but in the occlusocervical direction, they are also _____ .

Permanent
Maxillary
Right
1. Second Molar
2. First Molar
DISTAL

1   2

A notable difference between the maxillary first and second molars is that the cusp of
Carabelli is not present on the _____ surface of the _____ molar.

Permanent
Maxillary
Right
Second Molar
LINGUAL

M   D

distofacial

From the lingual view of the maxillary second molar, the _____ facial cusp is visible below the distolingual cusp.

Permanent
Maxillary
Right
Second Molar
LINGUAL

M   D

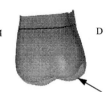

a. four;
b. faciolingual;
c. distolingual

The maxillary second molar generally resembles the maxillary first molar. Some of the essential differences are

a. The maxillary second molar has _____ cusps.
b. The second molar is generally smaller than the first molar except in the _____ direction.
c. The second molar has two common occlusal patterns, a variation largely due to the smaller size of the _____ cusp.

GO TO THE NEXT PAGE AND TAKE REVIEW TEST 4.4.

REVIEW TEST 4.4

Place an X on the lines that match the left-hand column with the top row.

	Maxillary First Molar	*Maxillary Second Molar*	*Neither or Both*
Shorter occlusocervically	_____	_____	_____
Longer faciolingually	_____	_____	_____
Wider mesiodistally	_____	_____	_____
Tooth which often has more supplemental grooves	_____	_____	_____

CHECK YOUR ANSWERS IN APPENDIX A.

4.5.0   PROXIMAL CONTACTS, EMBRASURES, AND CROWN CONTOURS: MAXILLARY SECOND MOLAR

middle

The first, second, and third molars of both arches have their mesial and distal contacts located occlusocervically approximately in the center of the _____ third of the crown.

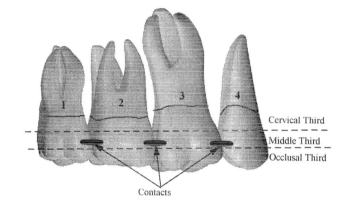

Permanent
Maxillary
Right
1. Third Molar
2. Second Molar
3. First Molar
4. Second Premolar
FACIAL

Cervical Third
Middle Third
Occlusal Third

Contacts

lingual, facial

Maxillary second molars, like the first and third molars, have the height of contour in the middle third on the _____ surface, and the cervical third on the _____ surface.

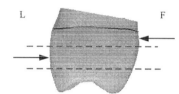

Permanent
Maxillary
Right
Second Molar
DISTAL

L   F

1/2

The lingual height of contour measures 1/2 mm. Similarly, the facial height of contour also measures _____ mm.

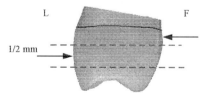

Permanent
Maxillary
Right
Second Molar
DISTAL

L   F

1/2 mm

facial

The proximal contacts on the maxillary second molar are located similarly to the first and third molars. That is, they are toward the _____ (facial, lingual) surface.

Because of this facial location, the _____ embrasures are deeper than the facial embrasures.

Permanent
Maxillary
Right
4. Second Premolar
3. First Molar
2. Second Molar
1. Third Molar
OCCLUSAL

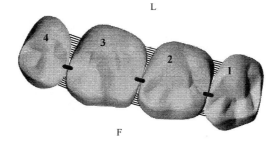

ROOT ANATOMY: MAXILLARY SECOND MOLAR

One general distinction between the root structures of the maxillary first and second molar is that the terminal roots lie closer together on the _____ _____

_____ .
                              (arch)   (tooth name)

Permanent
Maxillary
Right
1. First Molar
2. Second Molar
DISTOFACIAL

A second distinction between the maxillary first and second molars is the position of the apex of the lingual root in relation to the crown. In lingual view, the apex of the lingual root is centered over the distolingual developmental groove on the crown of the maxillary _____ molar.

Permanent
Maxillary
Right
1. First Molar
2. Second Molar
LINGUAL

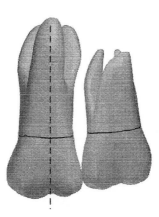

distolingual

On the maxillary second molar, the apex of the lingual root is centered over the _____ (mesiolingual/distolingual) cusp.

Permanent
Maxillary
Right
1. First Molar
2. Second Molar
LINGUAL

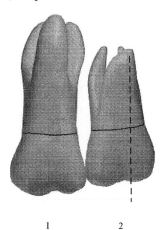

1   2

second molar

Fused and crooked terminal roots are two variations occurring on the root structures of the maxillary second molar. Which molar (maxillary first or second) has a root form that deviates more often from the average form? _____

less

The facial roots of the maxillary second molar have more surface irregularities (convexities and concavities) than the maxillary first molar. In relation to the first molar, however, the second molar has curvature of the terminal roots that is _____ (more/ less) divergent from the midline of the crown.

Permanent
Maxillary
Right
1. Second Molar
2. First Molar
FACIAL

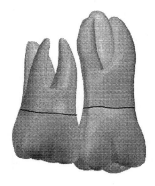

1   2

distal

In facial view, the two facial roots on the maxillary second molar have a slight deflection toward the center axis of the tooth in the apical third. Therefore, the larger of the two facial roots is initially straight, but near the apex it is inclined in the _____ direction.

Permanent
Maxillary
Right
Second Molar
FACIAL

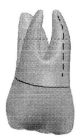

mesial

From the facial view, the apical third of the smaller root, the distofacial, has a slight deviation in the _____ direction.

Permanent
Maxillary
Right
Second Molar
FACIAL

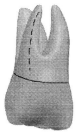

mesiofacial

In proximal view, one of the two facial roots of the maxillary second molar is nearly vertical in the cervicoapical direction. The other has a slight deviation to the facial. Which of the two facial roots is more nearly vertical? _____

Permanent
Maxillary
Right
Second Molar
DISTOFACIAL

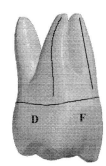

In distal view, the distofacial root of the maxillary second molar has a slight deflection in the _____ direction.

Permanent
Maxillary
Right
Second Molar
DISTOFACIAL

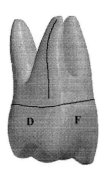

The cervicoapical curvature of the lingual root on the maxillary second molar is roughly similar to that of the maxillary first molar. Using your own words, describe the cervicoapical curvature of the lingual root on the maxillary second molar as viewed from the distolingual.

Permanent
Maxillary
Right
Second Molar
DISTOLINGUAL

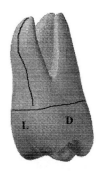

In lingual view, the lingual root may have a slight deflection toward the distal. More generally, however, it can be described as being relatively _____ .

Permanent
Maxillary
Right
Second Molar
LINGUAL

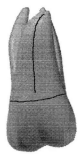

Of the three apexes on the maxillary first and second molars, one is blunt, one slightly blunted, and one pointed. The most blunt apex is on the _____ root; the most pointed is on the _____ root.

blunt (mesiofacial); pointed (distofacial)

Permanent
Maxillary
Right
Second Molar
FACIAL

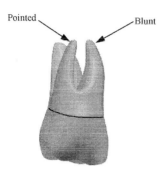

PULP ANATOMY: MAXILLARY SECOND MOLAR

4.5.2

The pulp cavity of the maxillary second molar is similar to that of the maxillary first molar. What are the names of the root canals in the most common form of the maxillary second molar? _____ , _____ , and _____

mesiofacial, distofacial, lingual (in any order)

Permanent
Maxillary
Right
Second Molar
MESIODISTAL SECTION

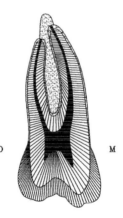

D   M

Due to the similarities between the first and second molars, the following three frames are a brief review of the maxillary first molar pulp anatomy.

The maxillary first molar has a pulp chamber with four major pulp horns corresponding to its four major cusps. These are called the _____ , _____ , _____ , and _____ pulp horns.

mesiofacial, distofacial, mesiolingual, distolingual (in any order)

Permanent
Maxillary
Right
First Molar
CROSS SECTION
OCCLUSAL

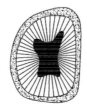

D   M

four

Surprisingly, given the number of roots in a maxillary molar, there are more often _____ (number) root canals.

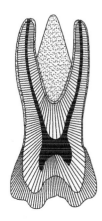

Permanent
Maxillary
Right
First Molar
MESIODISTAL SECTION

M   D

cervical

The two root canals present (with either one or two foramina) in the mesiofacial root, generally unite near the apical third of the root. A horizontal section showing two root canals in the mesiofacial root probably was taken in the _____ (cervical/ apical) portion of the root.

Permanent
Maxillary
Right
First Molar
1. FACIOLINGUAL SECTION
2. CROSS SECTION

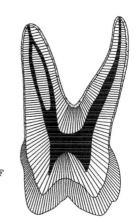

D

F   L

M

F   L

SUMMARY

Permanent Maxillary Right Second Molar OCCLUSAL - Summary

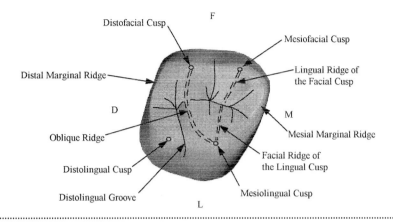

F

Distofacial Cusp

Mesiofacial Cusp

Lingual Ridge of
the Facial Cusp

Distal Marginal Ridge

D

M

Mesial Marginal Ridge

Oblique Ridge

Facial Ridge of
the Lingual Cusp

Distolingual Cusp

Distolingual Groove

Mesiolingual Cusp

L

Permanent Maxillary Right Second Molar FACIAL - Summary

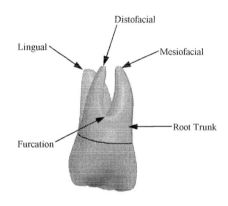

Distofacial

Lingual

Mesiofacial

Root Trunk

Furcation

Permanent Maxillary Second Molar Pulp Anatomy — Summary

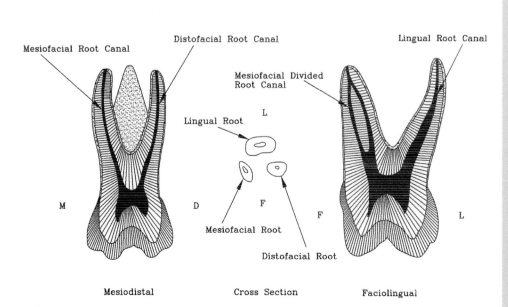

Mesiofacial Root Canal

Distofacial Root Canal

Lingual Root Canal

Mesiofacial Divided
Root Canal

L

Lingual Root

M

D

F

F

L

Mesiofacial Root

Distofacial Root

Mesiodistal

Cross Section

Faciolingual

TURN TO THE NEXT PAGE AND TAKE REVIEW TEST 4.5.

REVIEW TEST 4.5

1. The proximal contacts on the maxillary second molar are located _____ (a, b, or c) in the faciolingual direction?

   a. towards the lingual
   b. towards the facial
   c. in the middle 1/3 of the tooth

2. Which embrasures of the maxillary posteriors are larger?

   a. facial
   b. lingual

3. How many roots are present on the maxillary second molar?

   a. one
   b. two
   c. three
   d. four

4. Which root is the largest?

   a. mesiofacial
   b. distofacial
   c. lingual

5. Which root of the maxillary second molar is centered over the distolingual cusp?

   a. mesiofacial
   b. distofacial
   c. lingual
   d. none of these

6. Which root would have two root canals if there were two root canals present?

   a. mesiofacial
   b. distofacial
   c. lingual

7. The lingual root is widest in which direction?

   a. mesiodistal
   b. faciolingual

8. In which direction is the mesiofacial root the widest?

   a. mesiodistal
   b. faciolingual

9. The height of contour on the lingual surface of the crown is located in the

   a. cervical third
   b. middle third
   c. occlusal third

10. The lingual height of contour measures approximately

   a. 1 mm
   b. 1/2 mm

MAXILLARY THIRD MOLAR

The form of the third molar varies more than the form of any of the other teeth in the dental arch. The most common form of the maxillary third molar closely resembles the "heart-shaped" form of the maxillary second molar and has _____ (number) cusps.

Permanent
Maxillary
Right
Third Molar
OCCLUSAL
1–4 Variations
5. Typical Form

Generally, the distolingual cusp is absent on the maxillary third molar. The three remaining cusps maintain the names of the three largest cusps on the maxillary second molar; the _____ , _____ , and _____ cusps.

Permanent
Maxillary
Right
Third Molar
OCCLUSAL

Distofacial Cusp

Mesiofacial Cusp

D

M

Mesiolingual Cusp

Which of the well-developed cusps on the maxillary first and second molars does not develop on the most common form of the maxillary third molar? _____

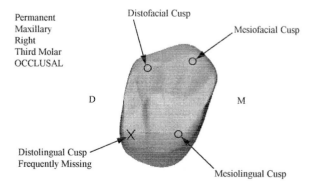

Permanent
Maxillary
Right
Third Molar
OCCLUSAL

Distofacial Cusp

Mesiofacial Cusp

D

M

Distolingual Cusp
Frequently Missing

Mesiolingual Cusp

second

Of the maxillary second and third molars, which has the larger facial cusps?

Permanent
Maxillary
Right
1. Third Molar
2. Second Molar
FACIAL

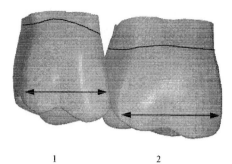

1   2

one

How many cusps are usually found on the lingual aspect of the third molar?

Permanent
Maxillary
Right
Third Molar
OCCLUSAL

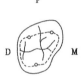

F

D   M

L

smaller

Compared to that of the maxillary second molar, the facial surface of the maxillary third molar is _____ (smaller/larger) in both directions.

Permanent
Maxillary
Right
1. Third Molar
2. Second Molar
FACIAL

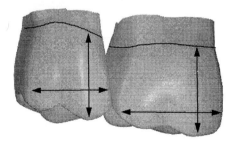

1   2

From the facial view, the facial groove of the maxillary third molar is less distinct than that of the maxillary second molar. Of the three maxillary molars, the molar with the most distinct facial groove is the first molar; the molar with the least distinct facial groove is the _____ _____ .

Permanent
Maxillary
Right
Third Molar
FACIAL

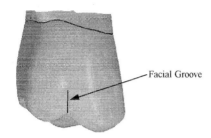

Facial Groove

Concerning cusp arrangement, one difference between the maxillary second and third molars is that the third molar frequently has only one _____ cusp.

Permanent
Maxillary
Right
Third Molar
OCCLUSAL

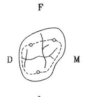

F

D   M

L

Similar to the maxillary first and second molars, when a small distolingual cusp is present on the third molar, as it is in the model tooth, it is separated from the mesiolingual cusp by the _____ groove.

Permanent
Maxillary
Right
Third Molar
OCCLUSAL

D   M

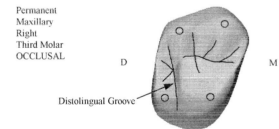

Distolingual Groove

Compared to that of the maxillary second molar, the lingual surface of the maxillary third molar has a mesiodistal convexity that is _____ _____ (more/less) pronounced.

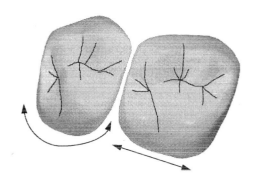

Permanent
Maxillary
Right
1. Third Molar
2. Second Molar
OCCLUSAL

Compared to those of the maxillary second molar, the measurements of the crown of the typical maxillary third molar are _____ (increased/reduced).

Sometimes, extra ridges descend from the cusp tips of the third molars onto the occlusal surface. Similar to the nomenclature for the shallow linear "extra" grooves on the occlusal surfaces of some teeth, these ridges are called _____ _____ .

Which proximal surface on the maxillary third molar is more uniformly convex? _____

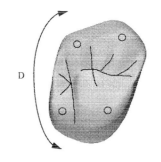

Permanent
Maxillary
Right
Third Molar
OCCLUSAL

D   M

Three significant features of the maxillary third molar are

a. The form of the third molar varies _____ (more/less) than any other tooth.
b. The typical form of the maxillary third molar has _____ cusps.
c. In all dimensions, the maxillary third molar is _____ (larger/smaller) than the second molar.

GO TO THE NEXT PAGE AND TAKE REVIEW TEST 4.6.

REVIEW TEST 4.6

1. In the "heart-shaped" variation of the second molar, which cusp is poorly developed?

   a. distolingual
   b. mesiolingual

2. Which is the most common form of the maxillary second molar?

   a. rhomboidal
   b. "heart shaped"

3. In the diagram, the arrow points to the _____ side of the tooth.

   a. mesial
   b. distal

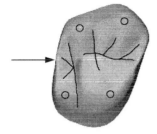

4. Which maxillary molar generally has the facial surface with the least distinct facial groove?

   a. second molar
   b. third molar

5. Which surface of the maxillary third molar is generally more uniformly convex?

   a. mesial
   b. distal

CHECK YOUR ANSWERS IN APPENDIX A.

4.7.0

PROXIMAL CONTACTS, EMBRASURES, AND CROWN CONTOURS: MAXILLARY THIRD MOLAR

middle, facially located

The mesial contact of the maxillary third molar is located in the _____ third in the occlusocervical direction. Faciolingually the contact is _____ (centered/facially located).

Permanent
Maxillary
Right
Third Molar
MESIAL

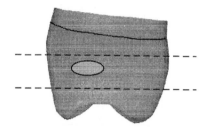

lingual

Again, the largest embrasure would be the _____ (facial/lingual).

Permanent
Maxillary
Right
4. Second Premolar
3. First Molar
2. Second Molar
1. Third Molar
OCCLUSAL

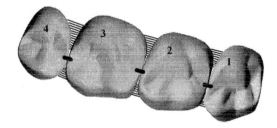

cervical, middle

The facial height of contour of the maxillary third molar is located in the _____ third, and the lingual height of contour is located in the _____ third.

Permanent
Maxillary
Right
Third Molar
MESIAL

F   L

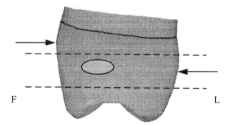

1/2

The facial and lingual heights of contour are approximately _____ mm.

ROOT ANATOMY: MAXILLARY THIRD MOLAR

The maxillary third molar presents too many variations in root form to be precisely described. Generally, however, it is similar to the maxillary first and second molars and has _____ (number) terminal roots.

three

Permanent
Maxillary
1. Right Third Molar
2. Left Third Molar
FACIAL

D

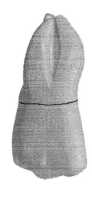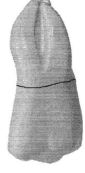

M   D

1   2

Frequently, the roots of the maxillary third molar are fused, forming one large root. Because of the fusion of the root structures, the root trunk of the maxillary third molar is usually _____ (longer/ shorter) than that on the other maxillary molars.

longer

Permanent
Maxillary
Right
Third Molar
MESIAL

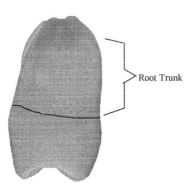

Root Trunk

The maxillary third molar may have as few as one fused root or as many as eight terminal roots. (The outline drawings are representative of the fused and multi-rooted teeth.)

Permanent
Maxillary
Right
Third Molar
MESIAL

4.7.2

roots

PULP ANATOMY: MAXILLARY THIRD MOLAR

The many different forms of the maxillary third molar make a detailed description of its pulp cavity impossible. Important to remember is that the root canals have the same general shape and number as the _____ .

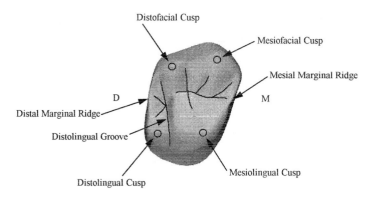

Permanent
Maxillary
Right
Third Molars
1. FACIAL
2. CROSS SECTIONS

SUMMARY

Permanent Maxillary Right Third Molar OCCLUSAL - Summary

Distofacial Cusp

Mesiofacial Cusp

Mesial Marginal Ridge

D

M

Distal Marginal Ridge

Distolingual Groove

Mesiolingual Cusp

Distolingual Cusp

Permanent Maxillary Right Third Molar OCCLUSAL

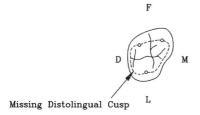

F

D   M

Missing Distolingual Cusp   L

Permanent Maxillary Third Molar FACIAL - Summary

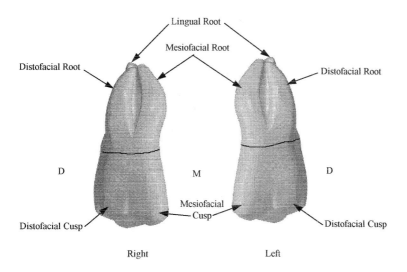

Lingual Root

Mesiofacial Root

Distofacial Root

Distofacial Root

D   M   D

Mesiofacial Cusp

Distofacial Cusp

Distofacial Cusp

Right   Left

TURN TO THE NEXT PAGE AND TAKE REVIEW TEST 4.7.

REVIEW TEST 4.7

1. The mesial contact of the maxillary third molar is occlusocervically located in the _____ third of the crown.
   a. occlusal
   b. middle
   c. cervical

2. Faciolingually the contact of the maxillary third molar is located
   a. facially
   b. lingually
   c. centered

3. The lingual height of contour of the maxillary third molar is approximately
   a. 1/2 mm
   b. 1 mm
   c. 3/4 mm

4. The maxillary third molar always has three roots and three root canals.
   a. True
   b. False

5. The universal code numbers for the maxillary third molars are
   a. 3 and 14
   b. 2 and 25
   c. 1 and 16
   d. 4 and 12

CHECK YOUR ANSWERS IN APPENDIX A.

MANDIBULAR FIRST MOLAR   4.8.0

The mandibular first molar is the largest, strongest tooth in the mandibular arch. It has _____ lobes.

five

Permanent
Mandibular
Right
First Molar
OCCLUSAL

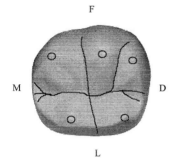

F

M   D

L

How many cusps (lobes) are located to the lingual? _____

two

Permanent
Mandibular
Right
First Molar
OCCLUSAL

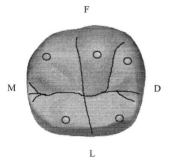

F

M   D

L

Similar to those of the maxillary second molar, the two lingual cusps of the mandibular first molar are called the mesiolingual and _____ cusps.

distolingual

Permanent
Mandibular
Right
First Molar
OCCLUSAL

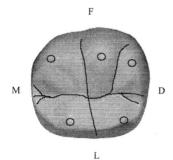

F

M   D

L

The three remaining cusps are the mesiofacial, distofacial, and distal cusps. Which of the five cusps on the mandibular first molar is the smallest? _____

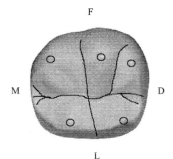

Permanent
Mandibular
Right
First Molar
OCCLUSAL

Which of the five cusps of the mandibular first molar is the widest? _____

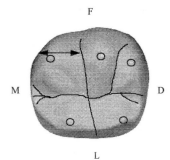

Permanent
Mandibular
Right
First Molar
OCCLUSAL

In which direction is the crown of the mandibular first molar wider? _____ (mesiodistal/faciolingual)

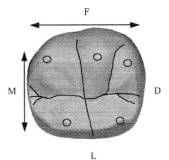

Permanent
Mandibular
Right
First Molar
OCCLUSAL

Similar to those of the mandibular first molar, the crowns of the mandibular second and third molars are wider in the mesiodistal direction than in the faciolingual direction.

Which of the following correctly describes the relationship between the mesiodistal and faciolingual measurements of the molars? _____

a. All molars, maxillary and mandibular, are wider mesiodistally than faciolingually.
b. Maxillary molars are wider faciolingually than mesiodistally, but the opposite is true for mandibular molars.

The relationship between the mesiodistal and faciolingual measurements of the crowns is one characteristic that differentiates maxillary from mandibular molars.

Remember that maxillary molars are wider faciolingually than mesiodistally, but on mandibular molars the crown is wider in the _____ direction.

mesiodistal

Permanent
1. Maxillary
2. Mandibular
Right
First Molar
OCCLUSAL

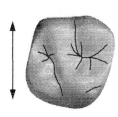

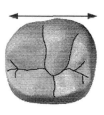

1   2

Another important difference between the maxillary and mandibular molars is in the pattern of their occlusal ridges. The maxillary molars have an _____ ridge and the mandibular molars do not.

oblique

Permanent
1. Maxillary
2. Mandibular
Right
First Molar
OCCLUSAL

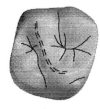

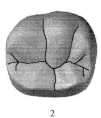

1   2

The occlusal surface of the mandibular first molar is divided into three fossae. Similar to the three fossae of the maxillary first molar, they are called the mesial, distal, and central fossae.

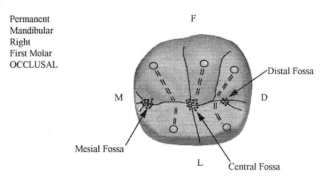

Permanent
Mandibular
Right
First Molar
OCCLUSAL

---

mesiofacial,
mesiolingual

The central fossa is the largest of the three and is separated from the mesial fossa by the triangular ridges of the _____ and _____ cusps.

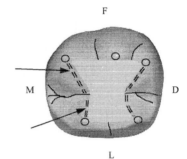

Permanent
Mandibular
Right
First Molar
OCCLUSAL

---

distal fossa

The triangular ridges of the distal and distolingual cusps separate the central fossa from the _____ _____ .

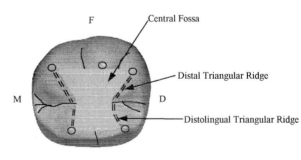

Permanent
Mandibular
Right
First Molar
OCCLUSAL

Which cusp of the mandibular first molar has a triangular ridge that does not form a part of the mesial or distal boundary of the central fossa? _____

Permanent
Mandibular
Right
First Molar
OCCLUSAL

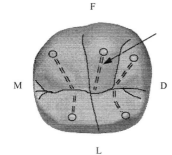

The triangular ridge of the distofacial cusp descends into the largest of the three fossae, the _____ fossa.

Permanent
Mandibular
Right
First Molar
OCCLUSAL

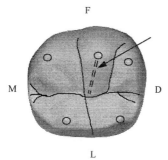

Four developmental grooves originate at the central pit in the central fossa. Of these four (the mesial, distal, facial, and lingual developmental grooves), which passes between the mesiolingual and distolingual cusps? _____

Permanent
Mandibular
Right
First Molar
OCCLUSAL

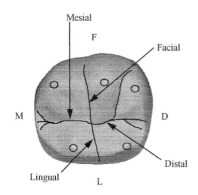

Name each of the developmental grooves of the mandibular first molar described.

a. The _____ groove originates at the central pit and terminates in the mesial fossa.

b. The _____ groove originates at the central pit and separates the mesiofacial and distofacial cusps.

c. The _____ groove originates at the central pit and terminates in the distal fossa.

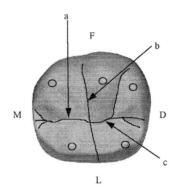

Permanent Mandibular Right First Molar OCCLUSAL

At a point slightly distal to the central pit, the distofacial developmental groove branches from the distal groove and passes between the distal and _____ cusps.

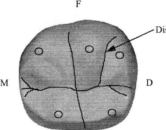

Permanent Mandibular Right First Molar OCCLUSAL — Distofacial Developmental Groove

Similar to the nomenclature for the maxillary molars, the union of the mesial and distal grooves on the mandibular first molar is called the _____ groove.

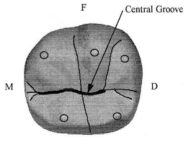

Permanent Mandibular Right First Molar OCCLUSAL — Central Groove

Additional shallow supplemental grooves are sometimes seen on the occlusal surface of the mandibular first molar. These supplemental grooves _____ (do/do not) mark the boundaries of the five lobes.

Permanent
Mandibular
Right
First Molar
OCCLUSAL

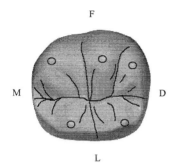

Use your note card mask to cover the next frame. Now, on this outline of the mandibular first molar, sketch the pattern formed by the ten developmental grooves. Use your own recall.

Permanent
Mandibular
Right
First Molar
OCCLUSAL

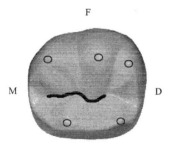

Check your drawing with this illustration.

Permanent
Mandibular
Right
First Molar
OCCLUSAL

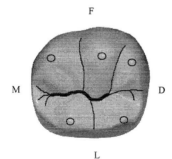

Here is an exercise in cusp and groove identification.

MANDIBULAR FIRST MOLAR

Name the cusps and grooves marked by the labels. Check your answers in the next frame.

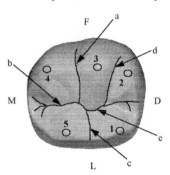

Cusps: 1. _____   4. _____
                2. _____   5. _____
                3. _____

Grooves: a. _____   b & e. _____
                b. _____
                c. _____
                d. _____
                e. _____

MANDIBULAR FIRST MOLAR: ANSWERS

If any items were missed, review the information until it is learned.

If all items are correct, continue with the next frame.

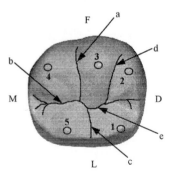

Cusps: 1. distolingual   4. mesiofacial
                2. distal   5. mesiolingual
                3. distofacial

Grooves: a. facial   b & e.   central
                b. mesial
                c. lingual
                d. distofacial
                e. distal

The "corners" of the occlusal view are _____ (sharply angled/rounded).

Permanent
Mandibular
Right
First Molar
OCCLUSAL

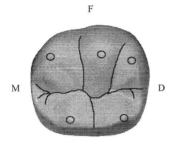

Unlike the maxillary first molar the mesial and distal surfaces of the mandibular first molar converge slightly toward the lingual. Which half of the mandibular first molar crown is wider in the mesiodistal direction? _____ (facial/lingual)

Permanent
1. Maxillary
2. Mandibular
Right
First Molar
OCCLUSAL

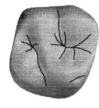 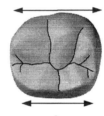

facial

The location of the distal cusp causes a problem in naming the four ridges. Because the mesial and distal ridges of other cusps help to form the borders of the occlusal surface, it is convenient to name the four ridges of the distal cusp as follows:

lingual ridge—descends onto the occlusal surface
facial ridge—descends onto facial surface very slightly distal to the distofacial line angle
mesial ridge—forms part of the faciocclusal line angle
distal ridge—blends with the distal marginal ridge

Name the ridges indicated by the labels.

1. _____
2. _____
3. _____
4. _____

Permanent
Mandibular
Right
First Molar
OCCLUSAL

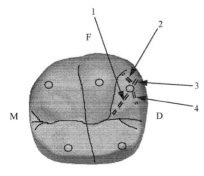

1. lingual; 2. mesial;
3. facial; 4. distal

How many cusps on the mandibular first molar have lingual ridges that are triangular ridges? _____

Permanent
Mandibular
Right
First Molar
OCCLUSAL

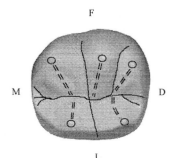

Similar to those of the maxillary molars, the mesial marginal ridge and the distal marginal ridge form two of the borders of the _____ _____ .

Permanent
Mandibular
Right
First Molar
OCCLUSAL

Distal Marginal
Ridge

Mesial Marginal
Ridge

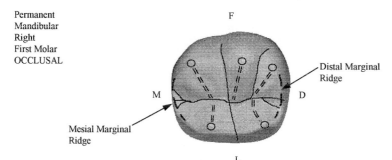

From the occlusal view, the linguocclusal line angle runs in a nearly straight line in the mesiodistal direction. The faciocclusal line angle is slightly more curved running in the mesiodistal direction; it is slightly convex toward the _____ direction.

Permanent
Mandibular
Right
First Molar
OCCLUSAL

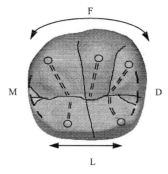

Of the five cusps, the _____ is the longest.

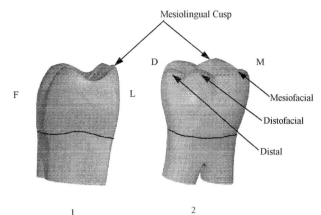

Permanent
Mandibular
Right
First Molar
1. MESIAL
2. FACIAL

Mesiolingual Cusp

F   L   D   M

Mesiofacial
Distofacial
Distal

1   2

The mesiolingual is slightly longer than the distolingual cusp, and the distofacial is slightly longer than the mesiofacial cusp. Which cusp of the mandibular first molar is the shortest? _____

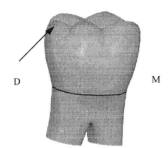

Permanent
Mandibular
Right
First Molar
FACIAL

D   M

TURN TO THE NEXT PAGE AND TAKE REVIEW TEST 4.8.

If three root canals are present, the larger, kidney-shaped canal is found in the _____ root, and the smaller, more circular canals are found in the _____ root.

Permanent
Mandibular
Right
Molar
CROSS SECTION

D   M

In some mandibular molars, the mesial root canals are not separate. Instead, there is a broad, ribbon-shaped root canal in the mesial root. When this occurs, the root canal is called the _____ root canal.

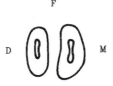

Permanent
Mandibular
Right
Molar
CROSS SECTION

F

D   M

The distal root canal in a mandibular molar usually is single and broad in a _____ direction.

Permanent
Mandibular
Right Molar
CROSS SECTION

F

D   M

L

In the margin: Figure 2, Figure 3 (in that order)

In a few cases, the distal root of a mandibular molar may have two root canals (Figure 3).

Of the three drawings, which illustrates the number of root canals that occurs most frequently in mandibular molars? _____ Which illustrates the number that occurs least frequently? _____

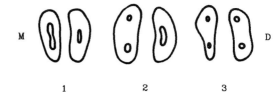

M   D

1   2   3

SUMMARY

Permanent Mandibular Left Third Molar - Summary

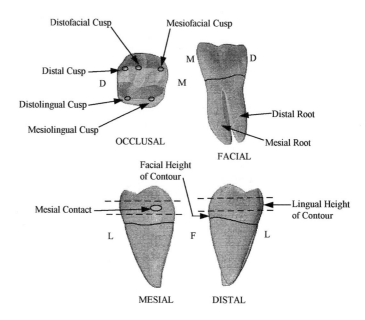

GO TO THE NEXT PAGE AND TAKE REVIEW TEST 4.14.

REVIEW TEST 4.14

Place an X on the lines that match the left-hand column with the top row.

Molars	Facial	Lingual	Mesial or Mesiofacial	Distal or Distofacial
Largest root of maxillary first molar	_____	_____	_____	_____
Inclination of lingual root apex, maxillary first molar	_____	_____	_____	_____
The smallest root of the maxillary first molar	_____	_____	_____	_____
Root with the sharpest apex, maxillary second molar	_____	_____	_____	_____
Largest root, mandibular first molar	_____	_____	_____	_____
Straighter root (occlusoapical direction) of mandibular first molar	_____	_____	_____	_____
Inclination of roots, mandibular third molar	_____	_____	_____	_____

1. What is the usual number of terminal roots of the molars in each arch?

   a. maxillary _____
   b. mandibular _____

2. Which of the following molars is most likely to have terminal roots that are fused?

   a. maxillary second molar
   b. maxillary third molar
   c. mandibular second molar

3. The mandibular first molar has a facial and a lingual root.

   a. true
   b. false

4. The distal root of the mandibular second molar has a cervicoapical curvature that

   a. inclines distally, with the apex usually deviated toward the mesial
   b. inclines distally, with (usually) no apical deviation

Write in the correct word(s) on the lines that matches the left-hand column with the top row.

Pulp of Posterior Teeth	*Maxillary First Molar*	*Mandibular First Molar*
Most common number of root canals	_____	_____
If the tooth has a less common number of root canals, what number of canals would that be?	_____	_____
Number of pulp horns in pulp chamber	_____	_____
Names of usual root canals (if more than one)	_____	_____

In order to end this chapter on a positive note, we have constructed a short, different test item with an interesting result.

1. Complete the following addition problems:

   a. Add the usual number of pulp horns on a mandibular second molar to the number of root canals it usually has.

   _____ + _____ = _____

   b. Add the most common number of root canals that every molar typically shows to the number of major pulp horns usually occurring on the maxillary first molar.

   _____ + _____ = _____

   c. Add the second most frequent number of root canals on mandibular molars to the number of pulp horns on the mandibular first molar.

   _____ + _____ = _____

CHECK YOUR ANSWERS IN APPENDIX A.

The Primary Dentition

THE PRIMARY DENTITION

Each quadrant of primary dentition consists of two incisors, a canine, and two molars. The total number of teeth in the primary dentition is _____ .

twenty, none

In contrast to the permanent dentition, how many premolar teeth are in the primary dentition? _____

Primary
Maxillary
Mandibular
OCCLUSAL

Universal Coding System

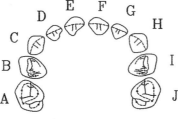
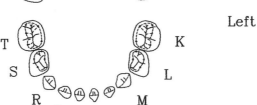

Right   Left

Because the anterior teeth consist of the incisors and canines and the posterior teeth of premolars and molars, each quadrant of the permanent dentition contains three anterior teeth and five posterior teeth. Each quadrant of the primary dentition contains _____ (number) anterior teeth and _____ (number) posterior teeth.

three, two
(in that order)

primary

Of the two, which dentition has crowns that are more bulbous or balloonlike? _____

Permanent
Maxillary
Right
1. Central Incisor
FACIAL
2. First Molar
MESIAL

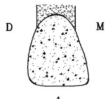
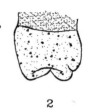

Primary
Maxillary
Right
3. Central Incisor
FACIAL
4. Second Molar
MESIAL

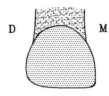
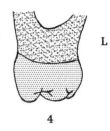

cervical line

The bulbous shape of the primary teeth is emphasized by a more pronounced constriction in the region of the _____ _____ .

constriction

The "pinched in" region in the area of the cervical line is called a cervical _____ .

Primary
Maxillary
Right
1. Central Incisor
MESIAL
2. Second Molar
MESIAL

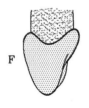
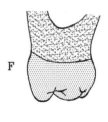

Makes it proportionately smaller than permanent molars S

A second feature contributing to the bulbous appearance of the crowns of primary molars is the strong occlusal convergence of the facial and lingual surfaces. What effect does the convergence have on the faciolingual measurement of the occlusal surface?

What is the universal code number for the tooth illustrated in Figure 2?_____

Primary
1. Maxillary Right
Second Molar
MESIAL
2. Mandibular Right
First Molar
MESIAL

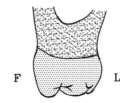
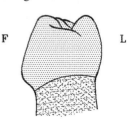

On primary crowns, the height of contour on the facial and lingual surfaces is more prominent than on permanent crowns.

The height of contour on the facial and lingual surfaces of the crown is sometimes called a
cervical or gingival ridge. Is "a" or "b" pointing to the cervical ridge? _____
What is the universal code for the tooth illustrated in Figure 1? _____
Figure 2? _____

Primary
Maxillary
Right
1. Central Incisor
MESIAL
2. Second Molar
MESIAL

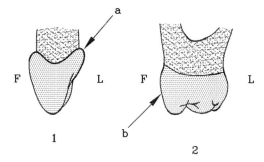

Compared to a permanent molar, the occlusal table of a primary molar is smaller in two
different ways: (1) it has less total area and (2) it is proportionately smaller in relation to
the total crown bulk.

The smaller total area of the occlusal table is the result of a smaller crown size and greater
convergence of the facial and lingual surfaces. The proportionately smaller occlusal table
on primary molars is related to only one of these two features, the _____
_____ .

1. Primary
Maxillary Right
First Molar
OCCLUSAL
2. Permanent
Maxillary Right
First Molar
OCCLUSAL

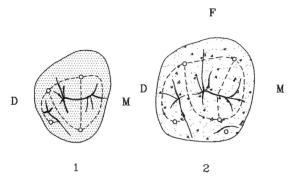

Examine this table and chart of approximate crown and root length of some of the primary and permanent teeth.

	PRIMARY TEETH				PERMANENT TEETH		
	Central Incisor	Canine	1st Molar		Central Incisor	Canine	1st Molar
Root Length	10	13.5	10	Root Length	13	17	12.5
Crown Length	6	6.5	5.1	Crown Length	10.5	10	7.5

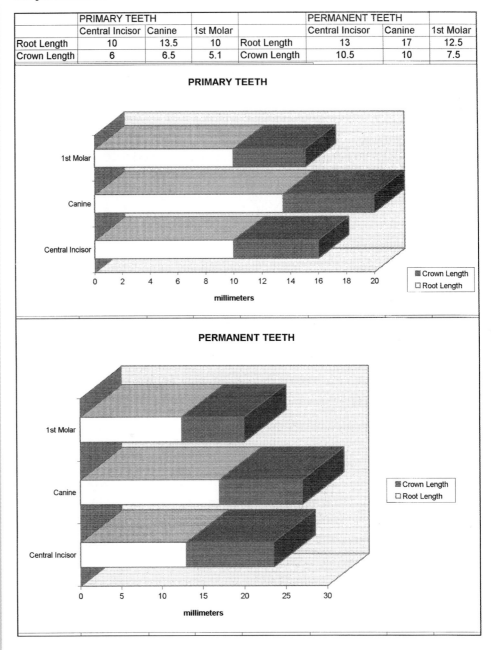

The primary central incisor has a root length of 10 and a crown length of 6. The ratio of these two lengths is 1.66, meaning that the root is, proportionately, one and two-thirds longer than the crown.

The permanent central incisor, on the other hand, has a root length of 13 and a crown length of 10.5. The ratio of root to crown length is, therefore, 1.24. This means that the root is proportionately longer than the crown by only one and one-quarter times.

This relationship between root and crown length in primary and permanent teeth holds true throughout the dentitions.

Examine the chart illustrating the root to crown ratio and answer the following question.

In which dentition is the ratio of root length to crown length greater? _____

a. primary
b. permanent

a. primary

In which dentition do the roots of the molars have a greater degree of divergence or outward flare? _____

1. Primary
Maxillary
First Molar
FACIAL
2. Permanent
Maxillary
First Molar
FACIAL

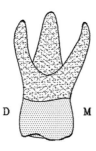 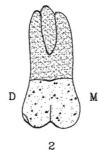

D   M   D   M

1   2

primary

The flare of the roots of primary molars provides space for the developing tooth buds of the _____ premolars.

permanent
(succedaneous)

Write a one- or two-word response that describes each of the following features of the primary dentition in relation to the permanent dentition.

A. Gross form of crown _____
B. Over-all crown size _____
C. Area of occlusal table in relation to crown size (posterior teeth only) _____
D. Degree of cervical constriction _____
E. Root length in relation to crown length _____
F. Relative amount of outward flare (divergence) of root structure (multirooted teeth only) _____
G. Convergence of the facial and lingual surfaces _____

A. more bulbous,
B. smaller,
C. proportionately
smaller,
D. greater
E. proportionately
longer,
F. greater,
G. greater

mandibular

The following graph represents a common eruption sequence for primary teeth. Differences among individuals is quite common. The chart offers a possible common eruption sequence.

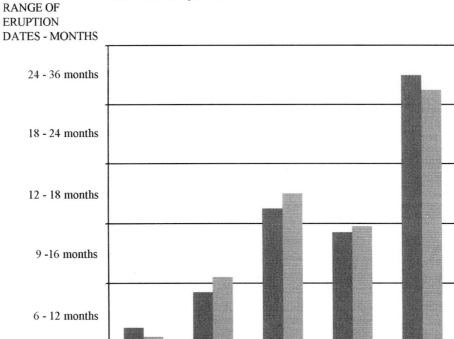

ERUPTION SEQUENCE AND DATES FOR PRIMARY TEETH

RANGE OF
ERUPTION
DATES - MONTHS

24 - 36 months

18 - 24 months

12 - 18 months

9 -16 months

6 - 12 months

CI   LI   C   1M   2M

CI - Central Incisor
LI - Lateral Incisor
C - Canine
1M - First Molar
2M - Second Molar

■ Maxillary
■ Mandibular

Though the eruption sequence is similar for each arch, the central incisors in the _____ arch normally precede their counterparts in the opposing arch.

first molar

Which permanent posterior tooth erupts prior to the eruption of one of the anterior teeth in each arch? _____ _____

A longitudinal section of a primary tooth reveals three anatomical features of significance in clinical dentistry. In relation to the corresponding features of the permanent teeth, (a) the enamel cap is thinner, (b) pulp cavities are relatively larger, resulting in proportionately thinner dentin, and (c) the pulp horns extend higher. Which of these three features makes the pulp of a primary tooth more susceptible to exposure by decay, cavity preparation, or fracture? _____

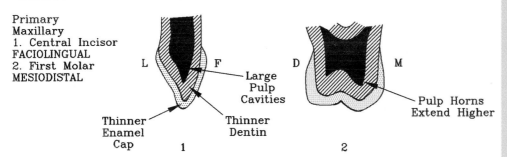

Primary
Maxillary
1. Central Incisor
FACIOLINGUAL
2. First Molar
MESIODISTAL

The dentin in primary teeth is generally less dense than in permanent teeth. Because a thicker, more dense dentin causes a darker color, will the primary teeth generally have a darker or lighter color than the permanent teeth? _____

The gross morphology of the primary dentition has many features common to that of the permanent dentition. Only the more important forms and critical differences will be described.

PRIMARY MAXILLARY CENTRAL INCISOR

On the facial surface of the primary maxillary central incisor, the mesiodistal width is _____ (greater/less) than the incisocervical length.

Primary
Maxillary
Right
Central Incisor
FACIAL

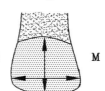

In other words, the crown of the primary maxillary central incisor is wider mesiodistally than it is long incisocervically. This "squatty," short appearance is characteristic of all primary anterior teeth, and is _____ (similar/dissimilar) to permanent anterior teeth.

1. Primary
Maxillary
Right
Central Incisor
FACIAL
2. Permanent
Maxillary
Right
Central Incisor
FACIAL

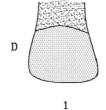

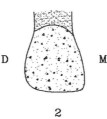

mesiodistal

The facial surface of the central incisor is convex in both the incisocervical and mesiodistal directions, but it is more convex in the _____ direction.

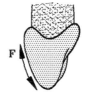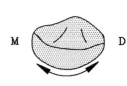

Primary
Maxillary
Central Incisor
1. MESIAL
2. INCISAL

A. mesial marginal ridge;
B. lingual fossa;
C. cingulum;
D. distal marginal ridge

The lingual features on the crown of a primary maxillary central incisor are smoothly contoured but have the same names as the corresponding features on a permanent central incisor. Identify each of the features labeled.

A. _____
B. _____
C. _____
D. _____

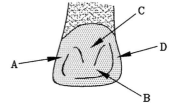

Primary
Maxillary
Right
Central Incisor
LINGUAL

conical

The root of a primary central incisor tends to be nearly circular in horizontal section and evenly tapered toward the apex in the longitudinal direction. Overall, the geometric form of the root can be described as _____ in shape.

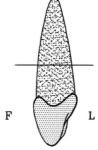

Primary
Maxillary
Right
Central Incisor
1. MESIAL
2. CROSS SECTION

The roof of the pulp chamber in a primary maxillary central incisor has three pulp horns. As with permanent incisors, the facial portion is described as having how many lobes?

Primary
Maxillary
Right
Central Incisor
MESIODISTAL SECTION

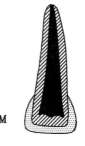

M   D

three

Since the cingulum of the primary incisor represents a single lobe, the tooth can be described as having a total of _____ lobes.

Primary
Maxillary
Right
Central Incisor
1. LINGUAL
2. MESIAL

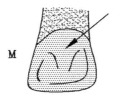   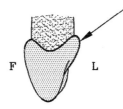

M   D   F   L

1   2

four

PRIMARY MAXILLARY LATERAL INCISOR

5.1.2

Of the two primary maxillary incisors, which is wider in the mesiodistal direction?

Primary
Maxillary
Right
1. Lateral Incisor
2. Central Incisor
FACIAL

D   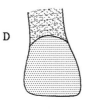   M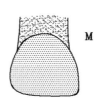

1   2

central

What is the incisocervical size relationship between the crowns of the primary maxillary central and lateral incisors? _____

Primary
Maxillary
Right
1. Lateral Incisor
2. Central Incisor
FACIAL

D   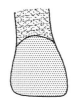   M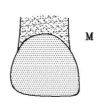

1   2

central is slightly larger

central

On the primary lateral incisor, the facial and lingual features are less prominent than those of the central incisor. Which primary incisor has the more prominent cingulum? _____

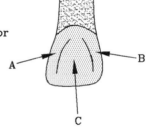

Primary
Maxillary
Right
1. Lateral Incisor
2. Central Incisor
LINGUAL

mesial marginal ridge

The primary lateral has more prominent marginal ridges. Which one is labeled "A"? _____ _____ _____ The lingual fossa, labeled C, is deeper due to the more prominent marginal ridges.

Primary
Maxillary
Right
Lateral Incisor
LINGUAL

Lateral is constricted more in the cervical area.

Illustrated is a difference between the cervical regions of the pulp cavity of the primary central and lateral incisors. What is the difference? _____

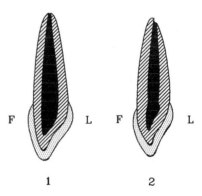

Primary
Maxillary
1. Central Incisor
2. Lateral Incisor
FACIOLINGUAL SECTIONS

Apart from this distinction, the root and pulp structures on the primary maxillary lateral incisors and central incisors are essentially _____ (similar/ dissimilar).

similar

Primary
Maxillary
1. Central Incisor
2. Lateral Incisor
FACIOLINGUAL SECTIONS

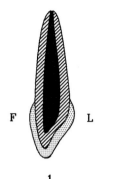 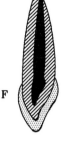

F   L   F   L

1   2

PRIMARY MANDIBULAR CENTRAL INCISOR

5.1.3

What is the size relationship between the maxillary and mandibular central incisors?

The mandibular are smaller.

Primary
1. Maxillary
Right
Central Incisor
LINGUAL
2. Mandibular
Right
Central Incisor
LINGUAL

M 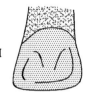 D   M 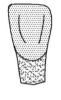 D

1   2

Although the facial surface on a mandibular incisor is convex in the mesiodistal direction, the degree of convexity progressively decreases from the _____ (cervical/incisal) border to the _____ (cervical/incisal) border.

cervical, incisal
(in that order)

Primary
Mandibular
Central Incisor
1. FACIAL
2. MESIAL

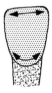 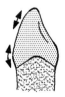

1   2

As with the other primary anterior teeth, but unlike the permanent mandibular anterior teeth, the primary mandibular central incisor has its incisal edge _____ (in line with/displaced from) the longitudinal axis of the tooth from a proximal view.

Primary
Mandibular
Right
Central Incisor
MESIAL

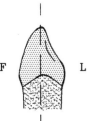

in line with

Similar to the permanent mandibular central incisor, the primary mandibular central incisor has mesioincisal and distoincisal angles that are approximately _____ (45°/right) angles.

Primary
Mandibular
Right
Central Incisor
FACIAL

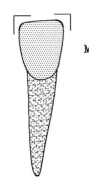

right

Compared to the maxillary incisor, the lingual contours of a mandibular incisor are reduced and smoothly curved. Therefore, the cingulum and marginal ridges will be _____ (distinct/indistinct).

Primary
1. Maxillary
Right
Central Incisor
LINGUAL
2. Mandibular
Right
Central Incisor
LINGUAL

1

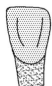

2

indistinct

PRIMARY MANDIBULAR LATERAL INCISOR

Of the two mandibular incisors, which crown has the greater incisocervical length?

_____ _____

Primary
Mandibular
Right
1. Central Incisor
2. Lateral Incisor
FACIAL

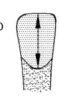 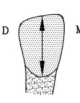

1   2

The crown of the mandibular lateral incisor compared to the mandibular central incisor, is longer and slightly _____ (narrower/wider).

Primary
Mandibular
Right
1. Central Incisor
2. Lateral Incisor
FACIAL

 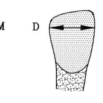

1   2

Of the two incisal angles on the mandibular lateral incisor, which is more rounded?

_____

Primary
Mandibular
Right
Lateral Incisor
FACIAL

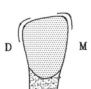

The cingulum and marginal ridges are a little larger; therefore the _____ _____ is a little deeper.

Primary
Mandibular
Right
Lateral Incisor
LINGUAL

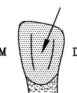

lateral incisor

Which incisor has the longer root? _____ _____

Primary
Mandibular
Right
1. Central Incisor
2. Lateral Incisor
FACIAL

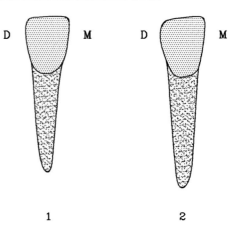

1   2

GO TO THE NEXT PAGE AND TAKE REVIEW TEST 5.1.

REVIEW TEST 5.1

Place an X on the lines that match the left-hand column with the top row.

	Both/ Neither	*Central*	*Lateral*
Primary maxillary incisor with the wider crown	_____	_____	_____
Primary maxillary incisor with the longer crown	_____	_____	_____
Primary mandibular incisor with the crown that appears slightly wider	_____	_____	_____
Mandibular incisor with a rounder distoincisal angle	_____	_____	_____

CHECK YOUR ANSWERS IN APPENDIX A.

5.2.0 PRIMARY MAXILLARY CANINE

C (all three directions)

The primary canines have considerably more bulk than the primary incisors. In the maxillary arch, in which directions are the measurements of the canines larger than those of the incisors? _____ (A/B/C)

A. mesiodistal and faciolingual only
B. mesiodistal and incisocervical only
C. mesiodistal, incisocervical, and faciolingual

Primary
Maxillary
Right
1. Canine
2. Lateral Incisor
3. Central Incisor
a. FACIAL
b. MESIAL

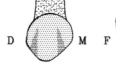

three, one
(in that order)

The number and position of the lobes that can be seen on a primary canine are similar to those of the incisors. Therefore, the facial portion is described as having _____ (number) lobes and the lingual portion as having _____ (number) lobe(s).

cusp, facial

The facial portion of the canine is "enlivened" by the well-developed central lobe area which forms two characteristic canine features, the _____ and its prominent _____ ridge.

Primary
Maxillary
Right
Canine
1. FACIAL
2. MESIAL

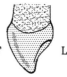

mesial

The cusp tip divides the incisal into the mesial cusp ridge and the distal cusp ridge. Which cusp ridge is longer? _____

Primary
Maxillary
Right
Canine
FACIAL

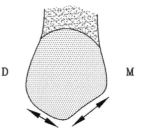

On the lingual, the prominent marginal ridges and the lingual fossae have the same names as the corresponding features on permanent canines. Name the features labeled in the drawing.

A. _____

B. _____

C. _____

D. _____

Primary
Maxillary
Right
Canine
LINGUAL

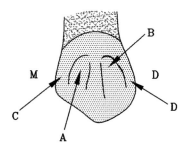

In the cervical third of the crown, the lingual ridge blends with the cingulum. The lingual ridge thus becomes less prominent as it runs in a _____ direction.

Primary
Maxillary
Right
Canine
LINGUAL

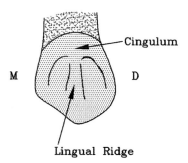

Cingulum

M   D

Lingual Ridge

Which of the following statements about the primary maxillary canine are true? _____

a. The root of the canine is longer than the root of the primary maxillary lateral and central.

b. The apex of the canine is pointed.

c. The root tapers sharply to a point.

Primary
Maxillary
Right
1. Canine
2. Lateral Incisor
3. Central Incisor
FACIAL

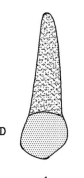
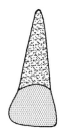

D   M

1   2   3

apex

The maxillary canine root is very gradually tapered. The root diameter is fairly constant throughout the cervical half, then tapers near the _____ .

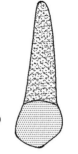

Primary
Maxillary
Right
Canine
FACIAL

D   M

central

The pulp chamber of the maxillary canine has three horns: the distal, central, and mesial. The largest is the _____ .

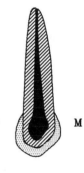

Primary
Maxillary
Right
Canine
MESIODISTAL SECTION

D   M

central, distal, mesial

The distal pulp horn is slightly larger and longer than the mesial horn. Rank the three pulp horns in the order of their size (largest to smallest).

_____ largest

_____

_____ smallest

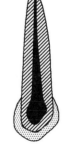

Primary
Maxillary
Right
Canine
MESIODISTAL SECTION

D   M

central

In the maxillary canine, there is little demarcation between the pulp chamber and the root canal. Thus, the pulp cavity of the canine is similar to that of the maxillary _____ incisor.

Primary
Maxillary
Right
Canine
MESIODISTAL SECTION

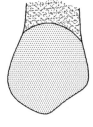

D   M

PRIMARY MANDIBULAR CANINE

5.2.1

distoincisal

The mandibular canine has essentially the same features and characteristics as the maxillary canine. One exception is the relative lengths of the mesioincisal and distoincisal edges (mesial cusp ridge and distal cusp ridge). On the mandibular canine, which incisal edge is longer? _____

Primary
1. Maxillary
2. Mandibular
Right Canine
FACIAL

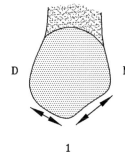

D   M   D   M

1   2

1. maxillary right
2. mandibular right

Indicate the quadrant to which each belongs. (Hint: measure the relative length of the mesial and distal cusp ridges.)

1. _____ _____ quadrant
2. _____ _____ quadrant

Primary
1. Maxillary
2. Mandibular
Canine
FACIAL

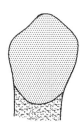

1   2

maxillary

Which of the two canine teeth is wider mesiodistally? _____

Primary
1. Maxillary
2. Mandibular
Right Canine
FACIAL

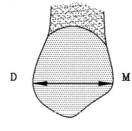
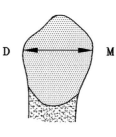

1   2

smaller

Compared to the maxillary canine, the lingual features of the primary mandibular canine are less prominent. The marginal ridges blend with the cingulum which is _____ (larger/smaller) than that of the maxillary canine.

Primary
Mandibular
Right
Canine
LINGUAL

M   D

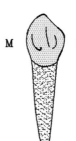

A. mesial marginal
ridge;
B. distal marginal
ridge;
C. cingulum

Although less prominent than on the maxillary canine, the usual features are present on the lingual portion of the mandibular canine. Identify each.

A. _____
B. _____
C. _____

Primary
Mandibular
Right
Canine
LINGUAL

M   D

B

A   C

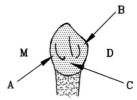

One difference between the root of the mandibular canine and the maxillary canine is the cervicoapical taper. Which canine has the more tapered root? _____
_____

Primary
1. Maxillary
2. Mandibular
Right Canine
FACIAL

1   2

The primary mandibular canine has no demarcation between the pulp chamber and root canal. In this regard, the mandibular canine is similar to most other primary anterior teeth except the _____ _____ _____ .

Mandibular
Right Canine
1. FACIOLINGUAL SECTION
2. MESIODISTAL SECTION

F   L   D   M

1   2

The primary canine with a mesioincisal edge longer than its distoincisal edge is found in the _____ arch.

TURN TO THE NEXT PAGE AND TAKE REVIEW TEST 5.2.

REVIEW TEST 5.2

Place an X on the lines that match the left hand column with the top row.

	Both/ Neither	Maxillary Canine	Mandibular Canine
Canine with a more tapered root	_____	_____	_____
Canine with the wider crown	_____	_____	_____
Canine with five lobes	_____	_____	_____
Canine with the less prominent mesial and distal marginal ridges	_____	_____	_____
Canine with its mesial cusp ridge longer than its distal cusp ridge	_____	_____	_____

1. The molars of the _____ dentition have the more narrow occlusal table (faciolingually) in proportion to the crown size.

   a. permanent
   b. primary

2. The greater dimension of the facial surface of the primary maxillary central incisor is the

   a. incisocervical
   b. mesiodistal

3. There is a conspicuous demarcation between the pulp chamber and the root canal in the

   a. primary maxillary central incisor
   b. primary maxillary lateral incisor

4. Which of the following is not a characteristic feature of the primary dentition?

   a. thin enamel cap
   b. thick and dense dentin
   c. large pulp chamber

5. In which dentition is the ratio of root length to crown length greater?

   a. primary
   b. permanent

6. Is this statement true or false?

   Whereas the incisocervical crown length of the maxillary lateral incisor is less than the length of the maxillary central incisor crown, the mandibular lateral incisor crown has a greater incisocervical length than the mandibular central incisor crown.

   a. true
   b. false

CHECK YOUR ANSWERS IN APPENDIX A.

PRIMARY MAXILLARY FIRST MOLAR

The maxillary first molar usually appears 3-cusped or 4-cusped. In any case, the geometric outline of the occlusal view is roughly _____ .

triangular

Primary
Maxillary
Right
First Molar
1. 3 cusps
2. 4 cusps
OCCLUSAL

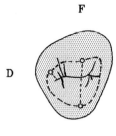
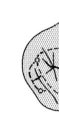

1   2

The tooth converges lingually which creates the triangular-shaped form. Which part of the crown is wider in the mesiodistal direction? _____ (facial/lingual)

facial

Primary
Maxillary
Right
First Molar
1. 3 cusps
2. 4 cusps
OCCLUSAL

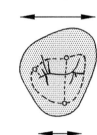
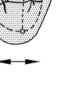
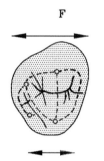

1   2

The cusps of the different forms of the maxillary first molar have similar names: (a) mesio-facial, (b) distofacial, (c) mesiolingual, and (d) distolingual. The more common 3-cusped form does not have a _____ cusp.

distolingual

Primary
Maxillary
Right
First Molar
1. 3 cusps
2. 4 cusps
OCCLUSAL

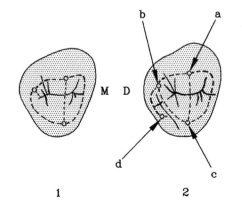

1   2

a. distofacial
b. lingual
c. mesiofacial

Name each of the three cusps of the 3-cusped maxillary first molar.

a. _____

b. _____

c. _____

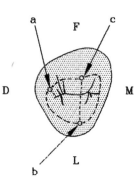

Primary
Maxillary
Right
First Molar
OCCLUSAL

distolingual

On the 4-cusped form, the smallest, least developed is the _____ cusp.

Primary
Maxillary
Right
First Molar
1. OCCLUSAL
2. LINGUAL

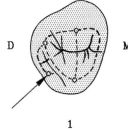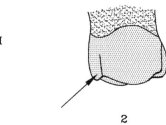

1   2

marginal ridges

Similar to the permanent molars, the occlusal surface (occlusal table) of a primary molar is surrounded by cusp ridges and the mesial and distal _____ _____ .

Primary
Maxillary
Right
First Molar
OCCLUSAL

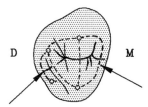

The oblique ridge that is characteristic of maxillary molars in the permanent dentition is also present on the maxillary molars of the primary dentition (Figure 2). However, on the 3-cusped form of the primary maxillary first molar (Figure 1), the oblique ridge blends with the _____ _____ ridge.

distal marginal

Primary
Maxillary
Right
First Molar
1. 3 cusps
2. 4 cusps
OCCLUSAL

D 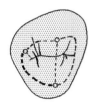   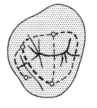 M

1   2

On either the 3-cusped or 4-cusped form of the primary maxillary first molar, the oblique ridge runs in an oblique direction, uniting the _____ and the _____ cusps.

mesiolingual
(lingual); distofacial

Primary
Maxillary
Right
First Molar
1. 3 cusps
2. 4 cusps
OCCLUSAL

D 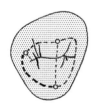   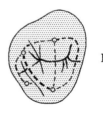 M

1   2

Of the two teeth adjacent to the maxillary first molar, the facial end of the oblique ridge is closest to the _____ _____ . The lingual end of the ridge ends on the lingual towards the mesial.

second molar

Primary
Maxillary
Right
First Molar
1. 3 cusps
2. 4 cusps
OCCLUSAL

D 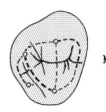   M

1   2

central

On the occlusal surface of the 3-cusped form, the mesial and central pits mark the confluence of developmental grooves. The confluence of the distal, facial, and mesial grooves is marked by the _____ pit.

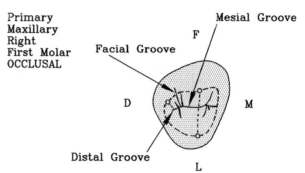

Primary
Maxillary
Right
First Molar
OCCLUSAL

Facial Groove

Mesial Groove

F

D

M

Distal Groove

L

mesial

The pit at the mesial end of the mesial groove is called the _____ pit.

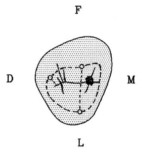

Primary
Maxillary
Right
First Molar
OCCLUSAL

F

D

M

L

A. distal;
B. facial;
C. mesial

The three grooves that originate in the central pit are named for the direction they run from that pit. As labeled, these grooves are the A. _____ , B. _____ , and C. _____ developmental grooves.

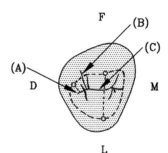

Primary
Maxillary
Right
First Molar
OCCLUSAL

F

(B)

(C)

(A)

D

M

L

The mesial pit marks the confluence of four developmental grooves: the mesial, mesiofacial triangular, mesial marginal, and mesiolingual triangular. The groove running between the mesial and central pits is the _____ groove.

Primary
Maxillary
Right
First Molar
OCCLUSAL

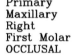
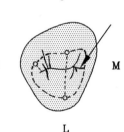

F

D   M

L

The groove previously described is often referred to as the central groove. Frequently, a structure will be identified using a different name. When using the other name, then, the groove running between the mesial fossa and central fossa would be the _____ groove.

The groove that originates at the mesial pit and ascends the slope of the mesial marginal ridge is the _____ _____ groove.

Primary
Maxillary
Right
First Molar
OCCLUSAL

F

D   M

L

A. mesial marginal;
B. mesiofacial
triangular;
C. mesiolingual
triangular;
D. facial

The mesiolingual triangular and mesiofacial triangular grooves originate at the mesial pit and run in the direction of the mesiolingual and mesiofacial line angles.

Name the developmental grooves labeled A, B, C, and D:

A. _____

B. _____

C. _____

D. _____

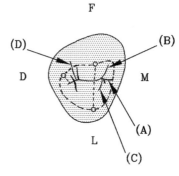

Primary
Maxillary
Right
First Molar
OCCLUSAL

central; distal
marginal ridge

The distal groove extends distally from the _____ pit, becoming indistinct as it reaches the _____ _____ _____ .

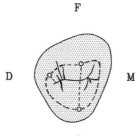

Primary
Maxillary
Right
First Molar
OCCLUSAL

central, distal

On the 4-cusped form of the primary maxillary first molar, three occlusal pits are present: mesial, central, and distal. The oblique ridge cuts across the occlusal surface and passes between the _____ and _____ pits.

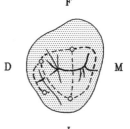

Primary
Maxillary
Right
First Molar
OCCLUSAL

With one exception, the four grooves that meet at the distal pit are named similar to those meeting at the mesial pit. The distolingual groove is not a triangular groove. Name the grooves in the drawing.

A. _____

B. _____

C. _____

D. _____

A. distofacial triangular;
B. distomarginal;
C. distolingual;
D. distal

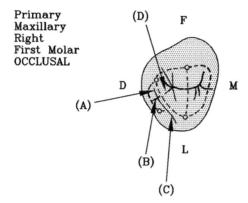

Primary
Maxillary
Right
First Molar
OCCLUSAL

Which groove on the 4-cusped form partially interrupts the oblique ridge? _____

distal

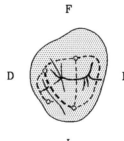

Primary
Maxillary
Right
First Molar
OCCLUSAL

The most common occlusal pattern found on the primary maxillary first molar is the _____-cusped form.

three

From the facial view, the mesiofacial cusp exhibits greater development than the distofacial cusp. When the mesiodistal width of the facial surface is divided into thirds, the mesiofacial cusp extends across the mesial _____ (1/3, 2/3) of the facial surface.

2/3

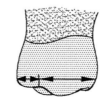

Primary
Maxillary
Right
First Molar
FACIAL

mesial

In addition, the mesiofacial cusp has a greater development in the occlusocervical direction. This cusp development gives the cervical line a skewed curvature and causes the greatest occlusocervical length on the facial surface to be located in the _____ half of the crown.

Primary
Maxillary
Right
First Molar
FACIAL

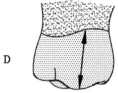

facial

Occasionally, a developmental groove may cross the faciocclusal line angle and extend onto the facial surface, separating the mesiofacial and distofacial cusps. This groove is called the _____ groove.

Primary
Maxillary
Right
First Molar
FACIAL

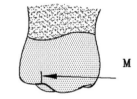

mesial

The mesial and occlusal views of the primary first molar illustrate the prominent height of contour on the facial surface (faciocervical ridge). The prominence of this ridge is characteristic of primary first molars, particularly the added thickness of this ridge toward the _____ (mesial/distal).

Primary
Maxillary
Right
First Molar
1. MESIAL
2. OCCLUSAL

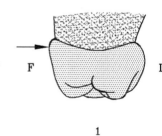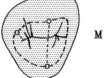

1   2

narrower (or synonym)

Compared to the mesiodistal width of the facial surface of this tooth, the lingual surface is _____ .

Primary
Maxillary
1. Left
2. Right
First Molar
1. LINGUAL
2. OCCLUSAL

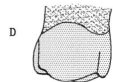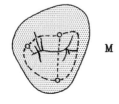

1   2

The lingual portion of the maxillary first molar contains the largest cusp on the tooth, the _____ .

Primary
Maxillary
Left
First Molar
LINGUAL

D   M

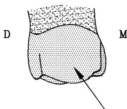

When a small distolingual cusp is present, it is partially separated from the mesiolingual cusp by a groove originating at the distal pit, the _____ groove.

Primary
Maxillary
Left
First Molar
LINGUAL

D   M

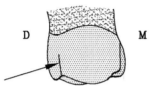

The roots of the primary maxillary first molar have the same names and relative positions as those of the permanent maxillary first molar. Name the roots in the drawing.

A. _____
B. _____
C. _____

Primary
Maxillary
Right
First Molar
FACIAL

(A)   (B)   (C)

D   M

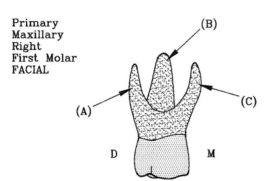

maxillary first premolar

The roots of the primary maxillary first molar are flared. This provides room for the tooth bud of which permanent tooth? _____ _____ _____

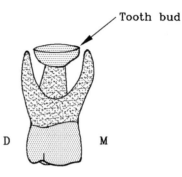

Primary
Maxillary
Right
First Molar
FACIAL

Tooth bud

D   M

---

lingual, mesiofacial,
distofacial
(in that order)

The mesiofacial root is second in size. List the three roots in the primary maxillary first molar in order of decreasing size.

_____ largest
_____
_____ smallest

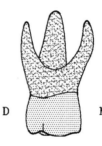

Primary
Maxillary
Right
First Molar
FACIAL

D   M

---

three, four

The roof of the pulp chamber follows the general form of the occlusal surface of the crown. Corresponding to the cusps, the primary maxillary first molar may have either _____ or _____ (number) pulp horns.

Primary
Maxillary
Right
First Molar
CROSS SECTIONS
OCCLUSAL

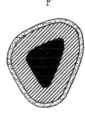

F   F

L   L

3 cusped   4 cusped

The pulp chamber of the primary maxillary first molar has a greater development facially than lingually, mesially than distally. Therefore, the largest and longest pulp horn is the _____ .

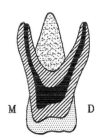

Primary
Maxillary
Left
First Molar
MESIODISTAL
SECTION
FACIAL

M   D

The names of three pulp horns of the 3-cusped maxillary first molar are

_____ largest

_____

_____ smallest

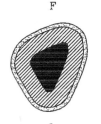

Primary
Maxillary
Right
First Molar
CROSS SECTION
OCCLUSAL

F

M

L

Give a short answer (one or two words) to these questions about the primary maxillary first molar.

1. How many cusps are present on the most common form? _____
2. Name the largest cusp. _____
3. Name the largest pulp horn. _____
4. How many developmental grooves meet at the central pit? _____
5. Of the facial and lingual end of the oblique ridge, which is located more toward the mesial? _____
6. A characteristic of this tooth is the development of the faciocervical ridge (buccogingival ridge) especially on one half of the crown. Which half? _____
7. The root canals correspond to the roots, one canal per root, making a total of _____ (number).

5.3.1 PRIMARY MAXILLARY SECOND MOLAR

permanent maxillary
first molar

Morphologically, the primary maxillary second molar strikingly resembles the permanent molar that erupts adjacent to it, the _____ _____ _____

(dentition)   (arch)   (tooth name)

_____ .

1. Primary
Maxillary
Right
Second Molar
OCCLUSAL
2. Permanent
Maxillary
Right
First Molar
OCCLUSAL

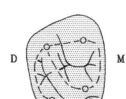

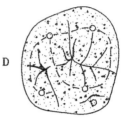

1   2

greater

In occlusal outline, the primary maxillary second molar is approximately rhomboid in appearance. However, as with the permanent maxillary first molar, the faciolingual measurement of the crown is _____ (greater/less than) the mesiodistal measurement.

Primary
Maxillary
Right
Second Molar
OCCLUSAL

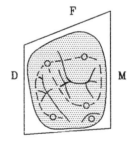

second molar

Of the two primary maxillary molars, which is larger? _____ _____

Primary
Maxillary
Right
1. Second Molar
2. First Molar
OCCLUSAL

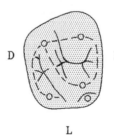

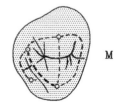

1   2

A small cusp is sometimes present on the lingual portion of the mesiolingual cusp. Thus, the number of cusps on the primary maxillary first molar is either _____ or _____ ; but the second molar has either _____ or _____ .

three, four; four, five (in that order)

Primary
Maxillary
Right
1. First Molar
2. Second Molar
OCCLUSAL

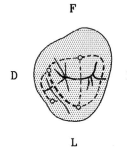

The small fifth cusp, the Carabelli cusp, and the four major cusps are named in a manner similar to those of the permanent maxillary first molar. Name the cusps of the primary second molar.

A. _____
B. _____
C. _____
D. _____
E. _____

A. mesiofacial;
B. mesiolingual;
C. Carabelli cusp;
D. distolingual;
E. distofacial

Primary
Maxillary
Right
Second Molar
OCCLUSAL

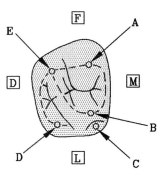

Of the four major cusps of the primary maxillary second molar, the widest is the _____ .

mesiolingual

Primary
Maxillary
Right
Second Molar
OCCLUSAL

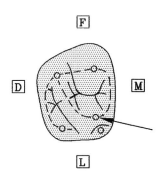

distolingual

The smallest of the four major cusps, also on the lingual portion of the crown, is the

_____ .

Primary
Maxillary
Right
Second Molar
OCCLUSAL

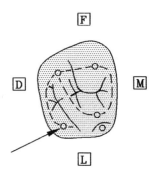

distal, central, mesial
(any order)

Three pits mark the intersections of the developmental grooves on the occlusal surface. As on the four-cusped form of the first molar, they are the _____ , _____ , and _____ pits.

Primary
Maxillary
Right
Second Molar
OCCLUSAL

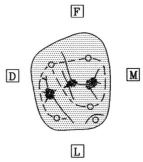

A. mesial marginal
B. facial
C. distal
D. distofacial triangular

The primary maxillary second molar has 11 developmental grooves. All but the three most lingually located (the distolingual triangular, distolingual, and mesiolingual) are positioned in a manner similar to those on the four-cusped primary maxillary first molar. Name the grooves labeled in the illustration.

A. _____
B. _____
C. _____
D. _____

Primary
Maxillary
Right
Second Molar
OCCLUSAL

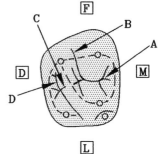

Of the distolingual, distolingual triangular, and mesiolingual grooves, only the triangular groove does not separate two cusps. Name the labeled grooves.

A. _____

B. _____

C. _____

Primary
Maxillary
Right
Second Molar
OCCLUSAL

On the primary maxillary second molar, the characteristic ridge of maxillary molars is well developed. It unites the _____ and _____ cusps and is named the _____ ridge.

Primary
Maxillary
Right
Second Molar
OCCLUSAL

Of the four cusps on the primary maxillary second molar, three are nearly equal in height. They are the _____ , _____ , and _____ .

Primary
Maxillary
Right
Second Molar
1. FACIAL
2. LINGUAL

longest

The mesiolingual is the _____ (longest/shortest) of the four major cusps on the maxillary second molar.

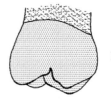

```
Primary
Maxillary
Right
Second Molar
1. FACIAL        D
2. LINGUAL
```

1   2

A. facial
B. mesiolingual
C. distolingual

From the facial and lingual views, three developmental grooves mark the boundaries of the lobes in the occlusal portion of the crown. Name these grooves.

A. _____

B. _____

C. _____

```
Primary
Maxillary
Right
Second Molar
1. FACIAL        D
2. LINGUAL
A
```

B

1   C   2

mesiofacial,
distofacial, lingual
(any order)

Similar to the other maxillary molars (primary and permanent), the primary maxillary second molar has three roots: the _____ , _____ , and _____ .

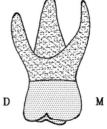

```
Primary
Maxillary
Right
Second
Molar
FACIAL

        D          M
```

The pulp cavity of the primary maxillary second molar has one pulp horn that corresponds to each cusp and one root canal that corresponds to each root. Therefore, it has _____ (number) root canals and either _____ or _____ pulp horns.

Primary
Maxillary
Right
Second Molar
1. Faciolingual Section
DISTAL
2. Faciolingual Section
MESIAL

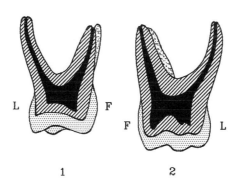

Similar to that of the primary maxillary first molar, the pulp cavity of the second molar shows more development facially and mesially. As a result, the largest and longest pulp horn is the _____ .

Primary
Maxillary
Right
Second Molar
1. Faciolingual Section
DISTAL
2. Faciolingual Section
MESIAL

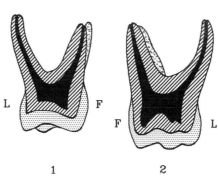

Give a short answer to these questions about the primary maxillary second molar.

1. What tooth in the human permanent dentition has a morphology similar to this tooth?
_____

2. If a cylindrical object, such as a pencil, is inserted into the mouth in a roughly anterior to posterior position, is the object more nearly parallel or perpendicular to the oblique ridge? _____

3. Name the widest and longest cusp. _____

5.3.2 PRIMARY MANDIBULAR FIRST MOLAR

Because of the extreme occlusal convergence of the facial surface, the occlusal table of the mandibular first molar is narrow in the _____ direction.

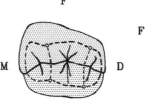
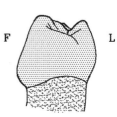

Primary
Mandibular
Right
First Molar
1. OCCLUSAL
2. MESIAL

F

M   D

L

F   L

1   2

From the mesial aspect, the prominent faciocervical ridge appears as a bulbous "overhang" and serves as an identifying feature. Which label (a or b) identifies this ridge in the drawing to the right? _____

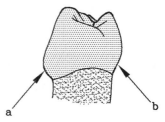

Primary
Mandibular
Right
First Molar
MESIAL

a   b

The facial view of this tooth is unusual. The faciocervical ridge is much more prominent at its _____ end.

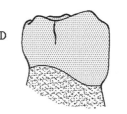

Primary
Mandibular
Right
First Molar
FACIAL

D   M

Of the two facial cusps (mesiofacial and distofacial) one is considerably wider but only slightly higher than the other. Which facial cusp is higher in the occlusocervical direction? _____

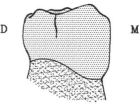

Primary
Mandibular
Right
First Molar
FACIAL

D   M

The facial groove may or may not be evident from the facial aspect. Whether or not the groove is present, the intersection of the facial lobes is suggested by the shallow, smoothly contoured facial concavity between the cusps. Because of the cusp development in the mesiodistal direction, the facial concavity is located in the _____ half of the crown.

distal

Primary
Mandibular
Right
First Molar
1. FACIAL
2. OCCLUSAL

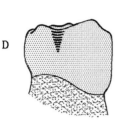

From the facial aspect, the skewed curvature of the cervical line is caused by the prominent mass formed by the highly developed _____ _____ .

faciocervical ridge

Primary
Mandibular
Right
First Molar
FACIAL

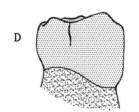

Seen from the mesial aspect, the occlusocervical curvature of the facial surface, from faciocervical ridge to cusp tip, is nearly _____ (convex/flat).

flat

Primary
Mandibular
Right
First Molar
MESIAL

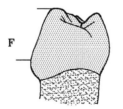

Two cusps are evident on the lingual portion of the crown of the mandibular first molar. Similar to the facial cusps, the wider and longer of the two lingual cusps is located toward the _____ .

mesial

Primary
Mandibular
Right
First Molar
LINGUAL

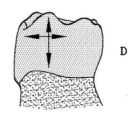

facial, mesiolingual

The relative sizes of the four cusps are shown in occlusal view. The two mesial cusps are larger than the distal cusps, the mesio-_____ cusp being slightly larger than the _____ cusp.

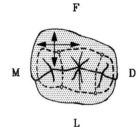

Primary
Mandibular
Right
First Molar
OCCLUSAL

mesiofacial,
mesiolingual

The distal portion of the occlusal surface has a deep occlusal sulcus. However, the mesial portion is marked by a distinct transverse ridge which runs across the occlusal surface between the _____ and _____ cusps.

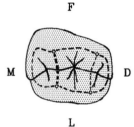

Primary
Mandibular
Right
First Molar
OCCLUSAL

oblique, transverse

In the maxillary arch, the ridge that crosses the occlusal surface of the molars is the _____ . On the primary mandibular first molar, the ridge crossing the occlusal surface is the _____ .

Primary
1. Maxillary
Right
Second Molar
OCCLUSAL
2. Mandibular
Right
First Molar
OCCLUSAL

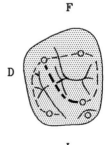

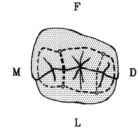

1

2

Three pits are formed by the intersection of the developmental grooves of the occlusal surface: the mesial, central, and distal pits. The transverse ridge divides the occlusal surface into two fossae, one containing the _____ pit, the other the _____ and _____ pits.

Primary
Mandibular
Right
First Molar
OCCLUSAL

The facial, mesial, lingual, and distal development grooves originate at the central pit. Name the grooves labeled in the illustration

A. _____

B. _____

C. _____

D. _____

Primary
Mandibular
Right
First Molar
OCCLUSAL

In addition to the distal groove, three grooves intersect at the distal pit: the distofacial triangular, distal marginal, and distolingual triangular. Name the grooves in the drawing.

A. _____

B. _____

C. _____

Primary
Mandibular
Right
First Molar
OCCLUSAL

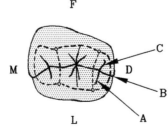

transverse ridge

The mesial groove is shallow and may fade out on the mesial and distal slopes of the
_____ _____ .

Primary
Mandibular
Right
First Molar
OCCLUSAL

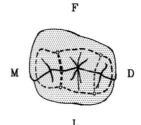

A. mesial marginal;
B. mesiofacial
triangular

Groove (A) is the _____ _____ , and groove (B) is the _____
_____ .

Primary
Mandibular
Right
First Molar
OCCLUSAL

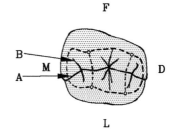

mesial, distal

Similar to the permanent mandibular molars, the primary mandibular molar has two roots,
the _____ and _____ roots.

Primary
Mandibular
Right
First Molar
1. FACIAL
2. MESIAL

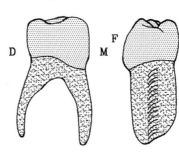

As was true on the roots of permanent mandibular molars, the mesial and distal roots of the primary mandibular first molar are narrow and convex in the _____ direction, but broad in the _____ direction.

Primary
Mandibular
Right
First Molar
1. FACIAL
2. MESIAL

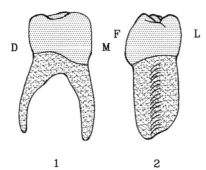

The pulp cavity of the primary mandibular first molar has three root canals. The larger of the two roots, corresponding to the two largest cusps, contains two canals. Following the established pattern for naming an entity of dental anatomy, the names of the three root canals are _____ , _____ , and _____ .

Primary
Mandibular
Right
First Molar
1. LINGUAL
2. CROSS SECTION

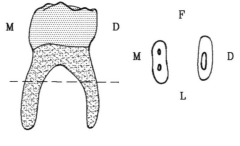

Corresponding to the number of cusps, the roof of the pulp chamber in the primary mandibular first molar has _____ (number) pulp horns.

Primary
Mandibular
Right
First Molar
FACIOLINGUAL
SECTIONS

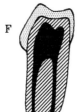
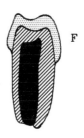

mesiofacial,
mesiolingual
(in that order)

Corresponding to the relative sizes of the cusps, the largest and second largest pulp horns are the _____ and _____ .

Primary
Mandibular
Right
First Molar
1. Faciolingual
MESIAL
2. Faciolingual
DISTAL

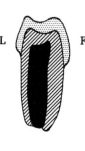
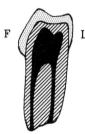

1   2

5.3.3   PRIMARY MANDIBULAR SECOND MOLAR

2, bulbous

The primary mandibular second molar has a morphology that closely resembles that of the permanent mandibular first molar. Specimens of the two teeth can be distinguished by their relative sizes and by the bulbous quality of the primary tooth. Although the drawing does not permit a size comparison, the primary molar is represented by drawing number _____ because it has the more _____ shape.

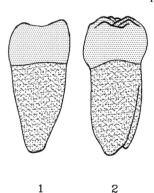

1   2

both

Additional distinctions between the morphology of the primary mandibular second molar and the permanent mandibular first molar include:

1. The relative size of the distal cusp.
2. Some slight differences in the groove patterns of the occlusal surfaces.
3. The ratio of the faciolingual to mesiodistal crown diameter.

On which of the two teeth (Figure 1/Figure 2) is the mesiodistal crown diameter greater than the faciolingual diameter as seen from an occlusal view? _____ (primary/permanent/both).

1. Permanent
Mandibular
Right
First Molar
OCCLUSAL
2. Primary
Mandibular
Right
Second Molar
OCCLUSAL

1   2

The cusps of the primary mandibular second molar may be identified by matching the letter in the illustration with the letter next to the cusp name.

Mesiofacial _____   A
Distofacial _____   B
Distal _____   C
Mesiolingual _____   D
Distolingual _____   E

The cusp labeled B is the _____ cusp

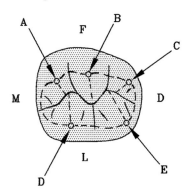

Primary
Mandibular
Right
Second Molar
OCCLUSAL

distofacial

Each cusp has a well-developed triangular ridge running from the cusp tip to the central portion of the _____ _____ .

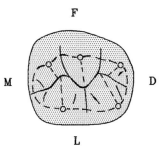

Primary
Mandibular
Right
Second Molar
OCCLUSAL

occlusal surface
(occlusal table)

The three major grooves that meet at the central pit are the lingual, mesiofacial, and distofacial. In the drawing, the mesiofacial groove is labeled _____ ; the lingual groove is labeled _____ .

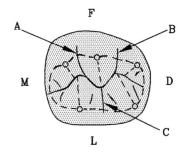

Primary
Mandibular
Right
Second Molar
OCCLUSAL

A, C (in that order)

mesiofacial, distofacial

The mesial (A) and distal (B) grooves of the primary mandibular second molar do not originate at the central pit, but branch from the _____ and _____ grooves.

Primary
Mandibular
Right
Second Molar
OCCLUSAL

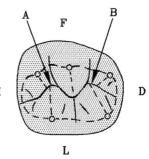

mesial pit, mesiofacial
groove (any order)

The mesial and distal grooves do not link the mesial and distal pits with the central pit. The mesial groove connects the _____ _____ and the _____ _____ .

Primary
Mandibular
Right
Second Molar
OCCLUSAL

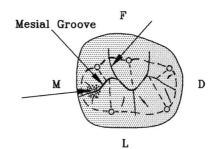

distofacial groove,
distal pit (any order)

Similarly, the distal groove runs from the _____ _____ to the _____ _____ .

Primary
Mandibular
Right
Second Molar
OCCLUSAL

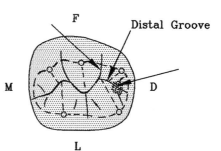

Six other grooves are evident: mesiofacial triangular, mesial marginal, mesiolingual triangular, distofacial triangular, distal marginal, and distolingual triangular.

Each of the six originates at either the mesial or distal pit. Name the four grooves labeled in the drawing.

A. _____
B. _____
C. _____
D. _____

Primary
Mandibular
Right
Second Molar
OCCLUSAL

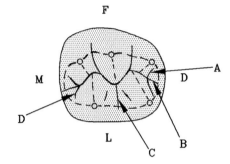

As seen from the facial and lingual views, the highest of the five cusps is the

_____ .

Primary
Mandibular
Right
Second Molar
1. FACIAL
2. LINGUAL

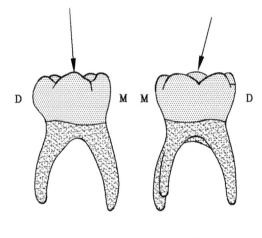

1   2

nearly equal
(or similar answer)

How do the two lingual cusps compare for height and size? _____

Primary
Mandibular
Right
Second Molar
1. FACIAL
2. LINGUAL

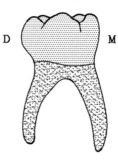
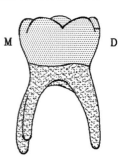

1   2

---

pit

In the occlusal portion of the facial and lingual surfaces are extensions of the developmental grooves that separate the cusps. The terminal end of the mesiofacial groove is often marked by a small, pointed depression called a _____ .

Primary
Mandibular
Right
Second Molar
1. FACIAL
2. LINGUAL

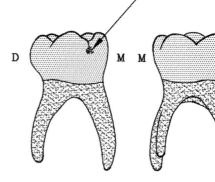

1   2

---

mesiofacial, distofacial

The facial pit on the primary mandibular second molar is generally located between the _____ and _____ cusps.

Primary
Mandibular
Right
Second Molar
FACIAL

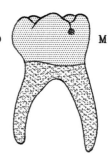

1

On the primary mandibular second molar, the characteristic bulbous form of the primary dentition is emphasized by the strong occlusal convergence of the facial surface. This convergence makes the _____ ridge more prominent.

Primary
Mandibular
Right
Second Molar
MESIAL

F   L

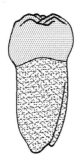

The flared roots provide space for the developing tooth bud of the permanent second premolar. The primary mandibular second molar has two roots: the _____ and _____ .

Primary
Mandibular
Right
Second Molar
1. LINGUAL
2. MESIAL

M   D   F   L

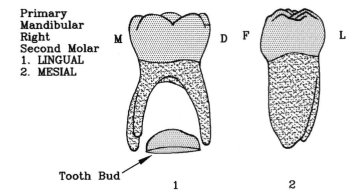

Tooth Bud

1   2

The roots of the primary mandibular second molar are generally similar to those of the mandibular first molar but _____ in size.

Primary
Mandibular
Right
1. First Molar
2. Second Molar
FACIAL

D   M   D   M

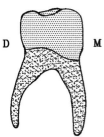
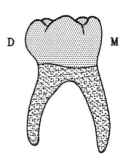

1   2

two, two

The pulp cavity of the primary mandibular second molar has either three or four root canals. In either case, the mesial root has _____ (number) root canals.

The number of root canals in the distal root of the primary mandibular second molar is either one or _____ .

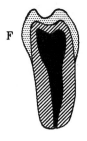

Primary
Mandibular
Left
Second Molar
CROSS SECTIONS

similar to

The mesial portion of the pulp chamber in the primary mandibular second molar is larger than the distal portion. The mesial horns are larger and higher than the distal horns; also, the mesial marginal border of the chamber is high and convex. This relative mesial to distal size differential of the pulp chamber is _____ (similar to/the opposite of) that in the primary mandibular first molar.

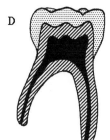

Primary
Mandibular
Right
Second Molar
Faciolingual
Section
1. MESIAL
2. DISTAL

pulp horns

As suggested by the number of cusps, the roof of the pulp chamber in the primary mandibular second molar has five _____ _____ .

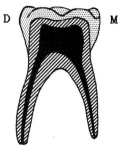

Primary
Mandibular
Right
Second Molar
1. FACIAL
2. LINGUAL

The contacts of the *primary* teeth are indicated in the illustration of the maxillary and mandibular right quadrants. The contacts are generally the same as the *permanent* teeth. The more posterior the tooth, the more _____ (cervical/incisal) the location of the contact.

Primary
Right Quadrant
1. Maxillary
2. Mandibular

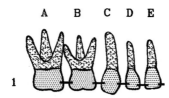

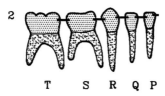

Give a short answer to each of these questions concerning the primary mandibular molars.

1. How many cusps are present on each tooth?
   a. First molar: _____
   b. Second molar: _____
2. Name the roots on a primary mandibular molar. _____ and _____
3. Which primary mandibular molar has a prominent transverse ridge that unites the mesiofacial and mesiolingual cusps? _____ _____
4. Which permanent tooth does each of the primary second molars most resemble?
   a. Maxillary second molar _____
   b. Mandibular second molar _____

....

PRIMARY DENTITION: SUMMARY

Primary Maxillary Central Incisor

	Right	*Left*
Universal code number	E	F
International code	5-1	6-1
Palmer notation	a⌋	⌊a

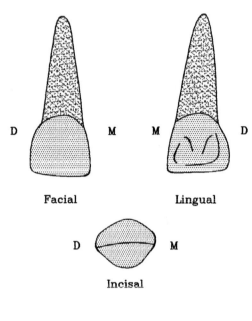

Facial   Lingual

Incisal

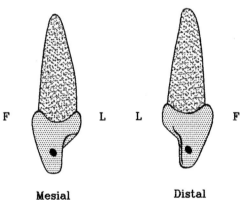

Mesial   Distal

The proximal contacts are marked on the mesial and distal views of the maxillary right central incisor in the illustration.

Features: The maxillary *primary* central, like the *permanent* central, has four lobes and three pulp horns.

Facial: From the facial view the primary maxillary central is wider mesiodistally than it is long incisocervically. It is more convex in the mesiodistal direction. It has a more rounded distoincisal angle.

Lingual: The lingual features include the mesial and distal marginal ridges, a lingual fossa, and a cingulum.

Root: Is has a conical-shaped root as seen in the facial view in the accompanying illustration.

Primary Maxillary Lateral Incisor

	Right	*Left*
Universal code number	D	G
International code number	5-2	6-2
Palmer notation	b⌋	⌊b

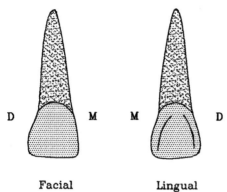

Facial   Lingual

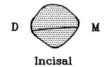

Incisal

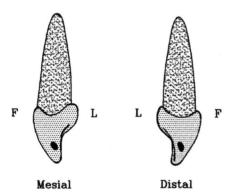

Mesial   Distal

The proximal contacts are marked on the mesial and distal views of the primary maxillary right lateral incisor in the illustration.

Features: The maxillary primary lateral incisor has four developemental lobes and three pulp horns.

Facial: It is smaller than the central incisor both mesiodistally and incisocervically. It has greater dimension incisocervically than mesiodistally. The distoincisal line angle is more rounded.

Lingual: The features are not as distinct. The marginal ridges are more prominent making the lingual fossa deeper.

Root: The root is longer than the primary maxillary central incisor and the apex less rounded.

Primary Maxillary Canine

	Right	*Left*
Universal code number	C	H
International code number	5-3	6-3
Palmer notation	c⌋	⌊c

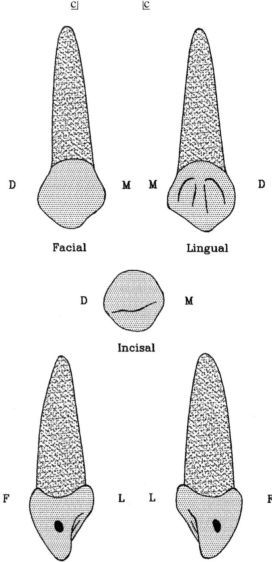

Facial   Lingual

Incisal

Mesial   Distal

The proximal contacts are marked on the mesial and distal views of the primary maxillary right canine in the illustration.

Features: The maxillary canine has a greater dimension in the incisocervical direction than the mesiodistal.

Facial: The mesioincisal cusp ridge has greater slope than the distoincisal as the cusp tip is distally located.

Proximal: The tooth is thicker faciolingually. The cervical line is less curved on the distal.

Lingual: There is a prominent lingual cingulum and lingual ridge. The mesiolingual and distolingual fossae are present.

Root: The root is similar to other maxillary anterior teeth except it is longer.

Primary Maxillary First Molar

	Right	*Left*
Universal code number	B	I
International code number	5-4	6-4
Palmer notation	d⌋	⌊d

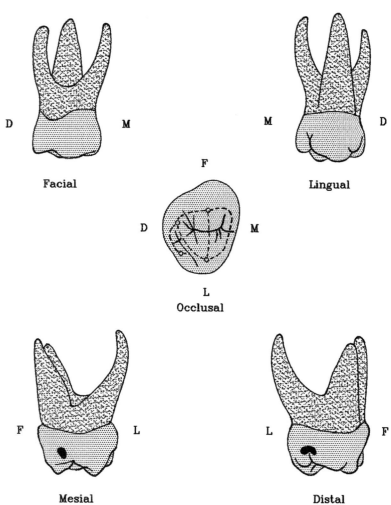

Facial

Lingual

Occlusal

Mesial

Distal

The proximal contacts are marked on the mesial and distal views of the primary maxillary right first molar in the illustration.

Features: The mesiodistal dimension is greater than the occlusocervical height. The facial is wider than the lingual.

Facial: The mesiofacial cusp has a greater occlusocervical length than the distofacial cusp, giving rise to a skewed cervical line. Sometimes a facial groove is present.

Proximal: This view reveals a prominent faciocervical ridge with added thickness toward the mesial. The distal surface is smaller than the mesial surface.

Lingual: The lingual surface is narrower than the facial surface. Of the two cusps, the *largest* is the mesiolingual and the *smallest* is the distolingual.

Occlusal surface: There is an oblique ridge present. Three or four cusps are possible. There are two fossae present on the three-cusped form, the mesial, and the central. On the four-cusped form, there are three fossae.

Roots: Three—from largest to smallest: lingual, mesiofacial, distofacial.

Pulp anatomy: Three or four pulp horns present depending on the number of cusps present. The largest pulp horn is the mesiofacial.

Primary Maxillary Second Molar

	Right	*Left*
Universal code number	A	J
International code	5-5	6-5
Palmer notation	e⌋	⌊e

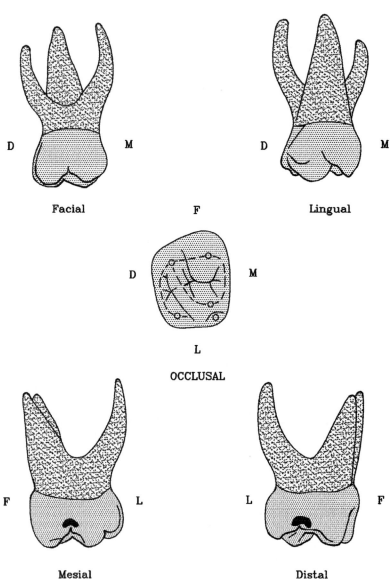

The proximal contacts are indicated on the mesial and distal views in the illustration.

Features: This tooth resembles the *permanent* maxillary first molar.

Occlusal: It has five cusps, an oblique ridge extending from the distofacial to the mesiolingual cusp, and the presence of facial, distolingual, and mesiolingual grooves. It has the same groove pattern as the *permanent* maxillary first molar. Within the mesial and distal fossae are the mesio/distofacial triangular grooves, the mesio/distolingual triangular grooves, and the mesial/distal marginal grooves. The mesial, distal, and facial grooves meet in the central fossa.

Facial: The facial features the mesiofacial cusp, distofacial cusp, and the facial groove.

Lingual: Features on the lingual include the mesiolingual cusp, distolingual cusp, cusp of Carabelli, and the mesiolingual and distolingual grooves. The longest cusp is the mesiolingual, while the other three, distolingual, mesiofacial, and distofacial, are nearly equal in height.

Roots: The three roots present from largest to smallest are: lingual, mesiofacial, distofacial.

Pulp anatomy: There are four or five pulp horns and three root canals. The longest and largest pulp horn is the mesiofacial.

Primary Mandibular Central Incisor

	Right	*Left*
Universal code number	P	O
International code number	8-1	7-1
Palmer notation	a̱|	|a̱

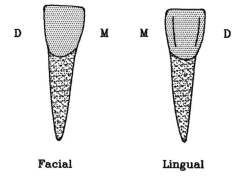

Facial   Lingual

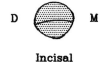

Incisal

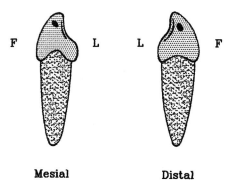

Mesial   Distal

The proximal contacts are indicated on the mesial and distal views in the illustration.

Features: It is generally smaller than the maxillary central incisor.

Facial: It is more convex at the cervical than the incisal. The mesioincisal and distoincisal angles are approximately right angles.

Lingual: The lingual surface is generally smooth making the marginal ridges and cingulum indistinct and the lingual fossa shallow.

Root: The root is single, slender, and long.

Primary Mandibular Lateral Incisor

	Right	*Left*
Universal code number	Q	N
International code number	8-2	7-2
Palmer notation	⌐⌐	⌐⌐

Facial   Lingual

Incisal

Mesial   Distal

The proximal contacts are marked on the mesial and distal views in the illustration.

Features: Generally larger than the mandibular central incisor.

Facial: The lateral has greater incisocervical and mesiodistal dimension. The distoincisal angle is more rounded than the mesioincisal angle.

Lingual: The lingual mesial marginal ridge and distal marginal ridge are more convex, making the lingual fossa deeper.

Root: The root is longer and thicker than the mandibular central incisor.

Primary Mandibular Canine

	Right	*Left*
Universal code number	R	M
International code number	8-3	7-3
Palmer notation	c̄⌋	⌊c̄

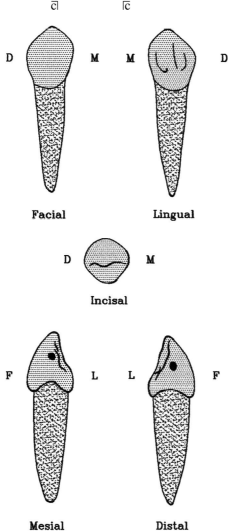

The proximal contacts are marked on the mesial and distal views in the illustration.

Features: The distoincisal edge of the mandibular canine is longer than the mesioincisal. The mandibular canine is narrower mesiodistally than the maxillary canine.

Lingual: The lingual features are less distinct on the mandibular canine than on the maxillary canine, however, the mesial and distal marginal ridges and cingulum are present.

Root: The root is more tapered than the maxillary canine.

Primary Mandibular First Molar

	Right	Left
Universal code number	S	L
International code number	8-4	7-4
Palmer notation	d⌋	⌊d

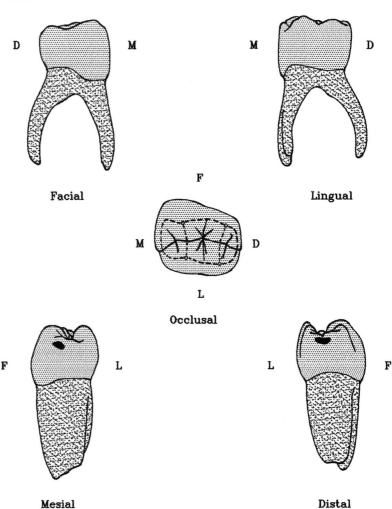

Facial   Lingual

Occlusal

Mesial   Distal

The proximal contacts are marked on the mesial and distal views in the illustration.

Features: The crown is wider mesiodistally than faciolingually which is similar to the permanent molars.

Facial: The two cusps present are the mesiofacial and distofacial. There is a facial depression between the two cusps, but usually no facial groove. The cervical line is deeper and more skewed on the mesial where the cervical ridge is more prominent.

Lingual: The two cusps present are the mesiolingual and distolingual. The mesiolingual cusp is the higher of the two cusps which are generally shorter than the facial cusps. The cervical line is straighter on the lingual than it is on the facial.

Mesial: Visible are the mesiofacial and distofacial cusps and the large cervical ridge.

Distal: All four cusps can be seen. The mesiofacial cusp is the longest. The distal marginal ridge is less prominent than the mesial marginal ridge, and located more cervically than the mesial marginal ridge.

Occlusal: The four cusps present are the mesiofacial, distofacial, mesiolingual, distolingual. The mesial cusps are larger than the distal cusps. The *transverse ridge* is formed by the facial ridge of the mesiolingual cusp and lingual ridge of the mesiofacial cusp. There are three *pits* present, the mesial, central, and distal. The four *grooves* originating at the central pit are the mesial, distal, facial, and lingual.

Intersecting in the distal pit are the distal groove, distolingual triangular groove, distal marginal groove, and the distofacial triangular groove. Within the mesial pit are the mesial marginal groove, and the mesiofacial triangular groove. The mesial groove frequently fades out in the transverse ridge.

Roots: There are two roots present, the mesial and distal. Similar to the permanent molars, the roots are wider faciolingually than mesiodistally. The mesial root is longer and wider than the distal root.

Pulp anatomy: The number of pulp horns corresponds with the number of cusps, therefore there are four pulp horns present. Similar to the permanent molars, there may be two root canals in the mesial root and one in the distal root. They would be the distal, mesiofacial, and mesiolingual. The two largest pulp horns are the mesiofacial, then the mesiolingual.

Primary Mandibular Second Molar

	Right	Left
Universal code number	T	K
International code number	8-5	7-5
Palmer notation	e̅|	|e̅

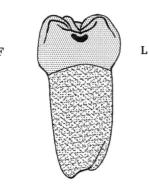

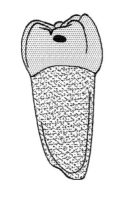

The proximal contacts are marked on the mesial and distal views in the illustration.

Features: The *primary* mandibular second molar closely resembles the *permanent* mandibular second molar.

Occlusal: Five *cusps* present: the mesiofacial, distofacial, distal, mesiolingual, and distolingual. There is a triangular ridge running from each cusp tip to the center of the occlusal surface. *Grooves* present are as follows: mesiofacial, distofacial, and lingual meet at the central pit. The mesial groove branches from the mesiofacial groove and the distal groove branches from the distofacial groove. The other six grooves are the mesial marginal and distal marginal, the mesiofacial triangular and the distofacial triangular, and the mesiolingual triangular and distolingual triangular.

Facial: Three cusps visible are the mesiofacial, distofacial, and distal, with the highest being the distofacial. Also visible are the extensions of the distofacial and mesiofacial grooves. The mesiofacial groove may terminate in a facial pit between the mesiofacial and distofacial cusps.

Lingual: All five cusps can be seen from the lingual.

Proximal: The occlusal convergence can be easily seen. This convergence makes the faciocervical ridge quite prominent.

Roots: The two roots present, mesial and distal, are larger than the primary mandibular first molar roots.

Pulp anatomy: There are five pulp horns to correspond with the five cusps. There are either three or four root canals, the most common being three. The root canals would be mesiofacial, mesiolingual, and distal.

TURN TO THE NEXT PAGE AND TAKE REVIEW TEST 5.3.

REVIEW TEST 5.3

1. The fifth cusp often found on the primary maxillary second molar is the

   a. distal cusp
   b. Carabelli cusp

2. The lingual surface of the primary maxillary second molar has two major cusps (distolingual and mesiolingual) separated by the

   a. distolingual groove
   b. mesiolingual groove

3. The most prominently convex portion of the faciocervical ridge on the primary mandibular first molar is the

   a. distal
   b. mesial

4. On the primary mandibular second molar, the distal cusp is separated from the distofacial cusp by the

   a. distal groove
   b. buccal groove
   c. distofacial groove

CHECK YOUR ANSWERS IN APPENDIX A.

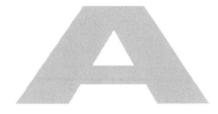

Review Test Answers

CHAPTER 1

REVIEW TEST 1.1 (page 12)

1. a. canine (p. 6)
   b. premolar (p. 9)
   c. incisors (p. 4)
2. b (p. 2)
3. c (p. 11)
4. a,b (p. 8)
5. b (p. 1, 2)
6. c (p. 8)
7. c (p. 10)
8. b (p. 9)

REVIEW TEST 1.2 (pages 33 and 34)

1. a (p. 13, 14)
2. b (p. 26, 21)
3. b, c (p. 31)
4. b (p. 13, 14)
5. **18**—Permanent mandibular left second molar
   I—Primary maxillary left first molar
   3—Permanent maxillary right first molar
   M—Primary mandibular left canine (p. 19, 20)
6. d (p. 22)
7. c (p. 22)
8. b, c (p. 26, 15)
9. c (p. 19)
10. b (p. 19)
11. c (p. 20)
12. a (p. 20)
13. a (p. 17)
14. d (p. 19, 20)
15. a (p. 17)

REVIEW TEST 1.3 (page 46 and 47)

1. c (p. 37)
2. b (p. 19)
3. a (p. 38)
4. b (p. 36)
5. d (p. 37)
6. a, c (p. 31)
7. c (p. 39)
8. a (p. 44, 45)
9. b, d (p. 37)
10. b (p. 37)

REVIEW TEST 1.4 (page 60)

1. f apical foramen
2. g pulp horn
3. I orifice
4. j pulp cavity

5. b accessory canal
6. h lymphatic vessels
7. c cementum (pp. 48-59)

True/False

8. F (p. 55)
9. T (p. 52)
10. F (p. 59)

REVIEW TEST 1.5 (page 71)

1. c (p. 67)
2. a (p. 65)
3. b (p. 61-72)

4. from top of illustration
to the bottom:
e
f
d
c
b
a (p. 70)

5. from top to bottom:
b (p. 72)
a
c
6. from top to bottom:
(p. 61)
cementum
dentin
pulp
enamel

REVIEW TEST 1.6 (page 86)

1. c (p. 74)
2. b (p. 77)

3. d (p. 81)
4. a (p. 73)

5. b (p. 83)

REVIEW TEST 1.7 (page 111)

1. b (p. 107)
2. b (p. 106)
3. c (p. 107)
4. c (p. 88)
5. a (p. 97)
6. I. b, II. c, III. a
(p. 91-93)

7. a, Angle Class III
b, Angle Class II
c, Angle Class I (p. 91-93)
8. a (p. 89, 90)
9. b (p. 92)
10. b (p. 92)

11. c (p. 89-91)
12. b (p. 94)
13. b (p. 99)
14. a (p. 97)
15. b (p. 97)

REVIEW TEST 1.8 (page 120)

1. c (p. 118)
2. a (p. 114)

3. a. I
b. J
c. M
d. I
e. M
f. M
g. M (p. 106)

4. c (p. 106)
5. b (p. 106)

CHAPTER 2

REVIEW TEST 2.1 (page 135)

1. b (p. 127)
2. a (p. 127)
3. b (p. 125)
4. b (p. 125)

5. a. cervical and
      middle
   b. cervical
   c. middle (p. 132-134)

6. b (p. 127)
7. b, c (p. 133)
8. b (p. 128)
9. a (p. 127)
10. b (p. 133)

REVIEW TEST 2.2 (page 143)

1. b (p. 136)
2. b (p. 137)
3. a (p. 137)

4. c (p. 139)
5. a (p. 139)

6. a (p. 134)
7. b (p. 136)

REVIEW TEST 2.3 (page 146)

1. b (p. 137)
2. a (p. 127)

3. c (p. 144)
4. b (p. 145)

5. c (p. 145)

REVIEW TEST 2.4 (page 154)

1. a. cingulum
   b. distal marginal ridge
   c. lingual fossa
   d. mesial marginal
      ridge
   e. lingual pit (p. 133-134)

2. c (p. 150)
3. b (p. 147)
4. b (p. 150)

5. a (p. 145)
6. a (p. 144)

REVIEW TEST 2.5 (page 170)

1. b (p. 156)
2. b (p. 159)
3. d (p. 160)
4. b (p. 157)

5. b (p. 162)
6. a (p. 164)
7. b (p. 164)
8. b (p. 167)

9. b (p. 167)
10. a (p. 168)

REVIEW TEST 2.6 (page 185)

1. a (p. 175)
2. a (p. 174)
3. a (p. 175)
4. a (p. 175)

5. a (p. 181)
6. a (p. 177)
7. attrition (p. 183)
8. c (p. 172)

9. a (p. 180)
10. a (p. 181)

REVIEW TEST 2.7 (page 195)

1. a (p. 177)
2. c (p. 186)
3. attrition (p. 183)

4. c (p. 172)
5. b (p. 188, 184)

6. a (p. 191)
7. c,d (p. 193)

REVIEW TEST 2.8 (page 200)

1. a (p. 175)
2. a, c, d, f (review)
3. c (p. 198)
4. a (p. 196)
5. a (p. 19)
6. b (p. 198)

REVIEW TEST 2.9 (page 208)

1. a (p. 205)
2. b (p. 206)
3. b (p. 201)
4. a (p. 201)
5. b (p. 203)
6. b (p. 204)

REVIEW TEST 2.10 (page 220)

1. a (p. 213)
2. a (p. 217)
3. b (p. 212)
4. c (p. 212)
5. b (p. 104, 213)
6. a (p. 215)
7. b (p. 215)
8. a (p. 216)
9. b (p. 213)

REVIEW TEST 2.11 (page 228)

1. b (p. 226)
2. c (p. 226)
3. c (p. 221)
4. c (p. 222)
5. b (p. 223)
6. a (p. 224)
7. a (p. 223)
8. a (p. 222)

REVIEW TEST 2.12 (page 236)

1. b (p. 233)
2. a (p. 234)
3. a (p. 234)
4. b (p. 229)

REVIEW TEST 2.13 (page 246)

1. a (p. 237)
2. b (p. 183)
3. c (p. 237)
4. b (p. 240)
5. c (p. 242)
6. distal (p. 241)
   mandibular (p. 241)
7. b (pp. 239-40)
8. permanent mandibular
   central
   permanent mandibular
   lateral
   permanent mandibular
   canine (review)
9. b (p. 243)
10. a. 1 (p. 225)
    b. 2 (p. 167)
    c. 3 (p. 167)

CHAPTER 3

REVIEW TEST 3.1 (page 265)

1. b (p. 257)
2. b (p. 263)
3. b (p. 256)
4. a (p. 251)
5. a (p. 256)
6. a (p. 262)
7. a (p. 254)
8. b (p. 251)
9. a (p. 258)
10. b (p. 260)

REVIEW TEST 3.2 (page 279)

Maxillary First Premolar	Mesial	Distal
Which ridge of the facial cusp is shorter and which is longer?	Longer (p. 268)	Shorter (p. 268)
Which surface has a cervical line with more curvature?	X (p. 274)	
Occlusocervical location of this contact area ...	Middle (p. 275)	Middle
Does the developmental groove extend onto this surface?	Yes (p. 274)	No

1. b (p. 273)
2. a (p. 273)
3. a (p. 273)
4. a (p. 276)

5. a. extension of mesial marginal ridge onto the mesial surface
   b. concavity cervical to the contact area
   c. lingual cusp shorter than facial cusp (p. 276)

6. a. middle (p. 276)
   b. cervical (p. 275)

REVIEW TEST 3.3 (page 289)

1. b (p. 282)
2. a (p. 282)
3. a (p. 283)
4. b (p. 285)

5. b (p. 285)
6. b (p. 286)
7. a (p. 274)
8. b (p. 276)

9. b (p. 276)
10. b (review)

REVIEW TEST 3.4 (page 295)

	First Premolar	Second Premolar	Neither/ Both
Longer buccal cusp ...	(p. 292) X		
Mesial marginal groove extends onto mesial surface ...	X (p. 292)		
More supplemental grooves ...		(p. 291) X	
Cervical line less contoured ...		(p. 294) X	
Mesial surface has less curvature ...		X (p. 293)	

1. b (p. 290)   3. a (p. 290)
2. b (p. 290)   4. a (p. 291)

REVIEW TEST 3.5 (page 302)

1. b (p. 297)   5. b (p. 298)   9. a (p. 282)
2. c (p. 297)   6. b (p. 299)   10. a (p. 274)
3. b (p. 301)   7. a (p. 300)
4. a (p. 298)   8. b (p. 290)

REVIEW TEST 3.6 (page 320)

1. a (p. 311)   4. a (p. 316)   7. a (p. 311)
2. b (p. 304)   5. b (p. 312)   8. a (p. 318)
3. a (p. 308)   6. b (p. 308)   9. b (p. 318)

REVIEW TEST 3.7 (page 329)

1. d (p. 321)   4. a (p. 323)   6. b (p. 326)
2. a (p. 321)   5. a (p. 323)   7. c (p. 326)
3. a (p. 322)

REVIEW TEST 3.8 (page 342)

Mandibular Second Premolar	Mesial	Distal
Occlusal fossae located at the ...	(p. 334) X	(p. 334) X
Larger of the two lingual cusps ...	(p. 338) X	
Marginal ridge at lower level ...		(p. 340) X
Central pit displaced toward the ...		(p. 340) X

1. a (review)   3. b (p. 334)   5. a, b, d, g (review)
2. b (p. 334)   4. a (p. 333)

REVIEW TEST 3.9 (page 351)

Pulp of Premolars	Max. First Premolar	Mand. First Premolar	Max. Second Premolar	Mand. Second Premolar
Most common number of root canals.	2	1	1	1
If the tooth has a less common number of root canals, what number of canals would that be?	1	2	2	2
Number of pulp horns in pulp chamber.	2	1	2	3 if 3 cusps, 2
Names of usual root canals (if more than one).	Facial Lingual	1	1	1
Universal code numbers..........	4, 12	28, 21	5, 13	29, 20

1. a (p. 349)	5. b (p. 344)	9. b (p. 346)
2. c (review)	6. b (p. 344)	10. b (review)
3. a (p. 344)	7. b (p. 345)	
4. b (p. 344)	8. a (p. 346)	

CHAPTER 4

REVIEW TEST 4.1 (page 368)

	Mesio facial	Mesio lingual	Disto lingual	Disto facial
Cusp with widest mesiodistal measurement		X (p. 358)		
Two cusps joined by oblique ridge		X (p. 359)		X (p. 359)
The cusp which is least developed of the four major cusps			X (p. 360)	
Cusp nearest the cusp of Carabelli		X (p. 356)		
Cusps with ridges that surround the central fossa	X (p. 362)	X (p. 362)		X (p. 362)

1. b (p. 354)
2. b (p. 357)
3. a (p. 365)
4. a (p. 361)
5. a. facial
   b. mesial
   c. mesial marginal
   d. mesiolingual
   e. distolingual
   f. distal marginal

g. distal
b & g. central
(pp. 364-367)
6. A. mesial
   B. central
   C. distal (p. 364)
7. A. distal marginal ridge
   B. distal ridge of the distolingual cusp

C. mesial ridge of the distolingual cusp
D. mesial ridge of the mesiolingual cusp
E. mesial marginal ridge
F. distal ridge of the mesiofacial cusp (p. 362)

REVIEW TEST 4.2 (page 379)

Maxillary First Molar	Facial	Lingual	Mesial	Distal
What surfaces are visible from the facial aspect? (complete or part)	X (p. 371)			X (p. 371)
What surfaces are visible from the lingual aspect? (complete or part)		X (p. 373)	X (p. 373)	
Which proximal view exposes more of the occlusal?				X (p. 377)
What surfaces have their widest measurement at the occlusal?	X (p. 373)	X (p. 373)		
Which surfaces are marked by a developmental groove that terminates in a pit?	X (p. 371)	X (p. 374)		

1. c (p. 374)　　　3. b (p. 372)
2. b (p. 373)　　　4. d (p. 377)

REVIEW TEST 4.3 (page 394)

1. b (p. 380)　　5. a (p. 380)　　9. a. mesial
2. a (p. 380)　　6. c (p. 381)　　　 b. distal
3. b (p. 380)　　7. c (p. 384)　　　 c. facial
4. a (p. 381)　　8. a (p. 388)　　　 d. there are only three
　　　　　　　　　　　　　　　　　　　　 (p. 383)
　　　　　　　　　　　　　　　　10. a (p. 384)

REVIEW TEST 4.4 (page 403)

	Maxillary First Molar	Maxillary Second Molar	Neither or Both
Shorter occlusocervically...		X (p. 395)	
Longer faciolingually... Wider mesiodistally...	X (p. 395)	X (p. 395)	
Tooth which often has more supplemental grooves...		X (p. 399)	

REVIEW TEST 4.5 (page 412)

1. b (p. 404)	5. c (p. 406)	9. b (p. 404)
2. b (p. 405)	6. a (p. 410)	10. b (p. 404)
3. c (p. 406)	7. a (p. 405)	
4. c (p. 405)	8. b (p. 407)	

REVIEW TEST 4.6 (page 417)

1. a (p. 413)	3. b (p. 413)	5. b (p. 416)
2. a (p. 413)	4. b (p. 415)	

REVIEW TEST 4.7 (page 422)

1. b (p. 418)	3. a (p. 418)	5. c (review)
2. a (p. 418)	4. b (p. 420)	

REVIEW TEST 4.8 (page 434)

Cusps of the Mandibular First Molar

	Mesio-facial	Disto-facial	Distal	Disto-lingual	Mesio-lingual
Widest cusp	X (p. 424)				
Smallest cusp			X (p. 424)		
Has triangular ridge that descends into the central fossa		X (p. 427)			
Connected by the oblique ridge		(no oblique ridge is present) (p. 425)			
Longest cusp					X (p. 433)

1. b (p. 426)
2. a (p. 425)

3. a. no oblique ridge (p. 425)
   b. maxillary is widest faciolingually—doesn't converge lingually (p. 425)

4. distofacial (p. 428)

REVIEW TEST 4.9 (page 443)

Mandibular First Molar	Facial	Lingual	Mesial	Distal
The views from which five cusps are visible...	X (p. 435)			X (p. 442)
The proximal surface with the more convex curvature in the faciolingual direction as seen from an occlusal view...				X (p. 441)
The portion of the crown with the two most pointed cusps...		X (p. 439)		

1. a (p. 437)
2. b (p. 438)
3. a (p. 440)

REVIEW TEST 4.10 (page 455)

1. b (p. 444)
2. a (p. 444)
3. c (p. 444)
4. a (p. 444)
5. b (p. 445)
6. b (p. 445)
7. d (p. 445)
8. b (p. 446)
9. a, b (p. 446)
10. a (p. 451)

REVIEW TEST 4.11 (page 463)

1. d (p. 456)
2. distal (p. 458)
3. d (p. 458)
4. a, b, c, d (p. 459)
5. a (review)

REVIEW TEST 4.12 (page 474)

1. b (p. 464)
2. a (p. 464)
3. c (p. 464)
4. a (p. 464)
5. b (p. 465)
6. b (p. 465)
7. d (p. 465)
8. b (p. 466)
9. a, b (p. 466)
10. a (p. 470)

REVIEW TEST 4.13 (page 478)

Mandibular Molars

Mandibular Molars	First	Second	Neither
The tooth with three lingual cusps...			X (review)
The tooth with the more symmetrical form...		X (review)	
The tooth with the smaller measurements in all dimensions...		X (p. 475)	
The tooth with the greater amount of lingual convergence on the mesial and distal surfaces...	X (review)		
The tooth with two developmental grooves of the facial surface...	X (review)		

1. b (p. 457)
2. b (p. 459)
3. b (p. 475)
4. b (p. 476)
5. b (p. 475)

REVIEW TEST 4.14 (page 483)

Molars	Facial	Lingual	Mesial or Mesio-facial	Distal or Disto-facial
Largest root of maxillary first molar.		X (p. 384)		
Inclination of lingual root apex, maxillary first molar.	X (p. 386)			
The smallest root of the maxillary first molar.				X (p. 384)
Root with the sharpest apex, maxillary second molar.				X (p. 409)
Largest root, mandibular first molar.			X (p. 447)	
Straighter root (occluso-apical direction) of mandibular first molar.				X (p. 449)
Inclination of roots, mandibular third molar.				X (p. 480)

1. a. Maxillary 3
   b. Mandibular 2
2. b
3. b
4. b

Pulp of Posterior Teeth	Maxillary First Molar	Mandibular First Molar
Most common number of root canals.	four (p. 409-410)	three (p. 450-452)
If the tooth has a less common number of root canals, what number of canals would that be?	four (p. 409-410)	four or two (p. 450-452)
Number of pulp horns in pulp chamber.	four (p. 409-410)	five (p. 450-452)
Names of usual root canals (if more than one).	Mesiofacial Distofacial Lingual (p. 409-410)	facial canal of Mesial, lingual canal of Mesial, Distal (p. 450-452)

1. a. 4 + 3 = 7
   b. 3 + 4 = 7
   c. 2 + 5 = 7

CHAPTER 5

REVIEW TEST 5.1 (page 499)

	Both/ Neither	Central	Lateral
Primary maxillary incisor with the wider crown.		X (p. 493)	
Primary maxillary incisor with the longer crown.		X (p. 493)	
Primary mandibular incisor with the crown that appears slightly wider.			X (p. 497)
Mandibular incisor with a rounder distoincisal angle.			X (p. 497)

REVIEW TEST 5.2 (page 506)

	Both/ Neither	Maxillary Canine	Mandibular Canine
Canine with a more tapered root.			X (p. 505)
Canine with the wider crown.		X (p. 504)	
Canine with five lobes.	(p. 500) X		
Canine with the less prominent mesial and distal marginal ridges.			X (p. 504)
Canine with its mesial cusp ridge longer than its distal cusp ridge.		X (p. 500)	

1. b (p. 487)   3. b (p. 484)   5. a (pp. 488-489)
2. b (p. 491)   4. b (p. 491)   6. a (review)

REVIEW TEST 5.3 (page 550)

1. b (p. 518)   3. b (p. 521)
2. a (p. 521)   4. c (p. 532)

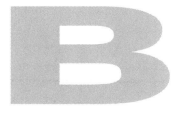

TABLE OF CODE CONVERSION
Universal and International Tooth Identification Codes

PERMANENT MAXILLARY		PERMANENT MANDIBULAR	
Universal	*International*	*Universal*	*International*
1	1-8 or 18	17	3-8 or 38
2	1-7 or 17	18	3-7 or 37
3	1-6 or 16	19	3-6 or 36
4	1-5 or 15	20	3-5 or 35
5	1-4 or 14	21	3-4 or 34
6	1-3 or 13	22	3-3 or 33
7	1-2 or 12	23	3-2 or 32
8	1-1 or 11	24	3-1 or 31
9	2-1 or 21	25	4-1 or 41
10	2-2 or 22	26	4-2 or 42
11	2-3 or 23	27	4-3 or 43
12	2-4 or 24	28	4-4 or 44
13	2-5 or 25	29	4-5 or 45
14	2-6 or 26	30	4-6 or 46
15	2-7 or 27	31	4-7 or 47
16	2-8 or 2i	32	4-8 or 48

PRIMARY MAXILLARY		PRIMARY MANDIBULAR	
Universal	*International*	*Universal*	*International*
A	5-5 or 55	K	7-5 or 75
B	5-4 or 54	L	7-4 or 74
C	5-3 or 53	M	7-3 or 73
D	5-2 or 52	N	7-2 or 72
E	5-1 or 51	O	7-1 or 71
F	6-1 or 61	P	8-1 or 81
G	6-2 or 62	Q	8-2 or 82
H	6-3 or 63	R	8-3 or 83
I	6-4 or 64	S	8-4 or 84
J	6-5 or 65	T	8-5 or 85

INDEX